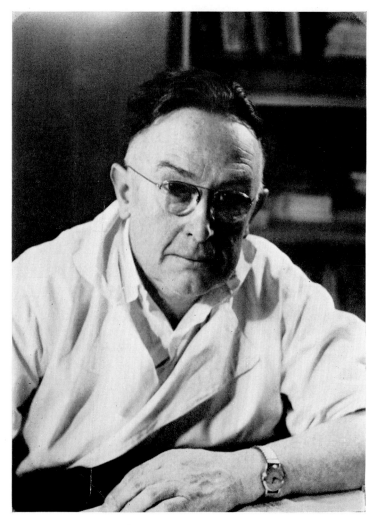

The Late Marcel Dargent

# Mammary Cancer and Neuroendocrine Therapy

# Mammary Cancer and Neuroendocrine Therapy

*Edited by*

**BASIL A. STOLL**

*Honorary Consultant to the Radiotherapy Departments, St. Thomas' Hospital and Royal Free Hospital, London*

**BUTTERWORTHS**

ENGLAND:        BUTTERWORTH & CO. (PUBLISHERS) LTD.
                LONDON: 88 Kingsway, WC2B 6AB

AUSTRALIA:      BUTTERWORTHS PTY. LTD.
                SYDNEY: 586 Pacific Highway 2067
                MELBOURNE: 343 Little Collins Street, 3000
                BRISBANE: 240 Queen Street, 4000

CANADA:         BUTTERWORTH & CO. (CANADA) LTD.
                TORONTO: 14 Curity Avenue, 374

NEW ZEALAND:    BUTTERWORTHS OF NEW ZEALAND LTD.
                WELLINGTON: 26–28 Waring Taylor Street, 1

SOUTH AFRICA:   BUTTERWORTH & CO. (SOUTH AFRICA) (PTY.) LTD.
                DURBAN: 152–154 Gale Street

Suggested U.D.C. Number: 618.19–006: 615.252.43
Suggested Additional Number: 618.19–006:615.357

I.S.B.N. 0 407 26440 X

*Printed in Great Britain by*
*The Camelot Press Ltd, London and Southampton*

# Contents

CONTENTS

# List of Contributors

R. Chemama, M.D., Physician to the Department of Medicine, Fondation Curie, Paris*

James A. Clemens, Ph.D., Research Physiologist, Department of Physiological Research, The Eli Lilly Research Laboratories, Indianapolis, Indiana.

A. T. Cowie, B.Sc., Ph.D., D.Sc., M.R.C.V.S., Head of the Physiology Department, National Institute for Research in Dairying, Shinfield, Reading, Berkshire

V. M. Dilman, M.D., Professor of Endocrinology, Petrov Research Institute of Oncology, Leningrad

A. Ennuyer, M.D., Head of the Department of Medicine, Fondation Curie, Paris

K. Fotherby, Ph.D., F.R.I.C., Reader in Biochemistry in the University of London at the Royal Postgraduate Medical School

H. G. Friesen, M.D., Professor of Experimental Medicine, McGill University, Montreal

H. J. Guyda, M.D., Assistant Professor of Pediatrics, McGill University, Montreal

M. Hayem, Associate Oropharyngeal Surgeon, Institut Gustave Roussy, Villejuif, France

J. C. Heuson, M.D., Deputy Director, Department of Medicine, Institut Jules Bordet, Brussels

P. Hwang, M.B., B.S., Research Fellow, McGill University, Montreal

Frances James, B.Sc., Ph.D., Research Fellow, Royal Postgraduate Medical School, London

M. F. Jayle, Professor of Biochemistry, U.E.R. Biomédicale des Saints—Pères, Paris

P. Juret, Chief of the Department of Medicine, Centre Françoise Baclesse, Caen, Frane

Howard D. Kolodny, M.D., Director of the Department of Medicine, Queens Hospital Center Affiliation of the Long Island Jewish–Hillside Medical Center, Jamaica, New York; Associate Professor of Medicine, School of Medicine, State University of New York at Stony Brook

* Deceased.

LIST OF CONTRIBUTORS

Robert M. MacLeod, B.S., M.S., Ph.D., Professor of Medicine, University of Virginia School of Medicine, Charlottesville, Virginia

Joseph Meites, Ph.D., Professor of Physiology, Michigan State University, East Lansing, Michigan

Charles S. Nicoll, Ph.D., Department of Physiology, University of California, Berkeley, California

Simone Saez, M.D., Department of Medical Biology, Centre Léon Bérard, Lyon, France

Lawrence Sherman, M.D., Associate Director, Department of Medicine, Queens Hospital Center Affiliation of the Long Island Jewish–Hillside Medical Center, Jamaica, New York; Associate Professor of Medicine, School of Medicine, State University of New York at Stony Brook

Basil A. Stoll, Honorary Consultant to the Radiotherapy Departments, St. Thomas' Hospital and Royal Free Hospital, London

Karen C. Swearingen, Ph.D., Department of Physiology, University of California, Berkeley, California

R. Tchao, B.Sc., Ph.D., Assistant Professor, Department of Pathology, Medical College of Pennsylvania, Philadelphia

L. Terenius, Ph.D., Associate Professor of Pharmacology, University of Uppsala

Clifford W. Welsch, Ph.D., Associate Professor of Anatomy, College of Human Medicine, Michigan State University, East Lansing, Michigan

# Tribute to Marcel Dargent (1908–1972)

The tragic news of the untimely passing of Marcel Dargent broke during the summer of 1972 while this Symposium was being written. It was thought appropriate that it should be dedicated to his memory.

Marcel Dargent was a man of enormously wide interests embracing science and literature, art and philosophy, but oncology was a field well suited to his talents, energy and enthusiasm. He was to reveal himself an extremely able administrator in the building up of the Centre Léon Bérard in Lyon. Under his leadership, and with the enthusiastic help of an outstanding team of co-workers whom he gathered around him, this centre rapidly grew from modest beginnings into one of the leading cancer institutes in Europe.

However, to ask such a man as Marcel Dargent to limit his activities to organization and administration would have been an impossible demand. He trained as a surgeon and its practice remained his vocation. He did not accept the popular concept of super-specialization in cancer surgery, but operated just as skilfully whether it was on the larynx, breast or abdomen. Nevertheless, he was not one to ignore the limitations of surgery, and this led him to familiarize himself with complementary and new approaches to cancer treatment, such as hormonal therapy, chemotherapy and immunotherapy.

He initiated a number of projects designed to combine these newly developing forms of therapy with surgery. He made his mark in the field of endocrine ablation therapy in breast cancer by being the first to carry out successfully, and to make a routine of, the portalization of the left adrenal gland. This procedure, which he performed on hundreds of patients with breast cancer, permitted many to enjoy the remission to be expected from standard bilateral adrenalectomy, without the burden of cortisone replacement therapy.

Those who had the privilege to be close to Marcel Dargent when he gave free rein to the flow of memory and fancy, quickly became aware of his cultural breadth. Served by a prodigious memory, a dazzling talent for story-telling and an incomparable sense of humour, he was an ideal companion at meetings and conferences. The pleasure of his companionship between and after the official sessions permitted a welcome escape from the rigours of oncology into the less austere world of witty anecdote and widely ranging speculation. He will be sadly missed both as a fighter and a teacher in the struggle against cancer, and also as a wonderful personality and companion.

Paul Juret

# Tribute to Dr. R. Chemama

Robert Chemama died tragically at the age of 50 during the compilation of this book to which he and his colleagues contribute an important chapter. His colleagues write the following tribute:

'A busy physician with four children must be a dedicated man to find the time to carry out research on an experimental and clinical level. Robert Chemama gladly accepted this challenge and was responsible for a research project at the Fondation Curie, aiming at the pharmacological inhibition of corticotrophin, gonadotrophin and thyrotrophin in the amelioration of mammary cancer in the human. The results of these investigations show considerable promise, and those of us who remain will reap the fruits of his labours. Robert Chemama was dedicated to his calling, devoted to his family, and a modest and kindly man. He will be missed.'

# Preface

The last few years have seen rapid advances in our knowledge of the hypothalamic neurohormones which control anterior pituitary secretion, and also of psychopharmacological agents able either to stimulate or depress the hypothalamic centres. New methods of radioimmunoassay of both polypeptide and steroid hormones have been developed, including the separation of prolactin from growth hormone in the human. This new knowledge has considerable bearing on the endocrine control of mammary cancer in the human.

Endocrine therapy of both experimental and human mammary cancer in the past 25 years has been characterized by a multiplicity of treatment methods, and no one hypothesis has been found satisfactory to explain the mechanism of all the methods used. A major reason for this is that the homeostatic mechanisms of the endocrine system create difficulty in distinguishing between the primary effects of additive or ablative hormonal manipulation and the secondary effects resulting from compensatory changes developing in the other endocrine glands. Furthermore, the evaluation of the cancer response in the human has been clouded by different methods of selecting cases for treatment and by different criteria of response.

Although still at an early stage, it is likely that pharmacological influences on the hypothalamus may simulate the effect of surgical ablation of the pituitary, *but in a selective fashion*. To clarify the possible mechanisms it appeared essential to bring together in one volume, relevant contributions from some research workers responsible for the advances in knowledge mentioned above. The Symposium might point the way to rational and effective therapy of hormone sensitive breast cancer in the human.

Basil A. Stoll

# PART I

# Endocrine Mechanisms in Normal and Malignant Mammary Growth

# 1

# Hormonal Factors in Mammary Development and Lactation

## A. T. Cowie

This chapter aims to review the relative roles, in laboratory animals and primates, of the anterior pituitary, ovarian and adrenal hormones, and of other factors in the normal growth and development of the mammary glands and in the control of milk secretion.

## MAMMARY DEVELOPMENT

Purified ovarian hormones became available in the 1930s and studies on a variety of laboratory animals soon showed that oestrogens and progesterone had the ability to induce duct growth and lobulo-alveolar development of the mammary gland. In some species oestrogens induced only duct growth while lobulo-alveolar development required a combination of oestrogen and progesterone, whereas in other species oestrogen alone could induce both duct and lobulo-alveolar development. It was then noted that the mammary glands of animals from which the pituitary had been surgically removed showed little or no growth response to the ovarian hormones, and it became apparent that one or more hormones from the anterior pituitary played an essential role in the induction of mammogenic (i.e. mammary growth-stimulating) effects in response to ovarian hormones. In the 1940s purified anterior pituitary hormones became available and Lyons and his colleagues initiated their classical studies on the analysis of the hormonal requirements for mammary duct growth and lobulo-alveolar development in rats; similar detailed studies were later carried out in mice by Nandi.

Attention also became focused on the placenta as an organ affecting mammogenesis when its ability in some species to secrete steroids became apparent in the 1940s. Over the last 20 years substances having mammotrophic (i.e. both mammogenic and lactogenic) activities have been detected in the placenta of rodents, ruminants and primates. A mammotrophic hormone has been isolated from human placenta and designated human placental lactogen or human chorionic somatomammotrophin.

In the early 1960s much research was centred on the preparation of human pituitary hormones. Attempts to isolate prolactin from primate pituitaries were initially unsuccessful. Human growth hormone, however, showed mammotrophic properties similar to those of ruminant prolactin. The belief grew that in primates the growth hormone with its intrinsic prolactin-like properties served the functions of both the growth hormone and the prolactin of non-primate mammals. However, in 1971 the existence of a separate prolactin was established in both human and monkey pituitaries.

From the above brief review of some of the more important landmarks in the study of the endocrine factors concerned in mammary growth it will be clear that the hormonal mechanisms concerned in mammary growth are complex (see reviews by Folley, 1952; Cowie and Tindal, 1971; Forsyth and Edwards, 1972).

It is now intended to examine selected aspects relative to the control of mammogenesis in the higher mammals and man.

## Mammogenesis in laboratory animals

Much of our information on the role of hormones in mammary growth in rodents derives from the studies of Lyons and of Nandi. Lyons recognized the futility of attempting to analyse the role of the various hormones in mammogenesis by injection of the hormones into intact animals (i.e. into animals whose endocrine glands were already secreting some or all of the hormones under study). He therefore used triply operated (i.e. hypophysectomized, ovariectomized, adrenalectomized) animals, since only when the animal was deprived of the endogenous hormones could interactions between injected and endogenous hormones be avoided, and responses in mammary growth be reliably related to the hormone(s) injected, or to their metabolites.

In triply-operated young rats, Lyons (1958) noted that normal mammary duct growth could be induced with bovine growth hormone + oestrone + adrenal steroids, but the addition of progesterone + sheep prolactin was necessary for lobulo-alveolar development. Such studies indicate that the mammary growth responses in the intact or ovariectomized rat in response to the administration of ovarian steroids are dependent on the presence of endogenous anterior pituitary and adrenal hormones. Subsequently Talwalker and Meites (1961) were able to induce moderate lobulo-alveolar development in triply-operated rats in the absence of ovarian or adrenal steroids by *thrice daily* injections of bovine growth hormone and sheep prolactin. These observations do not negate the role of steroid hormones in normal mammogenesis in rats but they do suggest that the steroids may sensitize the mammary tissue to the action of the pituitary hormones (see p. 11).

Nandi's studies (1958, 1959) revealed slightly different hormonal requirements for mammogenesis in mice. Some duct growth occurred in triply-operated mice in response to a combination of oestrogen and adrenal steroids (i.e. in the absence of growth hormone or prolactin)—a response which does not occur in the triply-operated rat. Nandi further observed that in this strain (C3H/HeCrgl) prolactin was not essential for lobulo-alveolar development although in other strains of mice prolactin was essential (Nandi and Bern, 1960).

Hormones of the thyroid gland play no essential role in mammary growth in the rat since ablation of the thyroid by surgery, or by radio-iodine or by a combination of these techniques did not, in triply-operated rats, affect lobulo-alveolar growth induced with the hormonal complexes already discussed (Chen et al., 1955). However, thyroid hormones may well *modify* the mammary growth response since there is evidence from *in vitro* studies on mouse mammary tissue that when levels of prolactin in the culture medium are optimal for lobulo-alveolar development then the addition of thyroxine inhibits this development; however, if levels of prolactin are suboptimal then thyroxine at low concentrations increases lobulo-alveolar development whereas at higher concentrations it again inhibits development (Singh and Bern, 1969). These observations may offer some explanation of the conflicting reports of the effects of thyroid hormones on mammary growth *in vivo* (for references see Singh and Bern, 1969).

Although the study of hormone administration to hypophysectomized rats and mice has permitted a much better understanding of the hormonal factors concerned in mammary growth by overcoming the difficulties of interaction with endogenous hormones, the technique may introduce other complications. The loss of the pituitary gland depresses a variety of essential metabolic processes which may affect the ability of the mammary gland to respond to exogenous hormones (Jacobson, 1958, 1961). Thus, treatment of the hypophysectomized rat with insulin will allow a limited growth-response of the duct system to steroid hormones, a response which can be enhanced with thyroxine but is counteracted by cortisone. The overall response is, however, small compared with that observed in intact rats.

The above studies have provided much information on the hormonal requirements for experimental mammary growth in rats and mice and undoubtedly reflect normal mechanisms. However, in pregnancy a mammotrophic hormone is known to occur in the placenta of both rats and mice (Cowie and Tindal, 1971) and no doubt supplements or synergises with the hormones from the anterior pituitary.

In the rat there is evidence that full lobulo-alveolar growth of pregnancy is dependent also on an intensified licking of the nipple skin over the mammary glands which is a behavioural characteristic of pregnant rats. If the rat is prevented from licking itself in this way then the normal mammary development of pregnancy is partially inhibited (Roth and Rosenblatt, 1968; McMurtry and Anderson, 1971). There is little doubt that this response is mediated through the release of anterior pituitary hormones. An allied reflexly-induced response is noted later in the non-pregnant human female (see page 7).

Limited attempts to analyse the hormonal requirements for mammary growth by replacement studies have been made in two other species—the rabbit and goat. Norgren (1968) has studied mammogenesis in the hypophysectomized rabbit: while the mammary parenchyma remained partially responsive to ovarian, adrenal and thyroid hormones, with no combination of these was the response comparable to that obtained in the presence of an intact pituitary. A study on a few hypophysectomized–ovariectomized goats by Cowie, Tindal and Yokoyama (1966) suggests that in the goat the ovarian hormones have little or no mammogenic effect in the absence of adenohypophysial or placental hormones.

## Mammogenesis in primates

Speert (1948), in an extensive study on normal and experimental mammary growth in intact and ovariectomized rhesus monkeys, showed that prolonged treatment with oestrogens alone can induce extensive lobulo-alveolar growth. The analysis of the hormonal requirements for developmental mammary growth in hypophysectomized monkeys using replacement therapy with anterior pituitary hormones has not, so far as I am aware, been carried out. Pituitary hormones are most probably involved in mammogenesis since atrophy of the mammary glands occurs in immature monkeys after destruction of the pituitary by deuteron irradiation (Simpson et al., 1959).

The existence of prolactin in the monkey pituitary has recently been established (Friesen et al., 1972a). In the monkey, however, levels of prolactin in the blood are low during pregnancy (Friesen et al., 1972a) suggesting an important role for the placental mammotrophic hormone (which has recently been obtained in a highly purified state by Shome and Friesen, 1971) in stimulating normal mammary growth; indeed, hypophysectomy of the pregnant monkey does not substantially affect mammary lobulo-alveolar development (Agate, 1952).

Information relevant to the endocrine control of mammary growth in man has necessarily to be derived from clinical observations. Oestrogens and progestagens have been widely used in therapeutic regimens for inadequate development in the size of the breasts (e.g., Bishop, 1969). The results of such therapy tend to be unsatisfactory, which is perhaps hardly surprising since in the non-pregnant woman breast size is likely to depend on the volume of stromal tissue present. In the young woman the mammary stroma is mainly fibrous tissue (Dabelow, 1957; Mayer and Klein, 1961; Sandison, 1962) and little information is available concerning the factors regulating the growth of this tissue. Only recently Paape and Sinha (1971) have made the somewhat unexpected observation that ovariectomy increases the rate of growth of the mammary fat pad in the rat! From reports in the literature on gynaeco-mastia it appears that the male breast readily increases in size in response to oestrogens (e.g. Bishop, 1969)

Prolactin is now known to occur in the human pituitary (Forsyth and Edwards, 1972; Friesen et al., 1972a) and since both it and human growth hormone are mammotrophic in laboratory animals, both hormones may well act in conjunction with the ovarian hormones in stimulating normal mammary growth. During pregnancy it is possible that placental lactogen plays an important role in lobulo-alveolar development although levels of prolactin in the blood are also high in women during the second half of pregnancy (Friesen et al., 1972a; Tyson et al., 1972b). In women it was noted many years ago that the presence of the ovaries is not essential for mammary growth during pregnancy (Halban, 1905). This is hardly surprising since it is now known that during gestation the placenta is the chief source of oestrogens and progesterone (Hytten and Leitch, 1971).

Numerous reports indicate that the suckling stimulus, if prolonged and repeated, may induce lobulo-alveolar proliferation in the breast and eventually milk secretion in non-pregnant, non-parturient women (Knott, 1907; Foss and Short, 1950; Deanesly and Parkes, 1951; Grishchenko and Grischenko, 1967; Cohen, 1971; Mobbs and Babbage, 1971). No doubt this response is mediated through a neuro-endocrine reflex leading to the release of anterior pituitary hormones. It may be relevant to note that lobulo-alveolar development and lactation can be induced in ovariectomized virgin goats by the repeated application of the milking stimulus and that this response is abolished when the pituitary stalk is surgically transected (Cowie et al., 1968; see also p. 18 for a discussion of the possible role of the cerebral cortex in prolactin release).

## Local mechanisms affecting mammary growth

So far we have discussed the hormones required for mammary growth and we have noted that lobulo-alveolar development, to the extent noted in pregnancy, can be induced experimentally in the virgin rodent by injecting the necessary hormones. There are, however, also local control mechanisms regulating mammary growth. In the cyclic female rodent the mammary duct system just before the onset of oestrus enters a phase of rapid growth when the ducts are growing at a rate some three to eight times that of the body surface as a whole (Cowie and Tindal, 1971). By the time the animal has reached three months of age the ducts have attained their maximum extension and duct proliferation virtually ceases. This phase of rapid growth is initiated and maintained by oestrogens from the ovary acting in conjunction with pituitary growth hormone; if the ovaries are removed before the onset of oestrous cycles, the phase of rapid proliferation does not occur; that is, the mammary ducts grow but only at the same rate as the body as a whole.

In the intact animal the phase of rapid growth ends at about three months of age although ovarian hormones are still present and the animal is still undergoing regular oestrous cycles. Some mechanism now overrules the hormonal stimulus. Studies in mice by Faulkin and DeOme (1960) have shown that it is the gland stroma which exerts this control and which regulates both the spacing of the ducts and the extent of their growth. In the infantile mouse it is possible to excise the mammary parenchyma from the stromal pad and later to transplant other mammary duct tissue into the empty pad. If a portion of duct tissue is taken from a gland which has attained maximum size (i.e. has ceased to grow) and is transplanted into an empty pad it will again respond to the circulating hormones and will proliferate until it fills the fat pad.

Although the mammary ducts in the virgin rodent appear to fill the fat pad, only a small portion of the total volume of the pad is occupied and the ducts do not touch one another except at their point of origin. It appears that there is a cylinder of stroma around each duct into which adjacent ducts do not enter. Thus the spacing of the ducts seems to be determined by some growth inhibiting factor imparted to the stroma by the existing ducts. Peripheral duct growth ceases at the border of the fat pad beyond which ducts do not grow.

The circulating hormones are thus the 'go' stimulus for mammary growth, but this stimulus can be superseded by a local duct-inhibiting 'stop' signal. When the animal becomes pregant, the hormonal environment changes and this local regulating system also appears to change; ductules and alveoli develop and occupy previously unoccupied interductal spaces until the whole stroma is almost entirely replaced by a tightly packed parenchyma.

Interesting effects of ageing on the mammary parenchyma and its responses to hormones have been noted in serial transplantation studies (Daniel et al., 1968, 1971; Hoshino, 1970; Daniel and Young, 1971) and also in mammary explants in organ culture, but there is little known about the relationship of the hormonal environment to the structural changes which occur in the human mammary gland with advancing age. These structural changes include atrophy of the lobules of parenchyma, a deposition of fat and a hyalinization of the fibrous tissue (see reviews by Geschickter, 1945; Dabelow, 1957).

## Proliferative changes in the mammary gland

### Cell division

Having discussed the hormonal and local mechanisms influencing mammary growth we can now look a little more closely at the proliferative process. It must be stressed that changes in the overall size of the gland may not indicate true growth, i.e. cell division. In late pregnancy, for example, the size of the mammary gland increases mainly because the individual cells increase in size and the alveoli fill up with secretion. In studying proliferative changes the problem is therefore one of recognizing increases in the number of parenchymal cells and in identifying the regions where the cells are actively dividing. Munford (1964) reviewed the various histological and biochemical techniques used to assess mammary growth such as numbers of alveoli and alveolar cells, frequency of mitosis, and estimations of deoxyribonucleic acid (DNA). Because of the tedious nature of the histological methods there has been a tendency for these to be replaced by biochemical procedures such as the DNA estimations. Unfortunately recent studies have shown that cellular DNA content may vary, and Simpson and Schmidt (1969) have concluded that the use of mammary DNA as a reliable index of the number of cells in the mammary gland must be rejected (see also Banerjee, Wagner and Kinder, 1971).

Bresciani (1971) has studied the fraction of cells engaged in DNA synthesis in the various parts of the mammary parenchyma during all stages of normal mammogenesis in the mouse as well as during the response to injections of oestrogen and progesterone.in ovariectomized mice. Although hypophysectomized mice were not included, Bresciani's studies were planned and interpreted on the basis of Nandi's analysis of the hormonal factors concerned in mammogenesis (see p. 5). During post-pubertal growth the cells engaged in DNA synthesis were located almost exclusively in the end-buds, i.e. at the tips of the ducts, suggesting that the growth of the ducts is effected by a process of elongation by division of the cells at the tip, and that the differentiation of an end-bud cell into a duct cell is associated with the arrest, at least for a time, of further reproductive activity of that cell.

The number of cells in the end-buds synthesizing DNA increases and decreases in a cyclic manner in phases of 5–7 days' duration. Ovariectomy results in the virtual disappearance within 3–5 days of DNA synthesis in the end-bud cells but this can be restored by physiological doses of oestradiol (1 μg/day). Despite a constant dosage with oestrogen, the cyclic pattern in DNA synthesis is also restored which Bresciani considers to be possibly associated with cyclic pituitary secretion of growth hormone.

Progesterone also induces DNA synthesis in the mammary glands of ovariectomized mice but in contrast to oestradiol it evokes DNA synthesis in the cells of the duct epithelium as well as in the cells of the end-buds (Banerjee and Rogers, 1971). The proliferation of the end-buds induced by progesterone, moreover, results in ramification of the ducts into finer ducts and terminal alveoli. These observations confirm that the lobulo-alveolar development and the further tortuosity of the duct system which occurs in pregnancy is associated with the increasing levels of progesterone in the blood. The role of metabolites of progesterone in mammotrophic effects has recently been discussed by Chatterton (1971).

Bresciani's studies show that the ovarian hormones, acting presumably in conjunction with growth hormone, or growth hormone + prolactin, have the effect both of increasing the percentage of parenchymal cells engaged in proliferation and of increasing the rate of cell replication. Bresciani distinguishes these two effects, indicating the first as an 'induction' and the second as a 'modulation' of the cell replication cycle.

## Organ culture studies

Numerous studies on the hormonal requirements for mammary growth have been carried out on mammary tissue explanted *in vitro*. For technical reasons the tissue has mainly come from mice and, to a lesser extent, rats. These studies are of great interest and have recently been the subject of an extensive review by Forsyth (1971). In general, studies on lobulo-alveolar growth have agreed remarkably well with those obtained *in vivo* in triply-operated animals; the presence of insulin in the culture medium in a concentration apparently considerably higher than that obtaining *in vivo* is, however, necessary. The significance of this observation is uncertain.

Glands taken from 5- to 7-week-old mice maintained as explants on a synthetic medium containing insulin, oestradiol, progesterone, aldosterone, prolactin and growth hormone grow and show lobulo-alveolar development. Glands from younger mice, however, do not grow unless the mice are pre-treated or primed with oestradiol + progesterone *in vivo* for a time sufficient to stimulate mammary duct growth and end-bud formation. The mammary glands will then respond in culture and full lobulo-alveolar development will occur, the minimal hormonal requirements for this being insulin + aldosterone + prolactin.

One cycle of cell division occurs in mouse mammary explants in response to the presence of insulin as the only hormone in the medium (Topper, 1970). This response does not occur, however, in rat mammary explants in which prolactin must be present for active cell division to occur (Dilley, 1971a, b). The insulin stimulated growth response seems to be associated with differentiation of the cells towards functional activity and not with lobulo-alveolar growth; it is important not to confuse these types of mammary differentiation (Cowie and Tindal, 1971). The regulation of gene expression during hormone-dependent cell differentiation in mouse mammary explants has been reviewed by Turkington and Kadohama (1972).

## Local action of hormones

We may now review briefly what is known of the modes of action of the hormones concerned in mammary development. In the intact rat it is clear that oestrogens can have an indirect action on mammogenesis by acting at hypothalamic and pituitary levels to release prolactin. However, the studies on triply-operated rodents, on mammary explants in organ culture, and other observations on local mammary responses to topical applications, indicate that the ovarian hormones also act directly on the mammary parenchyma. Although, as noted above, lobulo-alveolar development in the triply-operated rat can be induced with prolactin and growth hormone in the absence of steroids the pituitary hormones must then be given more frequently than is necessary when the steroids are present. This suggests that the steroids may in some way sensitize the parenchyma to the action of the pituitary hormones. Support for this view has come from recent observations by Nagasawa and Yanai (1971). They implanted small cholesterol pellets containing minute amounts of oestradiol (1 μg) over the mammary glands of ovariectomized rats. When the level of circulating prolactin was raised by implanting two homologous pituitaries under the kidney capsule, localized lobulo-alveolar development occurred in the immediate vicinity of the pellets, i.e. only the mammary parenchyma under the influence of oestrogen responded to the prolactin. On the other hand, if the level of oestrogen is too high, mammary growth may under some conditions be inhibited (Nagasawa and Yanai, 1972).

A clue as to the nature of the sensitizing effect of the ovarian steroids on mammary parenchyma has recently been provided by Banerjee and his colleagues (Banerjee and Rogers, 1971; Banerjee, Banerjee and Wagner, 1971) who studied the biochemical responses occurring in mouse mammary glands during the pre-treatment or priming process prior to explanting (see p. 10). Marked stimulation of the rate of synthesis of RNA, protein and DNA and the activation of DNA polymerase were noted and it is suggested that the end-bud cells enter a phase of rapid proliferation, thereby providing a pool of precursor cells for subsequent lobulo-alveolar differentiation (see also Bresciani, 1971). There is as yet no explanation as to why this priming process does not occur *in vitro*; possibly in the young mouse some ovarian steroid metabolite plays an essential role.

There is evidence that the mammary cells, like those of the uterus and vagina, can concentrate and retain oestradiol (Sander, 1968; Puca and Bresciani, 1969), progesterone (Lawson and Pearlman, 1964; Chatterton, Chatterton and Hellman, 1969; Chatterton, 1971) and cortisol (Paterson and Linzell, 1971), against large concentration gradients in the blood. It is suggested that the mammary cells contain receptor binding proteins responsible for carrying the steroids through the cytoplasm to the nuclear

11

membrane of the cell and thence to the nuclear effector sites on the genome (for review of mechanisms of steroid binding see Baulieu et al., 1971; King et al., 1971; Jensen and DeSombre, 1972). Although a high degree of specificity is a characteristic of the specific binding proteins, it is not absolute; for example, the oestrogen-binding protein of the endometrium has the same affinity to diethylstilboestrol and hexoestrol as to oestradiol but its affinity to oestrone is about 60 per cent of that to oestradiol; it does not bind corticoids or progesterone (Jungblut et al., 1970). Further studies are required on the nature and specificity of the steroid-binding macromolecules in the mammary cells but the possibility exists of competitive binding and of the blocking of the actions of one steroid by the presence of another. The recent observation of Slotin et al. (1970) that the mammary gland is capable of synthesizing progesterone adds to the complexity of the problem.

As yet little is known about the action of the anterior pituitary hormones at the cellular level. There is recent evidence that prolactin may bind to the alveolar-cell membranes and while so bound may exert its response without entering the cell (Falconer, 1972; Turkington, 1972a), and its half-life may be greatly increased (Birkinshaw and Falconer, 1972). The mechanisms of action of the steroid and of the protein hormones at cellular level are thus probably very different and it is perhaps unlikely that any competitive action exists between these two classes of hormones.

The question of changes in sensitivity of a target organ to its hormone has important implications, as recently stressed by Topper, Friedberg and Oka (1971). If a hormone has more than one target tissue and the sensitivity of each tissue remains steady, then alteration in the levels of the circulating hormone would not be expected to lead to very selective effects on a particular target tissue. If, however, the sensitivity of the target tissues varied under different physiological conditions then the selectivity of a hormone response could be much enhanced. It also follows that the plasma level of hormones need not necessarily be a reliable indication of hormone–tissue interaction. In short, responses in mammary growth and development, although induced essentially by anterior pituitary hormones, need not necessarily be associated with increased levels of these hormones in the blood.

Complexities in the control of mammogenesis and sensitivity of mammary target tissue additional to those discussed above may well exist in that the role of insulin remains to be fully elucidated. The parodox that insulin is mitogenic to mammary epithelium in vitro (see p. 10) but not in vivo, has recently been examined by Oka and Topper (1972) who suggest that the problem may be more apparent than real and that insulin may indeed be the physiological mitogenic agent in vivo but that prolactin is first essential to sensitize the epithelium to insulin, i.e. the mitogenic action of prolactin is an indirect effect. This concept, however, does not explain how mammary parenchyma may become sensitized in vitro to insulin in the absence of prolactin. Further studies on the local action of insulin in mammogenic mechanisms are required.

## MILK SECRETION

Lactation comprises two distinct physiological processes: *milk secretion* and *milk removal*. Milk secretion involves the synthesis within the alveolar cells of milk and its excretion into the alveolar lumen; milk removal concerns the transfer of milk from the alveoli and fine ducts into the large ducts, gland cistern or sinus. Milk secretion is regulated by hormones from the anterior pituitary although its initiation may in some species be aided by hormones from the placenta. Milk removal requires the operation of a neuro-endocrine reflex—the milk-ejection reflex—which involves the release of oxytocin from the posterior pituitary (Cowie and Tindal, 1971). In this review I shall deal only with milk secretion—its hormonal control, initiation (i.e. lactogenesis) and maintenance, stimulation and inhibition.

Milk secretion is considered in this review because most of the hormones involved are also concerned in mammary growth—as Lyons (1958) comments: 'lactogenesis may be considered as the final stage of mammogenesis'. Indeed there may be considerable overlap of these stages and in several species alveolar cell proliferation occurs in early lactation, while under experimental conditions in goats intense mammary growth and milk secretion can occur simultaneously within the same gland (Cowie et al., 1965, 1968).

### Hormonal requirements for its initiation

Prolactin has come to be regarded as *the* lactogenic hormone, but studies in species other than the rabbit have revealed that other pituitary hormones are equally essential (Cowie and Tindal, 1971). It is thus more correct to refer to a lactogenic complex of hormones. The components of this complex vary with the species. The studies of Lyons and of Nandi (pp. 4, 5) showed that in rats and mice both adrenocorticotrophin and prolactin were required to initiate milk secretion. In some strains of mice prolactin could be replaced by growth hormone (Nandi and Bern, 1960, 1961). In the hypophysectomized goat prolactin, growth hormone, adrenocortical and thyroid hormones are required for full milk secretion (Cowie and Tindal, 1971). In the triply-operated rabbit, however, prolactin alone is sufficient (Denamur, 1971).

So far as I am aware hormonal requirements for lactogenesis in primates have not been studied. Indeed it is only recently that the presence of prolactin in the primate pituitary has been established (Friesen et al., 1972a). Recent studies on the levels of prolactin and growth hormone in the blood of women who are breast feeding indicate that it is the prolactin levels alone that are raised in response to suckling so the role of growth hormone may be only minor (Frantz, Kleinberg and Noel, 1972; Forsyth, 1972). A mammotrophic hormone has been detected in the placenta of several species—including human and monkey placental tissue (Cowie and Tindal, 1971; Buttle, Forsyth and Knaggs, 1972). This hormone may participate in the initiation of milk secretion.

Oestrogens in low doses will induce mammary development and initiate milk secretion in virgin rabbits and ruminants (Cowie, 1961; Cowie and Tindal, 1971), but there is no evidence that oestrogen in the absence of prolactin exerts any direct lactogenic stimulus on the mammary epithelium. Its lactogenic effect is most probably mediated through the release of pituitary hormones (Cowie and Tindal, 1971) and recently it has been observed that oestradiol benzoate in low dosage (0·1–0·5 µg) administered to rats increases levels of circulating prolactin up to ten-fold (Chen and Meites, 1970; Voogt, Chen and Meites, 1970). The repeated application of the milking stimulus in the virgin goat, or suckling stimulus in the non-pregnant woman, may also induce mammary growth and milk secretion by releasing the necessary pituitary hormones (see p. 7).

An important question is 'how is lactogenesis effected at the end of normal pregnancy?' but only in the rat has an answer to this question been suggested. Kuhn (1969a) has shown that some 30 hours before parturition the progesterone level in the blood falls due to a change in the ovarian steroid metabolism, and he postulates that this fall in blood progesterone triggers off lactogenesis. The response can be mimicked by ovariectomy and can be inhibited by giving progesterone at the time of ovariectomy, although steroids closely related to progesterone are ineffective (Kuhn, 1969b).

It thus appears that, in the pregnant rat, milk secretion is inhibited during pregnancy by a direct action of progesterone on the alveolar cells which prevents them responding to the lactogenic effects of prolactin–adrenal steroid or placental lactogen–adrenal steroid complexes. The mode of action of progesterone is still obscure.

In ruminants there is also a decline in the levels of progesterone in the blood at the end of gestation but secretory activity is occurring in the mammary alveoli at mid-pregnancy and lactose is being synthesized long before the levels of progesterone decline (Jones, personal communication). It is possible that this early secretory activity is associated with rising levels of a placental lactogen now known to occur in ruminants (Buttle, Forsyth and Knaggs, 1972). There may thus be considerable species differences in the hormonal mechanisms regulating the initiation of milk secretion.

## Stimulation of milk secretion

Low milk yields in animals or man may be associated with anterior pituitary hormone deficiencies or imbalances resulting in a low rate of milk secretion, with malfunction of the milk-ejection reflex and inefficient milk removal, or with a combination of these factors. The failure of lactation in women can be due to a wide variety of psychological causes (Newton, 1961) and it may be optimistic to expect benefits from hormonal therapies in any but a small proportion of cases. Attempts to treat hypogalactia in women by administering ruminant prolactin have given unsatisfactory results (Cowie, 1966)—a finding that is not surprising in view of the now known species specificity of prolactin. Significant increases in the milk yield of women treated with human growth hormone have been reported (Lyons et al., 1968). Studies involving the administration of human prolactin must await the preparation of the hormone in suitable quantities. Peak levels of prolactin occurring in the blood of women in response to nursing decline as lactation proceeds (Tyson et al., 1972) and a syndrome of an isolated deficiency of prolactin secretion has been described in two patients with failure of lactation (Turkington, 1972b), so prolactin therapy may well be effective. In view of the scarcity of human prolactin, however, it may prove helpful in some types of hypogalactia to give thyrotrophin-releasing hormone to raise the levels of endogenous prolactin (see below).

The galactopoietic effects (i.e. stimulation of an existing lactation) of thyrotrophin, or of thyroxine or triiodothyronine, in lactating cows are well established (Cowie and Tindal, 1971) and beneficial effects of thyroid-active substances (iodinated proteins) on human lactation have also been reported (Lelong et al., 1950). Of considerable interest therefore is the recent finding that the hypothalamic thyrotrophin-releasing hormone (pyroglutamyl-histidyl-prolinamide), when injected intravenously in man, in doses of 100–800 µg, causes a marked and immediate rise in the prolactin levels in the blood (Bowers et al., 1971; Jacobs et al., 1971; L'Hermite et al., 1972) and an increase in milk yield in late lactation (Tyson, Friesen and Anderson, 1972). This response appears to be a direct action of the hypothalamic hormone on the pituitary cells; its physiological significance is as yet obscure.

Oestrogens in low doses may have galactopoietic effects in cows (Folley, 1952; Hutton, 1958) and tiny implants of oestrogen placed in the anterior pituitary of lactating rats increases milk yields (Bruce and Ramirez, 1970). As already noted (see p. 14) it is probable that lactogenic and galactopoietic responses to oestrogens depend largely on the hormone's ability to release prolactin and possibly other hormones from the anterior pituitary, either by acting on the pituitary itself or on the hypothalamic control mechanism (see also Clemens et al., 1971).

A variety of tranquillizer drugs exert both mammogenic and lactogenic effects and are sometimes the cause of galactorrhoea in patients. These responses are due to the ability of the drugs to release prolactin (Sulman, 1970; Forsyth and Edwards, 1972). There is, however, no evidence as yet that these drugs are galactopoietic, i.e. they do not increase milk yields.

## Inhibition of milk secretion

Milk secretion inhibits itself when milk removal ceases. For clinical reasons it may be necessary to suppress lactation either before it has become fully initiated or after it has become established; under such conditions hormonal therapy has been used in order to facilitate and speed up the natural inhibitory process and to relieve discomfort.

The administration of oestrogens in low doses to lactating mice or rats depresses the growth of the litter despite the continuance of nursing, but this does not occur if the mothers are first ovariectomized. The combined administration of oestrogen + progesterone, however, inhibits established lactation in ovariectomized rats, neither hormone being effective in the complete absence of the other. There is now clear evidence that the gonadal steroids can, at certain dose levels and in certain combinations, act directly on the mammary alveolar cells and render them less responsive to the *lactogenic* effects of prolactin (Cowie, 1961). This effect is in striking contrast to the sensitizing effect of ovarian hormones in respect of the *mammogenic* effects of prolactin already discussed (see p. 11). However, the antagonism may be relative and may be overcome either by increasing the dose of prolactin or reducing the levels of ovarian steroids (Cowie, 1961).

Recent studies in the rat have provided no support for the widely held view that large doses of oestrogen are inhibitory to prolactin synthesis and release. Even doses of $0 \cdot 1$–$0 \cdot 5$ mg oestradiol benzoate evoke some increase in prolactin levels in the blood although the increases are less than those obtained with much lower doses (see p. 14) (Chen and Meites, 1970). It is therefore interesting that for many years oestrogens have been prescribed to prevent the onset of milk secretion in women or to aid the suppression of an existing lactation. There is evidence that oestrogen therapy is effective because it prevents breast engorgement and breast pain but the efficacy of oestrogen in suppressing milk secretion has been much questioned (Cowie and Tindal, 1971). Recently satisfactory inhibition of the onset of milk secretion has been claimed from the use of a fat-stored oestrogen—quinestrol—given as a single dose (Brown and Snell, 1968; Cruttenden, 1971; Mann, 1971).

Studies on the effects of progestagens alone on milk secretion in women are few; 5–10 mg progesterone or 500 mg 17α-hydroxyprogesterone caproate given as single doses had little effect on milk secretion (for references see Toaff and Jewelewicz, 1963). However, 6α-methyl-17α-hydroxyprogesterone acetate (an oral progestagen without significant oestrogenic activity), given over a ten-day period in daily doses of 30 mg reducing to 10 mg, significantly depressed milk secretion and controlled pain engorgement but it was much more effective when supplemented with an oestrogen (Toaff and Jewelewicz, 1963). If nursing is continued even high doses of oestrogen–progestagen combinations will not completely inhibit milk secretion in women, while with lower dose levels,

16

comparable to those used in oral contraceptives, the milk yield is generally unaffected (Toaff et al., 1969).

## Prolactin inhibitors and milk secretion

The mammalian hypothalamus exerts an inhibitory influence on the synthesis of prolactin by means of a neurohumour—the prolactin-inhibiting factor (PIF)—which is released into the hypophysial portal system and carried to the anterior pituitary. This factor has not yet been isolated or characterized and there is recent evidence in favour of the occurrence also of a prolactin-releasing factor. Hypothalamic catecholamines apparently play an important role in regulating the PIF activity and prolactin release may be influenced by hormones or drugs acting on the hypothalamic control mechanisms or directly on the anterior pituitary (Nicoll, 1971; Cowie and Tindal, 1971; Meites, 1972). Certain ergot alkaloids depress the release of prolactin from the pituitary, the effect being apparently a direct one on the pituitary itself (Shaar and Clemens, 1972). One of these alkaloids, 2-Br-α-ergocryptine, has been used to suppress non-puerperal galactorrhoea and also unwanted lactation after childbirth (Lutterbeck et al., 1971; Besser et al., 1972; Wenner and Varga, 1972). It may also be of interest that the ergot alkaloids, ergocornine and ergocryptine, suppress the appearance of spontaneous mammary tumours in mice presumably by lowering the levels of prolactin in blood (Yanai and Nagasawa, 1971, 1972). These alkaloids are thought to block the stimulating effect of oestrogen on the release of prolactin by a direct action on the pituitary (Lu, Koch and Meites, 1971). No objective remission was observed, however, in 19 patients with advanced breast cancer treated with 2-Br-α-ergocryptine (Heuson, Coune and Staquet, 1972).

L-dopa, a metabolic precursor of dopamine and other catecholamines also suppresses prolactin release (Cowie and Tindal, 1971; Meites, 1972). It will lower prolactin levels in women with non-puerperal galactorrhoea (Malarkey, Jacobs and Daughaday, 1971; Turkington, 1972c) and in women treated with tranquillizers (Kleinberg, Noel and Frantz, 1971). Its efficacy in inhibiting milk secretion, however, requires further investigation (Friesen et al., 1972b).

These and other researches on hypothalamic control mechanisms and the studies in progress on the identification of the neurohumours regulating anterior pituitary function are likely to make available to the clinician powerful new ways and means for controlling the levels of the mammotrophic hormones (Stoll, 1972).

## Prolactin release and the cerebral cortex

It is customary to consider the control of the release of pituitary trophic hormones, amongst them prolactin, the preserve of the hypothalamus. As noted above, the hypothalamus exerts the final control over facilitation or inhibition of release by means of releasing or inhibiting factors. In addition it had been believed that appropriate stimuli, whether exteroceptive or interoceptive, pass direct to the hypothalamus to trigger the release mechanism. However, in the case of prolactin release recent work in this laboratory has indicated that higher neural centres may play a more important role than hitherto envisaged.

In the rabbit an ascending prolactin-release pathway has been traced in the brain stem to a region just in front of the lateral hypothalamus, the lateral preoptic area, and it is believed that this pathway is activated by the suckling stimulus to achieve release of prolactin. In the same series of experiments another pathway for prolactin release could be traced from the orbital part of the cerebral frontal cortex to the lateral preoptic area, and discrete electrical stimulation of this specific region of cortex caused a marked release of prolactin (Tindal and Knaggs, 1970, 1972).

Although as yet we have insufficient results to understand the significance of this finding, several facts are worthy of mention. Orbitofrontal cortex receives sensory inputs of spinothalamic, spinocervicothalamic, vagal and splanchnic origin, which are chiefly of a nociceptive nature (Korn, 1969) and also receives indirect sensory inputs from association cortex (Pandya and Kuypers, 1969); thus it receives sensory information of most modalities, except probably that of olfaction. Orbitofrontal cortex projects both to entorhinal cortex and hence to the limbic system and hypothalamus (Van Hoesen, Pandya and Butters, 1972) and more directly to the lateral preoptic and hypothalamic areas (Nauta, 1964) where it seems likely that information is finally integrated for triggering the release of prolactin (Tindal and Knaggs, 1972).

Cerebral cortical control may therefore play an important role in the regulation of prolactin secretion, a concept which carries with it the highly speculative implication for man that the psychiatric state of the individual may influence not only lactation but possibly the appearance of pathology associated with chronic hypersecretion of prolactin.

## REFERENCES

Agate, F. J. Jnr. (1952). 'The growth and secretory activity of the mammary glands of the pregnant rhesus monkey (*Macaca mulatta*) following hypophysectomy.' *Am. J. Anat.* **90**, 257.

Banerjee, D. N., Banerjee, M. R. and Wagner, J. (1971). 'DNA polymerase activity in mammary gland of virgin mice after ovarian hormone treatment.' *J. Endocr.* **51**, 259.

Banerjee, M. R. and Rogers, F. M. (1971). 'Stimulation of the synthesis of macromolecules by ovarian hormones during early development of the mouse mammary gland.' *J. Endocr.* **49**, 39.

Banerjee, M. R., Wagner, J. E. and Kinder, D. L. (1971). 'DNA synthesis in the absence of cell reproduction during functional differentiation of mouse mammary gland.' *Life Sci.* **10**, 867.

Baulieu, E-E., Alberga, A., Jung, I., Lebeau, M-C., Mercier-Bodard, C., Milgrom, E., Raynaud, J-P., Raynaud-Jammet, C., Rochefort, H., Truong, H. and Robel, P. (1971). 'Metabolism and protein binding of sex steroids in target organs: an approach to the mechanism of hormone action.' *Recent Progr. Hormone Res.* **27**, 351.

Besser, G. M., Parke, L., Edwards, C. R. W., Forsyth, I. A. and McNeilly, A. S. (1971). 'Galactorrhoea: successful treatment with reduction of plasma prolactin levels by brom-ergocryptine.' *Br. med. J.* **3**, 669.

Birkinshaw, M. and Falconer, I. R. (1972). 'The localization of prolactin labelled with radioactive iodine in rabbit mammary tissue.' *J. Endocr.* **55**, 323.

Bishop, P. M. F. (1969). 'Breasts of inappropriate size.' *Practitioner*, **203**, 171.

Bowers, C. Y., Friesen, H. G., Hwang, P., Guyda, H. J. and Folkers, K. (1971). 'Prolactin and thyrotropin release in man by synthetic pyroglutamyl-histidyl-prolinamide.' *Biochim. biophys. Acta* **45**, 1033.

Bresciani, F. (1971). 'Ovarian steroid control of cell proliferation in the mammary gland and cancer.' In *Basic Actions of Sex Steroids on Target Organs*, pp. 130–159, Ed. by P. O. Hubinont, F. Leroy and P. Galand. Basel; Karger.

Brown, D. and Snell, M. (1968). 'Inhibition of lactation with quinestrol.' *Br. med. J.* **4**, 326.

Bruce, J. D. and Ramirez, V. D. (1970). 'Site of action of the inhibitory effect of estrogen upon lactation.' *Neuroendocrinology*, **6**, 19.

Buttle, H. L., Forsyth, I. A. and Knaggs, G. S. (1972). 'Plasma prolactin measured by radioimmunoassay and bioassay in pregnant and lactating goats and the occurrence of a placental lactogen.' *J. Endocr.* **53**, 483.

Chatterton, R. T. Jnr (1971). 'Progesterone and mammary gland development.' In *The Sex Steroids, Molecular Mechanisms*, pp. 345–382, Ed. by K. W. McKerns. New York: Appleton-Century-Crofts.

— Chatterton, A. J. and Hellman, L. (1969). 'Metabolism of progesterone by the rabbit mammary gland.' *Endocrinology* **85**, 16.

Chen, C. L. and Meites, J. (1970). 'Effects of estrogen and progesterone on serum and pituitary prolactin levels in ovariectomized rats.' *Endocrinology* **86**, 503.

Chen, T. T., Johnson, R. E., Lyons, W. R., Li, C. H. and Cole, R. D. (1955). 'Hormonally induced mammary growth and lactation in the absence of the thyroid.' *Endocrinology* **57**, 153.

Clemens, J. A., Shaar, C. J., Tandy, W. A. and Roush, M. E. (1971). 'Effect of hypothalamic stimulation on prolactin secretion in steroid treated rats.' *Endocrinology* **89**, 1317.

Cohen, R. (1971). 'Breast feeding without pregnancy.' *Pediatrics* **48**, 996.

Cowie, A. T. (1961). 'The hormonal control of milk secretion.' In *Milk: The Mammary Gland and its Secretion*, Vol. 1, Chap. 4, pp. 163–203, Ed. by S. K. Kon and A. T. Cowie. New York and London; Academic Press.

— (1966). 'Anterior pituitary function in lactation.' In *The Pituitary Gland*, Vol. 2, Chap. 13, pp. 412–443, Ed. by G. W. Harris and B. T. Donovan. London; Butterworths.

Cowie, A. T., Cox, C. P., Folley, S. J., Hosking, Z. D., Naito, M. and Tindal, J. S. (1965). 'The effects of the duration of treatments with oestrogen and progesterone on the hormonal induction of mammary growth and lactation in the goat.' *J. Endocr.* **32**, 129.

— Knaggs, G. S., Tindal, J. S. and Turvey, A. (1968). 'The milking stimulus and mammary growth in the goat.' *J. Endocr.* **40**, 243.

— and Tindal, J. S. (1971). *The Physiology of Lactation.* London; Edward Arnold.

— — and Yokoyama, A. (1966). 'The induction of mammary growth in the hypophysectomized goat.' *J. Endocr.* **34**, 185.

Cruttenden, L. A. (1971). 'Inhibition of lactation.' *Practitioner* **206**, 248.

Dabelow, A. (1957). 'Die Milchdrüse.' In *Handbuch der mikroskopischen Anatomie des Menschen*, Vol. 3, Part 3, pp. 277–485, Ed. by W. von Möllendorf and W. Bargmann. Berlin, Göttingen and Heidelberg; Springer-Verlag.

Daniel, C. W., DeOme, K. B., Young, J. T., Blair, P. B. and Faulkin, L. J. Jnr. (1968). 'The *in vivo* life span of normal and preneoplastic mouse mammary glands: a serial transplantation study.' *Proc. natn. Acad. Sci. U.S.A.* **61**, 53.

— and Young, L. J. T. (1971). 'Influence on cell division on an aging process. Life span of mouse mammary epithelium during serial propagation *in vitro.*' *Expl Cell Res.* **65**, 27.

— — Medina, D. and DeOme, K. B. (1971). 'The influence of mammogenic hormones on serially transplanted mouse mammary gland.' *Exp. Geront.* **6**, 95.

Deanesly, R. and Parkes, A. S. (1951). 'Lactation: can we learn from primitive peoples?' *Colloques int. Cent. natn. Rech. scient.* No. 32, 173.

Denamur, R. (1971). 'Hormonal control of lactogenesis.' *J. Dairy Res.* **38**, 237.

Dilley, W. G. (1971a). 'Morphogenic and mitogenic effects of prolactin on rat mammary gland *in vitro.*' *Endocrinology* **88**, 514.

— (1971b). 'Relationship of mitosis to alveolar development in the rat mammary gland.' *J. Endocr.* **50**, 501.

Falconer, I. R. (1972). 'The distribution of $^{131}$I- or $^{125}$I-labelled prolactin in rabbit mammary tissue after intravenous or intraductal injection.' *J. Endocr.* **53**, lviii.

Faulkin, L. J. Jnr and DeOme, K. B. (1960). 'Regulation of growth and spacing of gland elements in the mammary fat pad of the C3H mouse.' *J. natn. Cancer Inst.* **24**, 953.

Folley, S. J. (1952). 'Lactation.' In *Marshall's Physiology of Reproduction*, 3rd edn., Vol. 2, Chap. 20, pp. 525–647, Ed. by A. S. Parkes. London; Longmans, Green.

Forsyth, I. A. (1971). 'Organ culture techniques and the study of hormone effects on the mammary gland.' *J. Dairy Res.* **38**, 419.

— (1972). 'Use of a rabbit mammary gland organ culture system to detect lactogenic activity in blood.' In *Lactogenic Hormones*, pp. 151–167, Ed. by G. E. W. Wolstenholme and J. Knight. Edinburgh and London; Churchill Livingstone.

— and Edwards, C. R. W. (1972). 'Human prolactin, its isolation, assay and clinical applications'. *Clin. Endocr.* **1**, 293.

Foss, G. L. and Short, D. (1950). 'Abnormal lactation'. *J. Obstet. Gynaec. Br. Commonw.* **58**, 35.

Frantz, A. G., Kleinberg, D. L. and Noel, G. L. (1972). 'Physiological and pathological secretion of human prolactin studied by *in vitro* bioassay.' In *Lactogenic Hormones*, pp. 137–150, Ed. by G. E. W. Wolstenholme and J. Knight. Edinburgh and London; Churchill Livingstone.

Friesen, H., Belanger, C., Guyda, H. and Hwang, P. (1972a). 'The synthesis and secretion of placental lactogen and pituitary prolactin'. In *Lactogenic Hormones,* pp. 83–103, Ed. by G. E. W. Wolstenholme and J. Knight. Edinburgh and London; Churchill Livingstone.

— Guyda, H., Hwang, P., Tyson, J. E. and Barbeau, A. (1972b). 'Functional evaluation of prolactin secretion: a guide to therapy.' *J. clin. Invest.* **51**, 706.

Geschickter, C. F. (1945). *Diseases of the Breast: Diagnosis, Pathology, Treatment,* 2nd Edn. Philadelphia; Lippincott.

Grischenko, I. I. and Grishchenko, M. P. (1967). 'Redkiĭ sluchaĭ poyavleniya laktatsii vne beremennosti i poslerodovogo perioda.' *Akush. Ginek.* **43**, 66.

Halban, J. (1905). 'Die innere Secretion von Ovarium und Placenta und ihre Bedeutung für die Function der Milchdrüse.' *Arch. Gynaek.* **75**, 353.

Heuson, J. C., Coune, A. and Staquet, M. (1972). 'Clinical trial of 2-Br-α-ergocryptine (CB154) in advanced breast cancer.' *Europ. J. Cancer* **8**, 155.

Hoshino, K. (1970). 'Indefinite *in vivo* life span of serially isografted mouse mammary gland.' *Experientia* **26**, 1393.

Hutton, J. B. (1958). 'Oestrogen function in established lactation in the cow.' *J. Endocr.* **17**, 121.

Hytten, F. E. and Leitch, I. (1971). *The Physiology of Human Pregnancy,* 2nd Edn. Oxford; Blackwell.

Jacobs, L. S., Snyder, P. J., Wilber, J. F., Utiger, R. D. and Daughaday, W. H. (1971). 'Increased serum prolactin after administration of synthetic thyrotropin releasing hormone (TRH) in man.' *J. clin. Endocr. Metab.* **33**, 996.

Jacobsohn, D. (1958). 'Mammary gland growth in relation to hormones with metabolic actions.' *Proc. R. Soc.* **B149**, 325.

— (1961). 'Hormonal regulation of mammary gland growth.' In *Milk: The Mammary Gland and its Secretion,* Vol. 1, Chap. 3, pp. 127–160, Ed. by S. K. Kon and A. T. Cowie. New York and London; Academic Press.

Jensen, E. V. and DeSombre, E. R. (1972). 'Estrogens and progestins.' In *Biochemical Actions of Hormones,* Vol. 2, pp. 215–255, Ed. by G. Litwack. New York and London; Academic Press.

Jungblut, P. W., McCann, S., Görlich, L., Rosenfeld, G. C. and Wagner, R. K. (1970). 'Binding of steroids by tissue proteins. Steroid hormone receptors.' *Research in Steroids* **4**, 213.

King, R. J. B., Gordon, J., Marx, J. and Steggles, A. W. (1971). 'Localization and nature of sex steroids receptors within the cell.' In *Basic Actions of Sex Steroids on Target Organs,* pp. 21–43, Ed. by P. O. Hubinont, F. Leroy and P. Galand. Basel; Karger.

Kleinberg, D. L., Noel, G. L. and Frantz, A. G. (1971). 'Chlorpromazine stimulation and L-dopa suppression of plasma prolactin in man.' *J. clin. Endocr. Metab.* **33**, 873.

Knott, J. (1907). 'Abnormal lactation: in the virgin; in the old woman; in the male; in the newborn of either sex ("witches' milk").' *Am. Med.* **13** (New Series 2), 373.

Korn, H. (1969). 'Splanchnic projection to the orbital cortex of the cat.' *Brain Res.* **16**, 23.

Kuhn, N. J. (1969a). 'Progesterone withdrawal as the lactogenic trigger in the rat.' *J. Endocr.* **44**, 39.

— (1969b). 'Specificity of progesterone inhibition of lactogenesis.' *J. Endocr.* **45**, 615.

Lawson, D. E. M. and Pearlman, W. H. (1964). 'The metabolism *in vivo* of progesterone-7-$^3$H; its localization in the mammary gland, uterus and other tissues of the pregnant rat.' *J. biol. Chem.* **239**, 3226.

Lelong, M., Giraud, P., Roche, J., Liardet, J. and Coignet, J. (1950). 'Sur l'action galactogène des proteines iodées chez la femme. Essais thérapeutiques.' *Archs fr. Pédiat.* **7**, 553.

L'Hermite, M., Vanhaelst, L., Copinschi, G., Leclercq, R., Golstein, J., Bruno, O. D. and Robyn, C. (1972). 'Prolactin release after injection of thyrotrophin-releasing hormone in man.' *Lancet* **1**, 763.

Lu, K-H., Koch, Y. and Meites, J. (1971). 'Direct inhibition by ergocornine of pituitary prolactin release.' *Endocrinology* **89**, 229.

Lutterbeck, P. M., Pryor, J. S., Varga, L. and Wenner, R. (1971). 'Treatment of non-puerperal galactorrhoea with an ergot alkaloid.' *Br. med. J.* **3**, 228.

Lyons, W. R. (1958). 'Hormonal synergism in mammary growth.' *Proc. R. Soc.* **B149**, 303.

— Li, C. H., Ahmad, N. and Rice-Wray, E. (1968). 'Mammotrophic effects of human hypophysial growth hormone preparations in animals and man.' In *Growth Hormone*, pp. 349–363, Ed. by A. Pecile and E. E. Müller. Excerpta Medica International Congress Series No. 158.

McMurtry, J. P. and Anderson, R. R. (1971). 'Prevention of self-licking on mammary gland development rats.' *Proc. Soc. exp. Biol. Med.* **137**, 354.

Malarkey, W. B., Jacobs, L. S. and Daughaday, W. H. (1971). 'Levodopa suppression of prolactin in nonpuerperal galactorrhea.' *New Engl. J. Med.* **285**, 1160.

Mann, C. W. (1971). 'Lactation inhibition in the Outer Hebrides. A trial of fat-stored oestrogen.' *Practitioner*, **206**, 246.

Mayer, G. and Klein, M. (1961). 'Histology and cytology of the mammary gland.' In *Milk: The Mammary Gland and its Secretion*, Vol. 1, Chap. 2, pp. 47–126, Ed. by S. K. Kon and A. T. Cowie. New York and London; Academic Press.

Meites, J. (1972). 'Hypothalamic control of prolactin secretion.' In *Lactogenic Hormones*, pp. 325-338, Ed. by G. E. W. Wolstenholme and J. Knight. Edinburgh and London; Churchill Livingstone.

Mobbs, G. A. and Babbage, N. F. (1971). 'Breast feeding adopted children.' *Med. J. Aust.* **2**, 436.

Munford, R. E. (1964). 'A review of anatomical and biochemical changes in the mammary gland with particular reference to quantitative methods of assessing mammary development.' *Dairy Sci. Abstr.* **26**, 293.

Nagasawa, H. and Yanai, R. (1971). 'Increased mammary gland response to pituitary mammotropic hormones by estrogen in rats.' *Endocr. jap.* **18**, 53.

— — (1972). 'Inhibitory effect of estrogen on mammary growth and its counteraction by pituitary isograft in mice.' *Endocr. jap.* **19**, 107.

Nandi, S. (1958). 'Endocrine control of mammary-gland development and function in the C3H/HeCrgl mouse.' *J. natn. Cancer Inst.* **21**, 1039.

— (1959). 'Hormonal control of mammogenesis and lactogenesis in the C3H/HeCrgl mouse.' *Univ. Calif. Publs Zool.* **65**, 1.

— and Bern, H. A. (1960). 'Relation between mammary-gland responses to lactogenic hormone combinations and tumor susceptibility in various strains of mice.' *J. natn. Cancer Inst.* **24**, 907.

Nandi, S. and Bern, H. A. (1961). 'The hormones responsible for lactogenesis in BALB/cCrgl mice.' *Gen. comp. Endocr.* **1**, 195.

Nauta, W. J. H. (1964). 'Some efferent connections of the prefrontal cortex in the monkey.' In *The Frontal Granular Cortex and Behavior*, Chap. 19, pp. 397–407, Ed. by J. M. Warren and K. Akert. New York; McGraw-Hill.

Newton, M. (1961). 'Human lactation.' In *Milk, The Mammary Gland and its Secretion*, Vol. 1, Chap. 7, pp. 281–320, Ed. by S. K. Kon and A. T. Cowie. New York and London; Academic Press.

Nicoll, C. S. (1971). 'Aspects of the neural control of prolactin secretion.' In *Frontiers in Neuroendocrinology 1971*, Chap. 10, pp. 291–330, Ed. by L. Martini and W. F. Ganong. New York; Oxford University Press.

Norgren, A. (1968). 'Modifications of mammary development of rabbits injected with ovarian hormones.' *Acta Univ. lund.* Section II, no. 4, 1.

Oka, T. and Topper, Y. J. (1972). 'Is prolactin mitogenic for mammary epithelium?' *Proc. natn Acad. Sci. U.S.A.*, **69**, 1693.

Paape, M. J. and Sinha, Y. N. (1971). 'Nucleic acid and collagen content of mammary glands between 30 and 80 days of age in normal and ovariectomized rats and during pregnancy.' *J. Dairy Sci.* **54**, 1068.

Pandya, D. N. and Kuypers, H. G. J. M. (1969). 'Cortico-cortical connections in the rhesus monkey.' *Brain Res.* **13**, 13.

Paterson, J. Y. F. and Linzell, J. L. (1971). 'The secretion of cortisol and its mammary uptake in the goat.' *J. Endocr.* **50**, 493.

Puca, G. A. and Bresciani, F. (1969). 'Interactions of 6,7-$^3$H-17β-estradiol with mammary gland and other organs of the C3H mouse *in vivo*.' *Endocrinology,* **85**, 1.

Roth, L. L. and Rosenblatt, J. S. (1968). 'Self-licking and mammary development during pregnancy in the rat.' *J. Endocr.* **42**, 363.

Sander, S. (1968). 'The uptake of 17-β oestradiol in breast tissue of female rats.' *Acta endocr. Copenh.* **58**, 49.

Sandison, A. T. (1962). 'An autopsy study of the adult human breast.' *National Cancer Institute Monograph*, No. 8, pp. 1–145.

Shaar, C. J. and Clemens, J. A. (1972). 'Inhibition of lactation and prolactin secretion in rats by ergot alkaloids.' *Endocrinology* **90**, 285.

Shome, B. and Friesen, H. G. (1971). 'Purification and characterisation of monkey placental lactogen.' *Endocrinology* **89**, 631.

Simpson, A. A. and Schmidt, G. H. (1969). 'Nucleic acid content of rat mammary gland nuclei during pregnancy, lactation and involution.' *Proc. Soc. exp. Biol. Med.* **132**, 978.

Simpson, M. E., Van Wagenen, G., Van Dyke, D. C., Koneff, A. A. and Tobias, C. A. (1959). 'Deuteron irradiation of the monkey pituitary.' *Endocrinology* **65**, 831.

Singh, D. V. and Bern, H. A. (1969). 'Interaction between prolactin and thyroxine in mouse mammary gland lobulo-alveolar development *in vitro*.' *J. Endocr.* **45**, 579.

Slotin, C. A., Heap, R. B., Christiansen, J. M. and Linzell, J. L. (1970). 'Synthesis of progesterone by the mammary gland of the goat.' *Nature, Lond.* **225**, 385.

Speert, H. (1948). 'The normal and experimental development of the mammary gland of the rhesus monkey, with some pathological correlations.' *Contr. Embryol.* **32**, 9.

Stoll, B. A. (1972). 'Brain catecholamines and breast cancer: a hypothesis.' *Lancet* **1**, 431.

Sulman, F. G. (1970). *Hypothalamic Control of Lactation*. Berlin, Heidelberg, New York; Springer-Verlag.

Talwalker, P. K. and Meites, J. (1961). 'Mammary lobulo-alveolar growth induced by anterior pituitary hormones in adreno-ovariectomized and adreno-ovariectomized-hypophysectomized rats.' *Proc. Soc. exp. Biol. Med.* **107**, 880.

Tindal, J. S. and Knaggs, G. S. (1970). 'Release of prolactin in the rabbit after electrical stimulation of the forebrain.' *J. Endocr.* **48**, xxxii.

— — (1972). 'Pathways in the forebrain of the rabbit concerned with the release of prolactin.' *J. Endocr.* **52**, 253.

Toaff, R. and Jewelewicz, R. (1963). 'Inhibition of lactogenesis by combined oral progestogens and oestrogens.' *Lancet* **2**, 322.

— Ashkenazi, H., Schwartz, A. and Herzberg, M. (1969). 'Effects of oestrogen and progestagen on the composition of human milk.' *J. Reprod. Fert.* **19**, 475.

Topper, Y. J. (1970). 'Multiple hormone interactions in the development of mammary gland *in vitro*.' *Recent Progr. Hormone Res.* **26**, 287.

— Friedberg, S. H. and Oka, T. (1971). 'On the development of insulin sensitivity by mouse mammary gland *in vitro*.' In *Changing Syntheses in Development* (Developmental Biology Supplement, Vol. 4, 1970), pp. 101–113, Ed. by M. N. Runner. New York and London; Academic Press.

Turkington, R. W. (1972a). 'Molecular biological aspects of prolactin.' In *Lactogenic Hormones*, pp. 111–127, Ed. by G. E. W. Wolstenholme and J. Knight. Edinburgh and London; Churchill Livingstone.

— (1972b). 'Phenothiazine stimulation test for prolactin reserve: the syndrome of isolated prolactin deficiency.' *J. clin. Endocr. Metab.* **34**, 247.

— (1972c). 'Inhibition of prolactin secretion and successful therapy of the Forbes–Albright syndrome with L-dopa.' *J. clin. Endocr. Metab.* **34**, 306.

— and Kadohama, N. (1972). 'Gene activation in mammary cells.' In *Gene Transcription in Reproductive Tissue*, pp. 346–368, Ed. by E. Diczfalusy. Stockholm; Karolinska Institutet.

Tyson, J. E., Friesen, H. G. and Anderson, M. S. (1972). 'Human lactational and ovarian response to endogenous prolactin release.' *Science, N.Y.* **177**, 897.

— Hwang, P., Guyda, H. and Friesen, H. G. (1972). 'Studies on prolactin secretion in human pregnancy.' *Am. J. Obstet. Gynec.* **113**, 14.

Van Hoesen, G. W., Pandya, D. N. and Butters, N. (1972). 'Cortical afferents to the entorhinal cortex of the rhesus monkey.' *Science, N.Y.* **175**, 1471.

Voogt, J. L., Chen, C. L. and Meites, J. (1970). 'Serum and pituitary prolactin levels before, during, and after puberty in female rats.' *Am. J. Physiol.* **218**, 396.

Wenner, R. and Varga, L. (1972). 'Prolactinhemmung mittels Ergocryptin.' *Acta endocr. Copenh.* **69**, Supplement 159, 40.

Yanai, R. and Nagasawa, H. (1971). 'Inhibition by ergocornine and 2-Br-α-ergocryptin of spontaneous mammary tumor appearance in mice.' *Experientia* **27**, 934.

— — (1972). 'Inhibition of mammary tumorigenesis by ergot alkaloids and promotion of mammary tumorigenesis by pituitary isografts in adreno-ovariectomized mice.' *J. natn. Cancer Inst.* **48**, 715.

# 2

# Neuroendocrine Control of Murine Mammary Carcinoma

## Clifford W. Welsch and Joseph Meites

Perhaps the most significant advance in endocrinology during the past 25 years has been the recognition that the endocrine system is mainly regulated by the central nervous system. Hormones associated with normal and neoplastic breast development are among those which appear to be markedly affected by changes in central nervous system activity. It seems to be a reasonable assumption, therefore, that a central nervous system–mammary tumorigenesis relationship exists, although few studies designed to verify this relationship have been initiated. In this chapter, we will present evidence which supports this relationship and demonstrates that regulation of mammary tumour development and growth can be achieved, at least in part, by application of techniques based on current neuroendocrine concepts and procedures.

## HORMONES IN THE INDUCTION AND GROWTH OF MURINE MAMMARY TUMOURS

The concept of hormonal involvement in mammary tumorigenesis in man and animals was derived, in part, from the classic studies of Beatson (1896) who in 1895 performed the first ovariectomy in human patients for the control of breast cancer, and from Lacassagne (1933) who demonstrated that chronic administration of oestrogen to mice resulted in a high incidence of mammary tumours. Following these early studies, experimental murine mammary tumour systems, particularly the spontaneous, virus-dependent, mouse mammary tumour and the carcinogen-induced rat mammary tumour, have been used most frequently as models for human breast cancer.

## Role of pituitary hormones

Strains of rats that are normally highly susceptible to spontaneous mammary tumorigenesis do not ordinarily develop mammary tumours if hypophysectomized (Moon et al., 1951). On the other hand, administration of

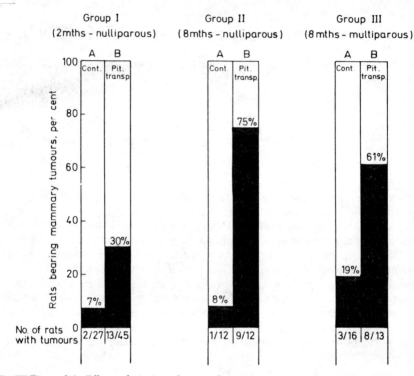

Figure 2.1. Effects of pituitary homografts on mammary tumour incidence nine months after grafting. Rats of Group I B (nulliparous) were grafted with pituitaries at two months of age. Rats of Group II B (nulliparous) and III B (multiparous) were grafted with pituitaries at eight months of age (Cont.=control) (after Welsch et al., 1970)

pituitary hormones to these animals markedly increases the incidence of mammary tumours. For example, transplantation of multiple pituitaries (Boot et al., 1962; Welsch, Jenkins and Meites, 1970) *(Figure 2.1)* or pituitary tumours (Haran-Ghera, 1961; Meites, 1972) to mice or rats significantly increased the incidence and decreased the latency period for development of spontaneous mammary tumours. Numerous neuroendocrine studies have demonstrated that the transplanted pituitary secretes large amounts of prolactin and greatly reduced amounts of all other pituitary hormones (Welsch et al., 1968), thus implicating prolactin as the principal pituitary hormone in development of murine mammary tumours. This concept is considerably strengthened by a report by Boot et al. (1962) of increased mammary tumour incidence in mice chronically injected with prolactin.

Pituitary hormones have emerged as the principal hormones in maintaining growth of carcinogen-induced rat mammary tumours. Growth of these tumours can be maintained or enhanced in ovariectomized rats by grafting prolactin and growth-hormone-secreting pituitary tumours (Kim and Furth, 1960) or by the concurrent administration of prolactin and growth hormone (Talwalker, Meites and Mizuno, 1964). That prolactin is the principal pituitary hormone in this growth-promoting process is further indicated by recent studies demonstrating enhanced growth of mammary tumours in ovariectomized–adrenalectomized rats injected daily with prolactin (Pearson et al., 1969; Nagasawa and Yanai, 1970). Administration of growth hormone alone was without any stimulatory effect. Hypophysectomy resulted in a marked regression of these tumours (Huggins, Briziarelli and Sutton, 1959).

## Role of ovarian hormones

If strains of mammary tumour-susceptible mice or rats are ovari- ectomized at an early age, mammary tumours seldom develop and, if ovariectomized–adrenalectomized, tumours very rarely develop (Durbin et al., 1966; Bittner and Cole, 1961; Terenius, 1971). The rare occurrence of spontaneous mammary tumours in ovariectomized mice is often accompanied by concurrent adrenal hyperplasia (Fekete, Woolley and Little, 1941; Richardson, 1967). Conversely, increased amounts of these hormones can enhance mammary tumorigenesis in intact mice and rats. Chronic administration of ovarian hormones, particularly oestrogen, to mice or rats has been a routine method for inducing mammary tumours in these species (Cutts and Noble, 1964; Huseby, 1965). Moderate dose levels of oestrogen also stimulate growth of existing carcinogen-induced rat mammary tumours, whereas large doses of oestrogen are inhibitory to tumour growth (Dao, 1964; Huggins, Moon and Morii, 1962). Ovariectomy of tumour-bearing rats also results in tumour regression (Daniel and Prichard, 1964; Young, Baker and Helfenstein, 1965; Dao, 1966; Welsch, 1971).

Hyperplastic alveolar nodules of the mammary gland have been described by a number of investigators and established by the Berkeley group (DeOme et al., 1962) as the precursors of many of the mammary tumours that occur in the mouse. These hyperplasias are considered precancerous because tumours arise from them much more frequently, and in less time, than from normal mammary tissue. The hormone dependency of these hyperplasias is shown in studies which demonstrate that hypophysectomy or ovariectomy of mammary tumour-susceptible mice suppresses their development and growth. Furthermore, their transformation to a carcinoma requires hormones from the ovary (or adrenals) and pituitary (Nandi, Bern and DeOme, 1960; Bern and Nandi, 1961). Recently, it was reported that prolactin appears to be the principal hormone necessary for the maintenance (Yanai and Nagasawa, 1971a) and transformation (Dux and Mühlbock, 1969) of these hyperplasias.

### Interaction of pituitary and ovarian hormones

It has been established that administered oestrogens markedly increase prolactin secretion, whereas ovariectomy decreases the secretion of this hormone (Meites and Nicoll, 1966), an observation which has led to the well-

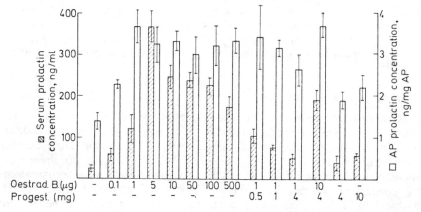

*Figure 2.2. Effects of different doses of oestradiol benzoate and/or progesterone on serum and anterior pituitary prolactin concentration in ovariectomized rats (five per group). The vertical bars indicate standard error of the mean (after Chen and Meites, 1970)*

known hypothesis that oestrogens are mammary oncogenic primarily because of their stimulatory effect on prolactin secretion (Furth, 1968). This concept is supported by studies such as those demonstrating the inability of oestrogen to reactivate or even maintain tumour growth in mammary tumour-bearing, hypophysectomized rats (Sterental et al., 1963) and a lack of detectable growth stimulatory effect of the steroid on growth of mammary tumour tissue *in vitro* (Welsch and Rivera, 1972). It is doubtful, however, that the mechanism of action of oestrogen in the genesis and maintenance of mammary tumours is solely indirect, i.e., via the pituitary. There is evidence that oestrogen can act directly on mammary tumour tissue increasing specific activity of certain enzyme systems (Hollander, Jones and Smith, 1958).

Although moderate dose levels of oestrogen are stimulatory to mammary tumour development and growth, large doses of the steroid inhibit growth of established mammary tumours in experimental animals as well as in man (Huggins, Moon and Morii, 1962; Stoll, 1969). It has been suggested that large doses of oestrogen inhibit mammary tumour growth by reducing prolactin secretion below normal levels (Kim, 1965). However, recent evidence (Chen and Meites, 1970) is to the contrary, as a wide range of doses of oestrogen, when administered to rats, have been found to elevate blood prolactin levels *(Figures 2.2)*. Moderate doses (5 µg) and high doses (500 µg) increase blood

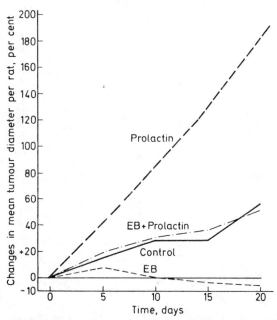

Figure 2.3. *Effects of daily injection of prolactin (1 mg NIH ovine prolactin, 28 i.u./mg), oestradiol benzoate (EB) (20 µg) or of both on growth of DMBA-induced mammary tumours in Sprague–Dawley rats. Note that EB inhibited tumour growth-stimulating action of prolactin and also prevented tumour growth in untreated tumour-bearing rats. The combination of prolactin and EB prevented the oestrogen from inhibiting mammary tumour growth (after Meites et al., 1971)*

prolactin levels from 10 to 20 times greater than that observed in the non-treated controls.

Recent studies have provided evidence that the inhibitory effect of large doses of oestrogen on mammary tumour growth may be primarily a result of direct action of the steroid on the tumour, directly interfering with the stimulatory effects of prolactin on cellular proliferation and perhaps also interfering with cellular metabolic processes. Meites, Cassell and Clark (1971) provide *in vivo* evidence that large doses of oestrogen directly inhibit stimulation by prolactin of carcinogen-induced mammary tumour growth. They demonstrate that large doses of prolactin could overcome the inhibitory effects of administered oestrogen, suggesting that the steroid interfered with the peripheral action of prolactin on the tumour tissue *(Figure 2.3)*.

Welsch and Rivera (1972) recently reported the results of a study designed

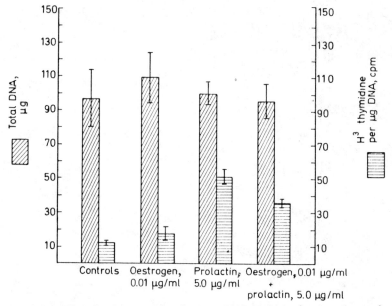

*Figure 2.4. Effect of oestrogen and prolactin on DNA synthesis of organ cultures of DMBA-induced rat mammary carcinoma: H³-thymidine incorporation per microgram of DNA; significance levels are: p < 0·01, controls (C)/P, C/P + E, E/P, and E/E + P; p < 0·05, P/E + P; p = NS, C/E. No significant difference among groups in total DNA was observed (after Welsch and Rivera, 1972)*

to determine and compare the capacity of oestrogen and prolactin to promote DNA synthesis in organ culture of carcinogen-induced rat mammary tumours. The results of this study demonstrated that prolactin stimulates DNA synthesis in organ cultures of rat mammary tumours *(Figure 2.4)*. Oestrogen, at moderate dose levels, was without effect but, at high dose levels, was inhibitory to DNA synthesis *(Figure 2.5)*. Oestrogen also suppressed prolactin-induced DNA synthesis *(Figure 2.4)*. Evidence, therefore, for an interaction of the steroid with the tumour either by directly interfering with DNA synthesis and/or by suppressing the prolactin stimulating effect is provided in this study. In accord, Turkington and Hilf (1968) have reported an oestrogen-induced inhibition of DNA synthesis by cultured C3H mouse mammary tumour. The observed stimulatory effect of prolactin on DNA synthesis (Welsch and Rivera, 1972) provides *in vitro* evidence that prolactin is an important hormone in promoting growth of rat mammary tumours, and

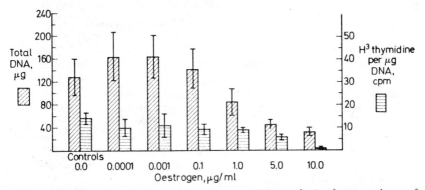

*Figure 2.5. Effect of varying levels of oestrogen on DNA synthesis of organ cultures of DMBA-induced rat mammary carcinoma: $H^3$-thymidine incorporation per microgram of DNA; and total DNA significance levels are: $p < 0.01$, controls/E (5.0 ug/ml) or E (10.0 ug/ml). No significant differences among other groups were observed (after Welsch and Rivera, 1972)*

the total lack of a stimulatory effect of oestrogen *in vitro* lends credence to the hypothesis that oestrogens are mammary oncogenic primarily as a result of their ability to influence prolactin secretion.

## INTER-RELATIONSHIP OF CENTRAL NERVOUS SYSTEM AND ENDOCRINE SYSTEM

It is now well established that the central nervous system significantly influences the activity of the endocrine system. A brief review of this area is intended solely to facilitate understanding of various experimental procedures and results discussed in subsequent sections of this chapter. A more comprehensive review of this subject is given in Chapters 7 and 8.

Numerous experiments have demonstrated that there are separate hypothalamic factors controlling each of the anterior pituitary hormones (Meites, 1970). Several of these factors (hypophysiotrophic hormones) have been extracted: corticotrophin-releasing factor (CRF), thyrotrophin-releasing factor (TRF), growth hormone-releasing factor (GRF), LRF–FRF and prolactin-release-inhibiting factor (PIF). Recent studies have suggested the possible existence of a prolactin-releasing factor (PRF) (Nicoll et al., 1970) and a growth hormone-inhibiting factor (GIF) (McCann, Dhariwal and Porter, 1968). Several laboratories have been actively pursuing the chemical identification of these hypothalamic hypophysiotrophic hormones (Schally et

31

al., 1970; Burgus and Guillemin, 1970). There is some disagreement among these laboratories on the precise chemical structure of several of the hormones, although general agreement exists that they are small polypeptides. For example, TRF is a tripeptide, L-pyroglutamyl-L-histidyl-L-proline amide (Burgus and Guillemin, 1970). LRF–FRF is a decapeptide with the ability to induce release of both LH and FSH (Matsuo et al., 1971). GRF is believed to be an acidic polypeptide with a molecular weight of 1600 (Schally et al., 1970). The chemical identity of the prolactin-release-inhibiting factor is unknown. The chemical nature of the hypophysiotrophic hormones is currently of great interest.

The hypophysiotrophic hormones are believed to be secreted by neurons which end on the capillary loops in the median eminence, from which the hypothalamic–pituitary portal vessels arise. Several studies have been designed to determine the hypothalamic site of origin of these hormones. Results of transplantation of pituitary tissue into different regions of the rat brain suggest that the medial–basal region of the hypothalamus (hypophysiotrophic area) is the principal area of hormone production. Several investigators have suggested that the control of the basal secretion of FSH, LH, TSH, ACTH, GH and prolactin is localized in this area and, to some extent, this area may be able to function independently of other hypothalamic areas (Szentagothai et al., 1968). However, this area does not control ovulation and environmental factors cannot influence anterior pituitary function unless neural connections to the medial–basal area remain intact.

Within and adjacent to the hypophysiotrophic area are hypothalamic nuclei which are believed to have a profound effect on synthesis and release of the hypophysiotrophic hormones. These nuclei may well be the specific sites of production of these hormones. Hypothalamic–anterior pituitary activity is also influenced and partly controlled by a variety of extra-hypothalamic afferent neural pathways arising principally from the limbic system, the habenular complex and the reticular formation. Although very little is known of the nature of these influences, electrolytic lesions in these neural structures result in marked changes in endocrine activity (Zoukar and deGroot, 1963; Elwers and Critchlow, 1966; Welsch, Clemens and Meites, 1969).

Hypophysiotrophic hormone secretion is believed to be largely regulated by negative feedback from: (1) target organ hormones (long loop); (2) anterior pituitary hormones (short loop); and perhaps (3) hypophysiotrophic hormones (ultra-short loop) (Meites, 1970). This concept has been developed from studies demonstrating that implantation of hormones into hypothalamic areas significantly influences hypophysiotrophic hormone concentration (Voogt et al., 1971; Welsch et al., 1968). In addition, radioautographic techniques have provided evidence that certain steroids concentrate in hypothalamic areas and extra-hypothalamic areas associated with the hypothalamus (Gorski, 1970). Considering the vast neuronal inter-relationships in the central nervous system, it is probable that many non-endocrine influences also can markedly influence hypophysiotrophic hormone secretions.

Catecholamines are present in the hypothalamus in relatively high concentrations and appear to be involved in the release of a number of anterior pituitary hormones. It has been reported that an adrenergic tonus stimulates the release of LH and FSH and inhibits prolactin release (Wurtman, 1970). It is probable that the catecholamines act as neuro-transmitters to induce the release of the hypothalamic hypophysiotrophic hormones. This is supported by studies demonstrating that the administration of drugs that increase hypothalamic catecholamines, e.g. dopamine, causes an increase in the release of LRF–FRF (Kamberi, Mical and Porter, 1970) and PIF (Kamberi, Schneider and McCann, 1970). The feedback mechanism of hormones on hypophysiotrophic hormone synthesis and release is probably mediated, at least in part, by influencing hypothalamic catecholamine activity.

## THE CENTRAL NERVOUS SYSTEM AND MAMMARY TUMORIGENESIS IN MICE AND RATS

Sufficient evidence is available to support the existence of a central nervous system–mammary tumorigenesis relationship in experimental animals as well as in man. Murine mammary tumour development and growth have been reported to be significantly influenced by a variety of factors that affect central nervous system activity, e.g. stress (Andervont, 1944; Reznikoff and Martin, 1957; Marchant, 1966), androgenization (Kovacs, 1965; Dao, 1966; Stern, Mickey and Osvaldo, 1966), hypothalamic implant of oestrogen (Nagasawa and Meites, 1970b) and constant light (Jull, 1966). A variety of psychological factors have also been reported to have a direct bearing on the incidence and progression of mammary cancer in man (for review, see LeShan, 1959). Experimentally, a more direct approach in evaluating this complex inter-relationship is to manipulate the brain using stereotaxic procedures or to administer drugs known to influence various aspects of brain activity and subsequently evaluate the effects of these procedures on the development and growth of mammary tumours.

### Effect of brain lesions

In one of the earliest attempts to more directly establish the influence of the central nervous system on mammary tumorigenesis, Liebelt (1959) induced hypothalamic damage in R111 X CBA virgin female mice by a single injection of gold thioglucose. All mice were treated at 70–80 days of age and developed a persistent obesity. Even though irregularities could not be detected in the oestrous cycle, these animals were incapable of reproduction. Mammary tumours developed in 100 per cent of the gold thioglucose-treated mice, in contrast to 85 per cent tumour incidence in the untreated virgins. Time of mammary tumour appearance was accelerated in the mice with hypothalamic damage, with 50 per cent developing tumours by 240 days as compared with 350 days in controls. Mammary tumours per animal averaged 3·2 in the gold thioglucose-treated mice, in contrast to 1·9 in the controls. Liebelt concluded that enhancement of mammary tumorigenesis in the mice bearing hypothalamic damage was associated with the hormonal imbalance initiated by an altered neuroendocrine mechanism.

Although there is sufficient evidence to demonstrate that mammary tumorigenesis is influenced by the central nervous system, few studies have been directed toward determining the role of *discrete areas* of the brain on mammary oncogenesis. One of the first studies designed to investigate this problem was by Clemens, Welsch and Meites (1968). Female Sprague–Dawley rats were given a single intravenous injection of 7,12-dimethyl-benzanthracene (DMBA) at 56 days of age and divided into four groups, as follows: (1) intact controls, no further treatment; (2) intact, bilateral electrolytic lesions in the median eminence area of the hypothalamus at 50 days of age; (3) ovariectomized at 64 days of age; and (4) placement of bilateral electrolytic lesions in the median eminence area of the hypothalamus at 50 days of age and ovariectomized at 64 days of age. Following carcinogen treatment, all animals were examined once weekly for development of mammary tumours.

Results (Table 2.1) demonstrated that lesions in the median eminence had a significant inhibitory effect on mammary tumour induction. In the intact controls (group 1), 95 per cent of the rats had mammary tumours when the experiment was terminated six months after carcinogen treatment, whereas intact rats with hypothalamic lesions (group 2) had only a 30 per cent incidence of mammary tumours. The ovariectomized controls (group 3) showed a 54 per cent tumour incidence, whereas ovariectomized rats with hypothalamic lesions (group 4) were completely free of mammary tumours six months after carcinogen treatment. The average number of tumours per tumour-bearing rat was significantly lower in the lesioned groups than in either of the control groups. These results were subsequently confirmed by Klaiber et al. (1969). They reported a 25 per cent incidence of mammary tumours in female Sprague–Dawley rats lesioned in the median eminence area of the hypothalamus prior to DMBA treatment, in contrast to 100 per cent tumour incidence in the sham-lesioned controls.

The decreased incidence of mammary tumours in rats with hypothalamic lesions placed prior to DMBA treatment is believed to be due to the increased release of prolactin, stimulating mammary growth but making the mammary tissue relatively refractory to the action of the carcinogen. We have observed that transplantation of pituitaries into intact rats (Welsch et al., 1968), treatment of rats with a norethynodrel–mestranol combination (Welsch and

## TABLE 2.1

### Effects of Median Eminence Lesions Placed in Rats before Treatment with DMBA

| Group and treatment* | Total no. of rats | No. and % of rats with tumours | Average no. of tumours/ tumour-bearing rat | Range and mean latency period (days) |
|---|---|---|---|---|
| (1) Control intact | 22 | 21 (95) | $3 \cdot 1 \pm 0 \cdot 11$† | 40–175 ( 78 $\pm$ 5)† |
| (2) Lesioned intact‖ | 20 | 6 (30) | $1 \cdot 16 \pm 0 \cdot 03$§ | 65–177 (104 $\pm$ 14)§ |
| (3) Control ovariectomized¶ | 13 | 7 (54) | $2 \cdot 33 \pm 0 \cdot 42$‡ | 102–186 (156 $\pm$ 7)‡ |
| (4) Lesioned ovariectomized | 20 | 0 (0) | 0 | 0 (0) |

After Clemens et al., 1968

* DMBA was administered on day 56.

†‡§ Groups possessing different superscripts are significantly different from each other ($p = 0.05$). Standard error of the mean is indicated for each group.

‖ ME lesion placed on day 50.

¶ ovariectomy performed on day 64.

Meites, 1969) or reserpine (Welsch and Meites, 1970) prior to DMBA treatment, similarly inhibits mammary tumorigenesis and at the same time stimulates mammary growth.

When female rats are lesioned in the median eminence area of the hypothalamus after carcinogen treatment, the results are markedly different as illustrated in the following studies (Welsch, Clemens and Meites, 1969; Klaiber et al., 1969). Female Sprague–Dawley rats, 55 days of age, were treated with DMBA: 70–90 days after carcinogen treatment, when all rats had at least one palpable mammary tumour, they were divided into groups and treated as follows: (1) intact controls, sham-operated; (2) intact and lesions placed in the median eminence area of the hypothalamus; (3) ovariectomized controls, sham-operated; (4) ovariectomized and lesions placed in the median eminence. At 0, 10 and 25 days after placement of the lesions, all rats were examined for number of palpable mammary tumours.

Intact rats bearing mammary tumours responded 10 and 25 days after lesions were placed in the median eminence with 138 and 200 per cent increases, respectively, in number of palpable mammary tumours/rat, in contrast to increases of only 23 and 27 per cent, respectively, in the intact controls (Table 2.2). A significant increase in mean mammary tumour diameter also was observed in the intact median eminence-lesioned rats. Rats with lesions placed in the median eminence and ovariectomized immediately thereafter responded 10 days later with a 25 per cent increase, and 25 days later with a 35 per cent decrease in number of palpable mammary tumours/rat in contrast to 40 and 58 per cent decreases at 10 and 25 days, respectively, in the ovariectomized controls. By contrast, when ovariectomy preceded the median eminence lesions by 10 days, no significant effect of the lesions was observed in the number of mammary tumours/rat or mean tumour diameter when compared to the ovariectomized controls (Welsch, Clemens and Meites, 1969).

These results are essentially in agreement with Klaiber et al. (1969) who reported that median eminence–hypothalamic lesions accelerated growth of established carcinogen-induced rat mammary tumours, and ovariectomy reduced this enhancing effect. In their study, the number of tumours/rat 21 days after placement of lesions was $9 \cdot 1$ in median eminence-lesioned intact rats in contrast to $5 \cdot 5$ in the intact controls. When ovariectomy and median eminence lesions were combined, $5 \cdot 4$ mammary tumours/rat were observed, as compared to $3 \cdot 2$ in the ovariectomized controls.

The effects of median eminence–hypothalamic lesions on pituitary function are, in many respects, qualitatively similar to those seen after stalk section or transplantation of the pituitary, i.e. increased secretion of prolactin and significantly reduced secretion of all other anterior pituitary hormones (Meites, 1966). Welsch et al. (1971) reported that placement of median eminence lesions in Sprague–Dawley female rats resulted in a ten-fold increase in serum

## TABLE 2.2

Effect of Median Eminence and Preoptic and Amygdaloid Lesions on Mammary Tumour Development and Growth in Intact Female Rats Treated with 7,12-Dimethylbenzanthracene (DMBA)

| Group | Treatment* | No. of rats | Average number of palpable mammary tumours | | | | |
|---|---|---|---|---|---|---|---|
| | | | At time of lesion | 10 days after lesion | % change | 25 days after lesion | % change |
| I | Intact + sham lesion | 22 | $3.0 \pm 0.3$† | $3.7 \pm 0.4^a$ | + 23 | $3.8 \pm 0.4^d$ | + 27 |
| II | Intact + median eminence lesion | 20 | $2.6 \pm 0.4$ | $6.2 \pm 0.8^b$ | +138 | $7.8 \pm 0.9^e$ | +200 |
| III | Intact + preoptic lesion | 11 | $3.7 \pm 0.8$ | $3.2 \pm 0.6^c$ | − 14 | $2.5 \pm 0.5^f$ | − 32 |
| IV | Intact + amygdaloid lesion | 12 | $4.8 \pm 0.6$ | $4.6 \pm 0.9$ | − 4 | $4.5 \pm 1.0$ | − 6 |

After Welsch et al., 1969.

a/b, d/e = $P < 0.001$; d/f = $P < 0.002$; a/c = $P < 0.05$.

* DMBA was administered at 55 days of age. Bilateral lesions were made 70–90 days after DMBA treatment.

† Standard error of the mean.

prolactin levels just 30 minutes after the lesion *(Figure 2.6)*. Serum prolactin levels remained significantly higher than control levels for a period of at least five months. The persistence of the increased serum prolactin levels constitutes further evidence that the predominant influence of the hypothalamus on

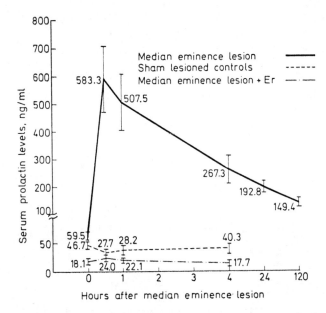

Figure 2.6. Effects of median eminence lesions on serum prolactin levels of female rats at 0·5, 1, 2, 4, 24, and 120 hours after placement of lesions; influence of ergocornine (Er) (after Welsch et al., 1971)

prolactin release is inhibitory. Lesions in the median eminence are believed to act, at least in part, by disrupting the hypothalamic–pituitary portal system, the final common vascular pathway from the hypothalamus to the pituitary, thereby preventing the prolactin-release-inhibiting factor from reaching the pituitary gland.

The striking increase in mammary tumour growth after median eminence–hypothalamic lesions provides further evidence that prolactin is the principal pituitary hormone in this growth process. Ovarian hormones, however, also appear to be involved, as a diminished growth response of the mammary tumours is observed in ovariectomized, median eminence-lesioned rats when compared to intact median eminence-lesioned rats (Welsch, Clemens and Meites, 1969; Klaiber et al., 1969). This is further supported by Sinha, Cooper and Dao (1972) who reported that growth of carcinogen-induced mammary tumours could be reactivated in ovariectomized, median eminence-lesioned rats by ovarian grafts. They also reported that mammary tumours continued to regress in the ovariectomized, median eminence-lesioned rats despite the presence of high levels of blood prolactin in these animals, results which were also observed in our laboratory (Welsch, 1972a). Although previous reports demonstrated increased growth of carcinogen-induced mammary tumours in ovariectomized–adrenalectomized rats injected daily with prolactin (Pearson et al., 1969; Yanai and Nagasawa, 1970), these treatments were only given for a limited duration and the effects observed may not have persisted over a longer period of time.

Few investigations have been initiated to evaluate the role of sites other than the median eminence area of the hypothalamus in tumorigenesis. Welsch, Clemens and Meites (1969) placed bilateral electrolytic lesions in the preoptic area of the hypothalamus or amygdaloid complex of female Sprague–Dawley rats bearing DMBA-induced mammary tumours. Rats with lesions in the preoptic area showed significant tumour regression for up to 25 days, as indicated by a decrease in the number of mammary tumours/rat and a marked decrease in the mean tumour diameter (Table 2.2). The mean tumour diameter in rats bearing amygdaloid lesions was also significantly decreased 25 days after lesion placement, but this treatment had no effect on the number of mammary tumours/rat. Unfortunately, an insufficient number of studies have been conducted adequately to analyse the precise hormonal alterations produced as a result of lesions in these areas.

The effect of median eminence-hypothalamic lesions on development of *spontaneous* mammary tumours was investigated by Welsch, Nagasawa and Meites (1970). Mature, multiparous, female Sprague–Dawley rats, free of palpable mammary tumours, were divided into two groups: one group was given bilateral electrolytic lesions in the median eminence, the other group served as sham-lesioned controls. Twenty-five weeks after placement of the lesions all rats were sacrificed, blood was withdrawn and assayed for prolactin, and the number of mammary tumours in each group was determined. Mammary tumour incidence in the median eminence-lesioned rats was 52 per cent in contrast to 19 per cent in the sham-lesioned controls (Table 2.3). Blood prolactin levels were more than three times greater in the rats bearing the hypothalamic lesions (179·8 ng/ml) than in the controls (50·9 ng/ml). It is clear from this study that an endocrine imbalance, consisting of elevated prolactin secretion and reduced secretion of all other anterior pituitary hormones, can be tumorigenic in the rat.

Bruni and Montemurro (1971) placed electrolytic lesions in the anterior, medial or posterior hypothalamus of nulliparous C302 F female mice. They observed that anterior and medial hypothalamic lesions significantly altered pituitary function to the extent that a number of mice in each of these groups were rendered permanently sterile. Concomitantly, these lesions increased the incidence of spontaneous mammary tumours and reduced the latency period

TABLE 2.3

Effects of Median Eminence Lesions on Development of Normal and Neoplastic Mammary Tissue and Serum Prolactin Levels in Female Rats

| Treatment* | Total no. of rats | Final body weight (g) | Serum prolactin levels (ng/ml) | Average mammary gland ratings | No. and % of rats with tumours | Total no. of tumours |
|---|---|---|---|---|---|---|
| Controls, sham lesion | 21 | $360 \pm 7^a$ | $50 \cdot 9 \pm 9 \cdot 6^a$ | $3 \cdot 1 \pm 0 \cdot 1^a$ | 4 (19%)[a] | 4[a] |
| Median eminence lesions | 23 | $451 \pm 19^b$ | $179 \cdot 8 \pm 23 \cdot 9^b$ | $4 \cdot 2 \pm 0 \cdot 2^b$ | 12 (52%)[b] | 20[b] |

After Welsch et al., 1970.
* All rats were sacrificed 25 weeks after placement of median eminence or sham lesions. Final body weight, serum prolactin levels, and average mammary gland ratings are represented as the mean value $\pm$ SE.
a/b = p < 0.001.

when compared with controls. Lesions placed in the posterior hypothalamus, as well as those in the anterior and medial hypothalamus that *did not* cause sterility, were essentially ineffective in influencing tumour incidence. Thus it appears that electrolytic lesions placed in the hypothalamus not only have a profound effect on growth of established mammary tumours but also markedly influence the genesis of these neoplasms. These results strongly support our hypothesis that certain alterations in function of the central nervous system may be one of the key aetiological factors in the development and progression of tumours of the mammary gland.

## Effect of drugs acting on the central nervous system

Numerous studies have indicated that hypothalamic catecholamines influence secretion of anterior pituitary hormones including prolactin. In general, an adrenergic tonus is believed to inhibit prolactin release and a reduction of hypothalamic catecholamines to promote prolactin secretion. Iproniazid, a monoamine oxidase inhibitor, is an effective inhibitor of prolactin secretion (Lu and Meites, 1971) (Table 2.4), presumably by interfering with the catabolism of catecholamines and thereby increasing their concentration in the hypothalamus. Nagasawa and Meites (1970a) investigated the effects of iproniazid on growth of DMBA-induced mammary tumours in female Sprague–Dawley rats. After these tumours reached approximately 1 cm in diameter, the rats were injected daily for 25 days with the drug. Iproniazid markedly suppressed mammary tumour growth and prevented development of new tumours whereas, in the controls, growth of the initial tumours increased about 100 per cent. Similarly, pargyline and L-dopa, drugs which also increase catecholamines, thus suppressing pituitary prolactin secretion (Lu and Meites, 1971) (Table 2.4), significantly inhibited DMBA-induced mammary tumour growth (Meites et al., 1972). *Figure 2.7* shows the effects of L-dopa and methyldopa on mammary tumour growth in rats.

In contrast, administration of reserpine, a tranquillizer which generally depresses central nervous system activity and reduces hypothalamic catecholamines, produced a rapid increase in pituitary prolactin secretion (Lu et al., 1970). Welsch and Meites (1970) administered reserpine to female rats bearing DMBA-induced mammary tumours and observed a marked stimulation of mammary tumour growth. Tumour-bearing rats treated with 100 µg reserpine per 100 g body weight for 10 and 25 days showed 58 and 115 per cent increases in tumour growth, in contrast to 18 and 61 per cent increases in the saline-treated controls (Table 2.5). Reserpine, however, could not reactivate growth of regressing mammary tumours in ovariectomized rats. Similarly, Pearson et al. (1969) administered perphenazine, a tranquillizer which also markedly enhances prolactin secretion, to DMBA-treated rats to determine whether this drug would influence the development of mammary

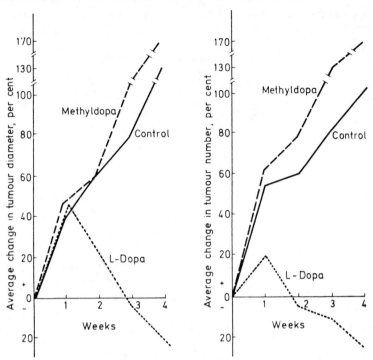

*Figure 2.7. Effects of L-dopa and methyldopa on change in mammary tumour diameter (left) and mammary tumour number (right) of DMBA-treated rats. At the end of one week the dose of L-dopa was increased and significantly depressed mammary tumour growth. Methyldopa significantly increased tumour growth (after Quadri, Kledzek and Meites, unpublished)*

tumours. After five months of treatment, 100 per cent of the perphenazine-treated animals developed mammary tumours, in contrast to 70 per cent of the saline-treated controls. The number and size of the tumours in the perphenazine-treated group exceeded that of the control group by a factor of two. Perphenazine was also administered to DMBA-treated, tumour-bearing rats following ovariectomy and adrenalectomy. After five months of treatment with the drug, 15 rats had a total of 15 mammary tumours, in contrast to none in the eleven saline-treated controls.

Perhaps the first group to investigate the effect of tranquillizers on the *genesis* of murine mammary tumours was Lacassagne and Duplan (1959). They reported that reserpine hastened the development of mammary tumours in C3H mice. Mice treated with reserpine developed mammary tumours in the eighth to the fifteenth months of life, in contrast to the controls which

## TABLE 2.4

Effects of a Single Intraperitoneal Injection of Drugs on Serum and Pituitary Prolactin Concentrations

| Treatment (7 rats/group) per rat | Pre-treatment | Serum prolactin (ng/ml) | | | AP prolactin conc (µg/mg of AP) |
|---|---|---|---|---|---|
| | | 30 min | 1 hour | 2 hours | |
| pH 2·8 solution, 0·3 ml (controls) | 158·6 ± 16·4* | 143·6 ± 12·0 | 146·0 ± 10·3 | 130·1 ± 9·7 | 10·34 ± 0·19 |
| L-dopa, 12 mg | 174·1 ± 12·7 | 85·1 ± 3·2‡ | 90·1 ± 8·8‡ | 66·7 ± 4·1‡ | 12·08 ± 0·79† |
| Methyldopa, 80 mg | 204·3 ± 21·8 | 955·3 ± 85·3‡ | 1319·1 ± 171·5‡ | 984·1 ± 188·1‡ | 8·19 ± 0·28‡ |
| Saline, 0·5 ml (controls) | 169·6 ± 10·1 | 193·1 ± 26·7 | 192·9 ± 24·6 | 181·9 ± 11·6 | 9·32 ± 0·29 |
| Pargyline, 15 mg | 187·4 ± 15·5 | 112·7 ± 7·0‡ | 107·1 ± 10·9‡ | 100·0 ± 11·1‡ | 9·35 ± 0·37 |
| Pargyline, 15 mg + L-dopa, 12 mg | 149·6 ± 13·3 | 66·7 ± 3·0‡ | 63·7 ± 6·0‡ | 70·1 ± 5·4‡ | 10·63 ± 0·11 |
| Lilly-15641, 8 mg | 208·0 ± 28·9 | 208·6 ± 32·9 | 173·1 ± 25·2 | 126·0 ± 21·7† | 11·63 ± 0·44‡ |
| Iproniazid, 40 mg | 195·6 ± 25·5 | 182·6 ± 40·0 | 168·7 ± 38·1 | 89·4 ± 13·8‡ | 8·89 ± 0·37 |
| d-Amphetamine, 1·2 mg | 142·9 ± 6·7 | 568·3 ± 126·1‡ | 1056·1 ± 211·4‡ | 956·1 ± 245·1‡ | 5·88 ± 0·32‡ |

After Lu and Meites, 1971.

* Mean ± standard error of mean.

† Significantly different from controls: $p < 0.05$; ‡ $p < 0.01$.

43

## TABLE 2.5

Effects of Reserpine on Growth and Development of DMBA-induced Mammary Tumours in Female Rats

| Group and treatment* | Total no. of rats | Average no. of palpable tumours/rat | | | | Change (%) | Average weight of tumours/rat (g) |
|---|---|---|---|---|---|---|---|
| | | Initial | 10 days after treatment | 25 days after treatment | 50 days after treatment | | |
| (1) Controls, intact | 16 | 3·3±0·5† | 3·9±0·6[a] | 5·3±0·8[d] | 6·9±1·0[g] | +109 | 12·0±3·8[j] |
| (2) Reserpine (10 µg), intact | 16 | 3·3±0·7 | 5·2±1·1[b] | 7·1±1·3[e] | 10·6±1·8[h] | +221 | 15·5±3·4 |
| (3) Controls, ovariectomized | 19 | 4·1±0·6 | 2·6±0·5[c] | 1·4±0·4[f] | 1·3±0·4[i] | −68 | 1·9±1·2[k] |
| (4) Reserpine (10 µg), ovariectomized | 16 | 4·0±0·7 | 2·4±0·4 | 1·6±0·4 | 1·3±0·4 | −68 | 1·4±0·7 |
| (5) Reserpine (100 µg), ovariectomized | 13 | 4·3±0·6 | 3·6±0·5 | 1·4±0·3 | — | — | — |

After Welsch and Meites, 1970.

* DMBA was administered at 55 days of age. The rats were treated with reserpine and/or ovariectomized approximately 75 days after DMBA treatment.

Dose levels of reserpine, per 100 g body weight.

† SE of the mean.

a, c; d, f; j, j; k = P < 0·01. a, b = < 0·02. d, e; h = P < 0·05.

developed mammary tumours in the eleventh to the seventeenth months. In mice of another strain, with little or no spontaneous mammary tumorigenesis, reserpine had no effect. In contrast, Cranston (1958) treated ZBC mice bearing transplants of mammary tumours with reserpine, chlorpromazine, promazine or promethazine and none of these central nervous system depressants significantly influenced growth of the tumour grafts. Dukor et al. (1966) reported that the maximally tolerated doses of reserpine given to C3H mice bearing spontaneous mammary tumours had a slight tumour-inhibiting effect that was correlated with the extent of body weight loss. This slight tumour-inhibiting effect was eliminated in mice treated simultaneously throughout the experiment with methylphenidate hydrochloride, a central nervous system stimulant. The probable explanation for the contrasting results of Lacassagne and Duplan (1959), Cranston (1958) and Dukor et al. (1966) is that the mouse spontaneous mammary tumour is not generally hormone-responsive in later stages of development, although they are hormone-responsive in the developmental stages (Dux and Mühlbock, 1969).

The regulation of mammary tumorigenesis by use of drugs which suppress prolactin secretion is receiving increased attention. Prolactin secretion can be significantly suppressed by the administration of certain ergot alkaloids in rats and mice as well as in man (Nagasawa and Meites, 1970a; Yanai and Nagasawa, 1970; Lutterbeck et al., 1971). Indirect evidence in rats, e.g. inhibition of pregnancy (Shelesnyak, 1958), of deciduoma formation (Shelesnyak, 1954) and of lactation (Zeilmaker and Carlsen, 1962), after administration of these ergots suggested that they reduce prolactin secretion. It was only recently that this was confirmed by radioimmunoassay (Nagasawa and Meites, 1970a). Investigations pertaining to the mechanism of action of these ergots indicate that at least one ergot drug, ergocornine, suppresses pituitary prolactin secretion by acting directly on the pituitary, thus mimicking the hypothalamic prolactin-release-inhibiting factor (Welsch et al., 1971; Lu, Koch and Meites, 1971), and also by acting at the hypothalamic level as well (Wuttke, Cassell and Meites, 1971).

Because of the marked suppressing activities of these ergots on prolactin secretion, their effects on murine mammary tumour development and growth have been well investigated. Ergocornine, or ergocryptine, administered to carcinogen-induced mammary-tumour-bearing rats (Nagasawa and Meites, 1970a; Heuson, Gaver and Legros, 1970; Cassell, Meites and Welsch, 1971) or to old rats bearing spontaneous mammary tumours (Quadri and Meites, 1971) caused significant regression of these tumours. When treatment with the ergots was withdrawn, prompt resumption of tumour growth was observed. Ergocornine-induced tumour regression paralleled that observed following ovariectomy and was more effective than ergocryptine treatment in these rats (Cassell, Meites and Welsch, 1971). Over 50 per cent of the palpable mammary tumours regressed so that they were no longer palpable after

TABLE 2.6

Effects of Ergocornine (Ec) and Ergocryptine (Ecy) on Mammary Tumour Growth

| Treatment | No. of rats | No. of tumours in each category at end of treatment | | | |
| | | Disappeared | Regressing | Unchanged | Progressing |
|---|---|---|---|---|---|
| Controls | 16 | 0 | 2 | 0 | 17 |
| Ec 0·4 and 0·2 mg | 13 | 11 | 18 | 1 | 4 |
| Ec 0·2 mg | 15 | 10 | 6 | 1 | 2 |
| Ecy 0·4 mg | 15 | 0 | 10 | 6 | 8 |
| Ovariectomized | 9 | 14 | 8 | 0 | 0 |

After Cassell et al., 1971.
These tumours initially were greater than 10 mm in diameter.
Dose levels, per 100 g body weight.

ergocornine treatment, whereas only 10 per cent of these tumours failed to be affected by this drug (Table 2.6). The rats continued to have a normal oestrous cycle, suggesting specificity of the drug for prolactin. Treatment with the drugs at the doses given had no adverse effects on body weights.

In view of the marked oncolytic effects of the ergots on rat mammary tumours, the effects of these drugs on growth of spontaneous mouse mammary tumours were recently evaluated. Treatment of C3H/HeJ tumour-bearing mice with maximally tolerated doses of ergocryptine failed to cause regression of these tumours (Welsch, 1972b). The lack of a significant effect of the ergots on established mouse mammary tumours is not surprising, as these tumours in their advanced state of development generally acquire hormone independence (Dux and Mühlbock, 1969). However, it has been acknowledged by several investigators that the early developmental phases of spontaneous mouse mammary tumorigenesis *are* markedly hormone responsive (DeOme et al., 1962; Bern and Nandi, 1961). It was of interest, therefore, to determine whether or not treatment of mice with ergocryptine could reduce the incidence and/or promote the regression of mammary hyperplastic alveolar nodules, as these hyperplasias have been reported to antedate the tumour (DeOme et al., 1962).

Five-week-old, nulliparous mice were injected subcutaneously daily for 10 months with 0·1 mg ergocryptine suspended in saline. Saline-treated mice served as controls. Ergocryptine significantly reduced the mean incidence of hyperplastic alveolar nodules when compared with the controls (Table 2.7). Furthermore, 70 per cent of the ergocryptine-treated mice were completely free of the pre-cancerous outgrowths after the treatment period. Fecundity of the ergot-treated mice was determined midway through the treatment period. It was found that mice rarely became pregnant while being treated with ergocryptine, when mated with males of the same strain, but upon drug withdrawal, normal fecundity was quickly re-established (Welsch, 1972b). In the second phase of the study, 20 eight-month-old, multiparous C3H/HeJ female mice were treated daily for 30 days with 0·1 mg ergocryptine. Forty mice served as controls, 20 sacrificed at day 0 and 20 at day 30. Ergocryptine significantly reduced the mean number of hyperplastic nodules when compared to the controls, day 0 and day 30 (Table 2.8). Ergocryptine, at the dose level used in both of these studies, did not alter the oestrous cycle, i.e. the mice continued to cycle normally, and it had no effect on body weight (Welsch, 1972b). In agreement with these results, Nagasawa and Yanai (1970, 1971) reported that treatment of mice with either ergocryptine or ergocornine promoted regression of existing hyperplastic alveolar nodules and reduced the incidence of mammary tumours in mice bearing pituitary homografts. Similarly, ergocornine has been reported to suppress the induction of mammary tumours in rats treated with DMBA (Clemens and Shaar, 1972).

These studies provide evidence that mammary tumorigenesis can be

TABLE 2.7

Effect of 10 Months of Treatment of C3H/HeJ Nulliparous Mice with 2-bromo-α-ergocryptine (CB-154) on Degree of Mammary Gland Development and Number of Mammary Hyperplastic Alveolar Nodules

| Group[†] | Treatment | Number of mice | Mean* inguinal mammary gland development | Mean* number of hyperplastic alveolar nodules inguinal mammary glands | Number of mice free of hyperplastic alveolar nodules inguinal mammary glands |
|---|---|---|---|---|---|
| I | Controls | 10 | $4.3 \pm 0.2^a$ | $3.0 \pm 0.5^a$ | 1 |
| II | CB–154 | 10 | $1.0 \pm 0.0^b$ | $0.4 \pm 0.2^b$ | 7 |

After Welsch, 1972.
* Mean ± standard error.
† All mice were 5 weeks of age at the beginning of treatment. CB–154 dose level, 0·1 mg/mouse/day.
a/b = P < 0·001.

TABLE 2.8

Effect of 30 Days of Treatment of C3H/HeJ Multiparous Mice with 2-bromo-α-ergocryptine (CB–154) on Degree of Mammary Gland Development and Number of Mammary Hyperplastic Alveolar Nodules

| Group[†] | Treatment | Number of mice | Mean* inguinal mammary gland development | Mean* number of hyperplastic alveolar nodules inguinal mammary glands | Number of mice free of hyperplastic alveolar nodules inguinal mammary glands |
|---|---|---|---|---|---|
| I | Controls, day 0 | 20 | $4 \cdot 6 \pm 0 \cdot 3^a$ | $6 \cdot 0 \pm 0 \cdot 8^a$ | 2 |
| II | Controls, day 30 | 20 | $4 \cdot 1 \pm 0 \cdot 2^a$ | $6 \cdot 6 \pm 0 \cdot 8^a$ | 3 |
| III | CB–154, day 30 | 20 | $2 \cdot 8 \pm 0 \cdot 1^b$ | $1 \cdot 7 \pm 0 \cdot 3^b$ | 8 |

After Welsch, 1972.
* Mean ± standard error.
† All mice were 8 months of age at the beginning of treatment. CB–154 dose level, 0.1 mg/mouse/day.
a/b = P < 0.001.

49

significantly influenced in rats and mice by the use of drugs which produce profound changes in the neuroendocrine system. These drugs effectively interfere with both the *development* and *growth* of mammary tumours by suppressing pituitary prolactin secretion, acting either at the hypothalamic and/or pituitary level. A logical consequence of these studies is the possible application of these procedures to the management of human breast cancer. Although prolactin has long been accepted as a distinct pituitary hormone in most animals, it is only recently that sufficient evidence has accumulated to confirm its separate existence in man (Friesen, 1971). Furthermore, the neuroendocrine factors associated with the regulation of prolactin secretion in lower animals appear to be the same as those operating in man (Eckles, Ehni and Kirschbaum, 1958; Brauman, Brauman and Pasteels, 1964; Sherwood, 1971; Friesen, 1971). In preliminary work L-dopa in combination with large doses of oestrogen has been reported to be effective in suppressing the progression of metastatic breast cancer in man (Stoll, 1972), and other investigators have recently reported that L-dopa alone may induce remission of breast cancer in some patients (Murray et al., 1972; Frantz et al., 1973). There is a preliminary report that ergocryptine may be effective in the treatment of some breast cancer patients (Schulz et al., 1973). An important consideration in such cases is prior determination of whether the tumour is prolactin responsive by means of *in vitro* testing of biopsy specimens.

## SUMMARY

Hormonal imbalances have long been recognized as a major causative factor in mammary tumorigenesis. The triggering mechanism for abnormalities in hormonal secretory patterns appears to lie within the central nervous system, as this immensely complex system has a major regulatory influence on the endocrine system. It is conceivable, therefore, that many endocrine-responsive mammary neoplasms may ultimately arise as a result of a disturbance or malfunction in the central nervous system. This concept is supported by several laboratory studies demonstrating that agents that influence central nervous system activities—e.g. brain lesions, drugs and stress—also significantly influence mammary tumour development.

Prolactin appears to be the key hormone in murine mammary tumorigenesis, although oestrogen is also involved under most conditions. The application of neuroendocrine techniques for regulating the secretion of prolactin and also oestrogen for the purpose of controlling development and growth of mammary tumours appears to have extraordinary potential. As our understanding of the complex central nervous system–endocrine system–mammary tumorigenesis inter-relationships increases, this potential may be realized.

## ACKNOWLEDGMENTS

Work supported in part by National Science Foundation Research Grant GB-17034 and National Institutes of Health Research Grant CA-35027 to Dr. Welsch and National Institutes of Health Research Grants AM-4784 and CA-10771 to Dr. Meites. Clifford W. Welsch is National Institutes of Health—National Cancer Institute Research Career Development Awardee.

## REFERENCES

Andervont, H. B. (1944). 'Influence of environment on mammary cancer in mice.' *J. natn Cancer Inst.* **4**, 579.

Beatson, G. T. (1896). 'On the treatment of inoperable cases of carcinoma of the mamma: Suggestions for a new method of treatment, with illustrative cases.' *Lancet* **2**, 104.

Bern, H. A. and Nandi, S. (1961). 'Recent studies of the hormone influence in mouse mammary tumorigenesis.' *Prog. expl Tumor Res.* **2**, 90.

Bittner, J. J. and Cole, H. L. (1961). 'Induction of mammary cancer in agent-free mice bearing pituitary isografts correlated with inherited hormonal mechanism.' *J. natn Cancer Inst.* **27**, 1273.

Boot, L. M., Mühlbock, D., Ropche, G. and van Ebbenhorst Tengbergen, W. (1962). 'Further investigations on induction of mammary cancer in mice by isografts of hypophyseal tissue.' *Cancer Res.* **22**, 713.

— — — (1962). 'Prolactin and the induction of mammary tumours in mice.' *Gen. Comp. Endocrinol.* **2**, No. 6.

Brauman, J., Brauman, H. and Pasteels, J. L. (1964). 'Immunoassay of growth hormone in cultures of human hypophysis by the method of complement fixation: comparison of the growth hormone secretion and the prolactin activity.' *Nature, Lond.* **202**, 1116.

Bruni, J. E. and Montemurro, D. G. (1971). 'Effect of hypothalamic lesions on the genesis of spontaneous mammary gland tumours in the mouse.' *Cancer Res.* **31**, 854.

Burgus, R. and Guillemin, R. (1970). 'Chemistry of thyrotropin-releasing factor (TRF).' In *Hypophysiotropic Hormones of the Hypothalamus: Assay and Chemistry*, p. 227, Ed. by J. Meites. Baltimore; Williams and Wilkins.

Cassell, E. E., Meites, J. and Welsch, C. W. (1971). 'Effects of ergocornine and ergocryptine on growth of 7,12-dimethylbenzanthracene-induced mammary tumors in rats.' *Cancer Res.* **31**, 1051.

Chen, C. L. and Meites, J. (1970). 'Effects of estrogen and progesterone on serum and pituitary prolactin levels in ovariectomized rats.' *Endocrinology* **86**, 503.

Clemens, J. A., Welsch, C. W. and Meites, J. (1968). 'Effects of hypothalamic lesions on incidence and growth of mammary tumors in carcinogen-treated rats.' *Proc. Soc. expl Biol. Med.* **127**, 969.

— and Shaar, C. J. (1972). 'Inhibition of ergocornine of initiation and growth of 7,12-dimethylbenzanthracene-induced mammary tumors in rats: effect of tumor size.' *Proc. Soc. expl Biol. Med.* **139**, 659.

Cranston, E. M. (1958). 'Effects of some tranquilizers on a mammary adeno-carcinoma in mice.' *Cancer Res.* **18**, 897.

Cutts, J. H. and Noble, R. L. (1964). 'Estrone-induced mammary tumors in the rat. I. Induction and behavior of tumors.' *Cancer Res.* **24**, 1116.

Daniel, P. M. and Prichard, M. M. L. (1964). 'The response of experimentally induced mammary tumors in rats to ovariectomy.' *Br. J. Cancer* **17**, 687.

Dao, T. L. (1964). 'Carcinogenesis of mammary gland in rat.' *Prog. expl Tumour Res.* **5**, 157.

— (1966). 'Mammary tumorigenesis in female rats receiving androgen neonatally.' *Proc. Am. Ass. Cancer Res.* **7**, 54.

— (1969). 'Studies on mechanism of carcinogenesis in the mammary gland.' *Prog. expl Tumor Res.* **11**, 235.

DeOme, K. B., Nandi, S., Bern, H. A., Blair, P. B. and Pitelka, D. (1962). 'The preneoplastic hyperplastic alveolar nodule as the morphological precursor of mammary cancer in mice.' In *The Morphological Precursors of Cancer,* Perugia.

Dukor, P., Salvin, S. B., Dietrich, F. M., Gelzer, J., Hess, R. and Loustalat, P. (1966). 'Effect of reserpine on immune reactions and tumor growth.' *Europ. J. Cancer* **2**, 253.

Durbin, P. W., Williams, M. H., Jeung, N. and Arnold, J. S. (1966). 'Development of spontaneous mammary tumors over the life-span of the female Charles River (Sprague–Dawley) rat: The influence of ovariectomy, thyroidectomy, and adrenalectomy-ovariectomy.' *Cancer Res.* **26**, 400.

Dux, A. and Mühlbock, O. (1969). 'Enhancement by hypophyseal hormones on the malignant transformation of transplanted hyperplastic nodules of the mouse mammary gland.' *Europ. J. Cancer* **5**, 191.

Eckles, N. E., Ehni, G. and Kirschbaum, A. (1958). 'Induction of lactation in the human female by pituitary stalk section.' *Anat. Rec.* **130**, 295.

Elwers, M. and Critchlow, B. V. (1966). 'Precocious ovarian stimulation following hypothalamic and amygdaloid lesions in rats.' *Am. J. Physiol.* **198**, 381.

Fekete, E., Woolley, G. and Little, C. C. (1941). 'Histological changes following ovariectomy in mice. I. dba high tumor strain.' *J. expl Med.* **74**, 11.

Frantz, A. G. et al. (1973). 'Physiological and pharmacological factors affecting prolactin secretion, including its suppression by L-dopa in the treatment of breast cancer.' In *International Symposium on Human Prolactin,* p. 120, Ed. by J. L. Pasteels and C. Robyn. Amsterdam; Excerpta Medica.

Friesen, H. G. (1971). 'Human placental lactogen and human pituitary prolactin.' *Clin. Obstet. Gynec.* **14**, 669.

Furth, J. (1968). 'Hormones and neoplasia.' In *Cancer and Aging.* Stockholm; Nordiska Bokhandelns Forlag.

Gorski, R. A. (1970). 'Localization of hypothalamic regulation of anterior pituitary function.' *Am. J. Anat.* **129**, 219.

Haran-Ghera, N. (1961). 'The role of mammotrophin in mammary tumor induction in mice.' *Cancer Res.* **21**, 790.

Heuson, J. C., Gaver, W. and Legros, N. (1970). 'Growth inhibition of rat mammary carcinoma and endocrine changes produced by 2-br-α-ergocryptine, a suppressor of lactation and nidation.' *Europ. J. Cancer* **6**, 353.

Hollander, V. P., Jonas, H. and Smith, D. E. (1958). 'Estradiol-sensitive isocitric dehydrogenase in non-cancerous and cancerous human breast tissue.' *Cancer* **11**, 803.

Huggins, C., Briziarelli, G. and Sutton, H. (1959). 'Rapid induction of mammary carcinoma in the rat and the influence of hormones on the tumors.' *J. expl Med.* **109**. 25.

— Moon, R. C. and Morii, S. (1962). 'Extinction of experimental mammary cancer. I. Estradiol-17B and progesterone.' *Proc. natn Acad. Sci.* **48**, 379.

Huseby, R. A. (1965). 'Steroids and tumorigenesis in experimental animals.' In *Methods in Hormone Research,* Chap. 6, p. 123, Ed. by R. I. Dorfman. New York; Academic Press.

Jull, J. W. (1966). 'The effect of infection, hormonal environment, and genetic constitution in mammary tumor induction in rats by 7,12-dimethylbenzanthracene.' *Cancer Res.* **26**, 2368.

Kamberi, I. A., Mical, R. S. and Porter, J. C. (1970). 'Intraventricular $(V_3)$ injection or pituitary perfusion of catecholamines and prolactin (LtH) release.' *Fedn Proc.* **29**, 378.

— Schneider, H. P. G. and McCann, S. M. (1970). 'Action of dopamine to induce release of FSH-releasing factor (FRF) from hypothalamic tissue in vitro.' *Endocrinology* **86**, 278.

Kim, U. (1965). 'Pituitary function and hormonal therapy of experimental breast cancer.' *Cancer Res.* **25**, 1146.

— and Furth, J. (1960). 'Relation of mammary tumors to mammotropes. II. Hormone responsiveness of 3-methylcholanthrene induced mammary carcinomas.' *Proc. Soc. expl Biol. Med.* **103**, 643.

Klaiber, M. S., Gruenstein, M., Meranze, D. R. and Shimkin, M. B. (1969). 'Influence of hypothalamic lesions on induction and growth of mammary cancers in Sprague-Dawley rats receiving 7,12-dimethylbenzanthracene.' *Cancer Res.* **29**, 999.

Kovacs, K. (1965). 'Effect of androgenisation on the development of mammary tumors in rats induced by the oral administration of 9,10-dimethyl-1,2-benzanthracene.' *Brit. J. Cancer* **19**, 531.

Lacassagne, A. (1933). 'Apparition de cancers de la mamelle chez la souris mâle a des injections de folliculine.' *Compt. Rend. Acad. Sci.* **195**, 630.

— and Duplan, A. F. (1959). 'Le mécanisme de la cancerisation de la mamelle chez la souris, considéré d'après les résultats d'expériences au moyen de la reserpine.' *Compt. Rend. Acad. Sci.* **249**, 810.

LeShan, L. (1959). 'Psychological states as factors in the development of malignant disease: a critical review.' *J. natn Cancer Inst.* **22**, 1.

Liebelt, R. A. (1959). 'Effects of goldthioglucose-induced hypothalamic lesions in mammary tumorigenesis in R 111 × CBA mice.' *Proc. Am. Ass. Cancer Res.* **3**, 37.

Lu, K. H., Amenomori, Y., Chen, C. and Meites, J. (1970). 'Effects of central acting drugs on serum and pituitary prolactin levels in rats.' *Endocrinology* **87**, 667.

— Koch, Y. and Meites, J. (1971). 'Direct inhibition by ergocornine of pituitary prolactin release.' *Endocrinology* **89**, 229.

— and Meites, J. (1971). 'Inhibition by L-dopa and monoamine oxidase inhibitors of pituitary prolactin release; stimulation by methyldopa and d-amphetamine.' *Proc. Soc. expl Biol. Med.* **137**, 480.

McCann, S. M., Dhariwal, A. P. S. and Porter, J. C. (1968). 'Regulation of adenohypophysis.' *Ann. Rev. Physiol.* **30**, 589.

53

Marchant, J. (1966). 'The effect of methylcholanthrene and different social conditions on the appearance of breast tumours in NZY mice.' *Br. J. Cancer* **20**, 210.

Matsuo, H., Arimura, A., Nair, R. M. G. and Schally, A. V. (1971). 'Synthesis of the porcine LH- and FSH-releasing hormone by the solid-phase method.' *Biochem. Biophys. Res. Commun.* **45**, 822.

Meites, J. (1966). 'Control of mammary growth and lactation.' In *Neuroendocrinology*, p. 669, Ed. by L. Martini and W. F. Ganong. New York; Academic Press.

— (Ed.) (1970). 'Direct studies of the secretion of the hypothalamic hypophysiotropic hormones (HHH).' In *Hypophysiotropic Hormones of the Hypothalamus; Assay and Chemistry*, p. 261. Baltimore; Williams and Wilkins.

— (1972). 'The relation of estrogen and prolactin to mammary tumorigenesis in the rat.' In *Estrogen Target Tissue and Neoplasia*, Chap. 17, p. 275, Ed. by T. L. Dao. University of Chicago Press.

— and Nicoll, C. S. (1966). 'Adenohypophysis: Prolactin.' *Ann. Rev. Physiol.* **28**, 57.

— Cassell, E. and Clark, J. (1971). 'Estrogen inhibition of mammary tumor growth in rats; counteraction by prolactin.' *Proc. Soc. expl Biol. Med.* **137**, 1225.

— Lu, K. H., Wuttke, W., Welsch, C. W., Nagasawa, H. and Quadri, S. K. (1972). 'Recent studies on functions and control of prolactin secretion in rats.' *Recent Progr Hormone Res.* **28**, 471.

Moon, H. D., Simpson, M. E., Li, C. H. and Evans, H. M. (1951). 'Neoplasms in rats treated with pituitary growth hormone. V. Absence of neoplasms in hypophysectomized rats.' *Cancer Res.* **11**, 535.

Murray, R. L. M. et al. (1972). 'Prolactin levels with L-dopa treatment in metastatic breast carcinoma.' In *Prolactin and Carcinogenesis*, p. 158, Ed. by A. R. Boyns and K. Griffiths. Cardiff; Alpha Omega Alpha.

Nagasawa, H. and Meites, J. (1970a). 'Suppression by ergocornine and iproniazed of carcinogen-induced mammary tumors in rats: Effects on serum and pituitary prolactin levels.' *Proc. Soc. expl Biol. Med.* **135**, 469.

— — (1970b). 'Effects of a hypothalamic estrogen implant on growth of carcinogen-induced mammary tumors in rats.' *Cancer Res.* **30**, 1327.

— and Yanai, R. (1970). 'Effects of prolactin or growth hormone on growth of carcinogen-induced mammary tumors of adreno-ovariectomized rats.' *Int. Jl Cancer* **6**, 488.

Nandi, S., Bern, H. A. and DeOme, K. B. (1960). 'Effect of hormones on growth and neoplastic development of transplanted hyperplastic alveolar nodules of the mammary gland of C3H/Crgl mice.' *J. natn Cancer Inst.* **24**, 883.

Nicoll, C. S., Fiorinda, R. P., McKennee, C. T. and Parsons, J. A. (1970). 'Assay of hypothalamic factors which regulate prolactin secretion.' In *Hypophysiotropic Hormones of the Hypothalamus: Assay and Chemistry*, p. 115, Ed. by J. Meites. Baltimore; Williams and Wilkins.

Pearson, O. H., Llerena, O., Llerena, L., Molina, A. and Butler, T. (1969). 'Prolactin-dependent rat mammary cancer: A model for man?' *Trans. Ass. Am. Phys.* **82**, 225.

Quadri, S. K. and Meites, J. (1971). 'Regression of spontaneous mammary tumors in rats by ergot drugs.' *Proc. Soc. expl Biol. Med.* **138**, 999.

Reznikoff, M. and Martin, D. E. (1957). 'The influence of stress on mammary cancer in mice.' *J. Psychosom. Res.* **2**, 56.

Richardson, F. L. (1967). 'Effect of ovariectomy at different ages on development of mammary tumors in (C3H × R111) F mice.' *J. natn Cancer Inst.* **39**, 347.

Schally, A. V., Arimura, A., Wokabayash, I., Sawano, S., Barrett, J. F., Bowers, C. Y., Redding, T. W., Mettler, J. C. and Saito, M. (1970). 'Chemistry of hypothalamic growth hormone-releasing hormone (GRH).' In *Hypophysiotropic Hormones of the Hypothalamus: Assay and Chemistry,* p. 208, Ed. by J. Meites. Baltimore; Williams and Wilkins.

Schulz, K. D. et al. (1973). 'Varying response of human metastasizing breast cancer to the treatment with 2-Br-α-ergocryptine (CB-154).—case report.' In *International Symposium on Human Prolactin,* Ed. by J. L. Pasteels and C. Robyn. Amsterdam; Excerpta Medica.

Shelesnyak, M. C. (1954). 'Ergotoxine inhibition of deciduoma formation and its reversal by progesterone.' *Am. J. Physiol.* **179**, 301.

— (1958). 'Maintenance of gestation in ergotoxine-treated pregnant rats by exogenous prolactin.' *Acta endocr.* **27**, 99.

Sherwood, L. M. (1971). 'Human prolactin.' *New Engl. J. Med.* **284**, 774.

Sinha, D., Cooper, D. and Dao, T. L. (1972). 'The relationship of estrogen and prolactin in mammary tumorigenesis in rats.' *Proc. Am. Ass. Cancer Res.* **13**, 10.

Sterental, A., Dominquez, J. M., Weissman, C., and Pearson, O. H. (1963). 'Pituitary role in the estrogen dependency of experimental mammary cancer.' *Cancer Res.* **23**, 481.

Stern, E., Mickey, M. R. and Osvaldo, L. (1966). 'Tumorigenesis in the androgen-sterile rat: Reciprocal incidence of carcinogen induced mammary gland and ovarian tumors.' First International Symposium on Biorhythms in Clinical and Experimental Endocrinology, Florence, Italy.

Stoll, B. A. (1969). 'Hormonal management of advanced breast cancer.' *Br. med. J.* **2**, 293.

— (1972). 'Brain catecholamines and breast cancer. A hypothesis.' *Lancet,* **1**, 431.

Szentogothai, J., Flerko, B., Mess, B. and Halasz, B. (1968). *Hypothalamic Control of the Anterior Pituitary.* Budapest; Akademiai Kiodo.

Talwalker, P. K., Meites, J. and Mizuno, H. (1964). 'Mammary tumor induction by estrogen or anterior pituitary hormones in ovariectomized rats given 7,12-dimethylbenzanthracene.' *Proc. Soc. expl Biol. Med.* **116**, 531.

Terenius, L. (1971). 'Effect of anti-oestrogens on initiation of mammary cancer in the female rat.' *Europ. J. Cancer* **7**, 65.

Turkington, R. W. and Hilf, R. (1968). 'Hormonal dependence of DNA synthesis in mammary carcinoma cells in vitro.' *Science* **160**, 1457.

Voogt, J. L., Clemens, J. A., Negro-Vilar, A., Welsch, C. W. and Meites, J. (1971). 'Pituitary GH and hypothalamic GH RF after median eminence implantation of ovine or human GH.' *Endocrinology* **88**, 1363.

Welsch, C. W. (1971). 'Growth inhibition of rat mammary carcinoma induced by cis-platinum diamminodichloride-II.' *J. natn Cancer Inst.* **47**, 1071.

— (1972a). 'Effect of brain lesions on mammary tumorigenesis.' In *Estrogen Target Tissues and Neoplasia,* Chap. 20, p. 317, Ed. by T. L. Dao. University of Chicago Press.

— (1972b). 'Reduced incidence of hyperplastic alveolar nodules in C3H/HeJ female mice treated with 2-bromo-α-ergocryptine.' *Proc. Am. Ass. Cancer Res.* **13**, 98.

— and Meites, J. (1969). 'Effects of a norethynodrel-mestranol combination (Enovid) on development and growth of carcinogen-induced mammary tumors in female rats.' *Cancer* **23**, 601.

— — (1970). 'Effects of reserpine on development of 7,12-dimethylbenzanthracene induced mammary tumors in female rats.' *Experientia* **26**, 1133.

— and Rivera, E. M. (1972). 'Differential effects of estrogen and prolactin on DNA synthesis in organ cultures of DMBA-induced rat mammary carcinoma.' *Proc. Soc. expl Biol. Med.* **139**, 623.

— Clemens, J. A. and Meites, J. (1968). 'Effects of multiple pituitary homografts or progesterone on 7,12-dimethylbenzanthracene-induced mammary tumors in rats.' *J. natn Cancer Inst.* **41**, 465.

— — — (1969). 'Effects of hypothalamic and amygdaloid lesions on development and growth of carcinogen-induced mammary tumors in the female rat.' *Cancer Res.* **29**, 1541.

— Negro-Vilar, A. and Meites, J. (1968). 'Effects of pituitary homografts on host pituitary prolactin and hypothalamic PIF levels.' *Neuroendocrinology* **3**, 238.

— Sar, M., Clemens, J. and Meites, J. (1968). 'Effects of estrogen on pituitary prolactin levels of female rats bearing median eminence implants of prolactin.' *Proc. Soc. expl Biol. Med.* **129**, 817.

— Jenkins, T. W. and Meites, J. (1970). 'Increased incidence of mammary tumors in the female rat grafted with multiple pituitaries.' *Cancer Res.* **30**, 1024.

— Nagasawa, H. and Meites, J. (1970). 'Increased incidence of spontaneous mammary tumors in female rats with induced hypothalamic lesions.' *Cancer Res.* **30**, 2310.

— Squiers, M. D., Cassell, E., Chen, C. L. and Meites, J. (1971). 'Median eminence lesions and serum prolactin: influence of ovariectomy and ergocornine.' *Am. J. Physiol.* **221**, 1714.

Wurtman, R. J. (1970). 'Brain catecholamines and the control of secretion from the anterior pituitary gland.' In *Hypophysiotropic Hormones of the Hypothalamus: Assay and Chemistry,* p. 184, Ed. by J. Meites. Baltimore; Williams and Wilkins.

Wuttke, W., Cassell, E. and Meites, J. (1971). 'Effects of ergocornine on serum prolactin and LH and on hypothalamic content of PIF and LRF.' *Endocrinology* **88**, 737.

Yanai, R. and Nagasawa, H. (1970). 'Suppression of mammary hyperplastic nodule formation and pituitary prolactin secretion in mice induced by ergocornine or 2-bromo-α-ergocryptine.' *J. natn Cancer Inst.* **45**, 1105.

— — (1971a). 'Enhancement by pituitary isografts of mammary hyperplastic nodules in adreno-ovariectomized mice.' *J. natn Cancer Inst.* **46**, 1251.

— — (1971b). 'Inhibition by ergocornine and 2-br-α-ergocryptin of spontaneous mammary tumor appearance in mice.' *Experientia* **27**, 934.

Young, S., Baker, R. A. and Helfenstein, J. E. (1965). 'The effects of androgens on induced mammary tumours in rats.' *Br. J. Cancer* **19**, 155.

Zeilmaker, G. H. and Carlsen, R. A. (1962). 'Experimental studies of the effect of ergocornine methanesulphonate on the luteotropic function of the rat pituitary gland.' *Acta endocr.* **41**, 321.

Zoukar, R. L. and deGroot, J. (1963). 'Effects of limbic brain lesions on aspects of reproduction of female rats.' *Anat. Rec.* **145**, 358.

# 3

# Tumour Regression Following Ovarian Steroid Therapy

### Basil A. Stoll

## INTRODUCTION

The use of ovarian hormones in the treatment of advanced human cancer originated in 1941 with reports on the successful palliation of prostatic cancer by treatment with phenolic oestrogens (Huggins and Hodges, 1941). It was soon extended in an empirical manner to the use of synthetic oestrogens in breast cancer (Haddow et al., 1944), and has since been extended, equally empirically, to the use of synthetic progestins in the treatment of endometrial, kidney and breast cancer. It is intended, in this section, to review some recent additions to our knowledge, particularly of hypothalamic feedback mechanisms and of steroid uptake in target cells, which throw light on the mechanisms involved in the regression of hormone-*responsive* breast cancer after administration of ovarian steroids. (It may be useful at this point to distinguish the term hormone-*dependent* which is usually reserved for those tumours regressing after endocrine ablation.)

In recent years, the presence of high affinity oestradiol receptor protein has been shown in the cytoplasm and nucleus of about half of breast cancer specimens examined. If receptor binding of oestrogen is a major factor in determining hormonal dependence, then those tumours showing high specific binding activity *in vitro* or high uptake of oestradiol *in vivo* should be the ones to show evidence of response to endocrine ablation. Such a relationship has recently been claimed in two series of patients with breast cancer regressing after various methods of endocrine ablation (Folca, Glascock and Irvine, 1961; Jensen et al., 1972), although not confirmed in a third (Braunsberg et al., 1973).

It cannot be assumed, however, that because of these findings, response by the tumour cell to high dosage oestrogen therapy must be mediated by the specific receptor binding sites. The last report (Braunsberg et al., 1973) found that tumour response to oestrogen therapy could not be correlated with either a low or high oestradiol uptake by the tumour *in vivo*. It is possible for oestrogen administration to damage tumour cells without binding sites through other cell mechanisms (see Chapter 4). In addition, oestrogen can exert

57

indirect effects on breast cancer growth, either by stimulating the immune response mechanisms or by an effect on the secretion of the anterior pituitary gland.

It cannot be assumed either that hormonal dependence is synonymous with oestrogen dependence. It is true that oestrogen receptor protein has been demonstrated to a greater extent in those dimethylbenzanthracene-induced rat mammary carcinomas which are hormone-dependent, and to a lesser extent in those which are autonomous. Nevertheless, it has been concluded from extensive experimental observations that prolactin plays the major role in maintaining the activity of the DMBA-induced tumour, although the effect of oestrogen may be synergistic in this respect (see Chapter 2).

There are obvious dangers in extrapolating conclusions derived from experimental murine mammary carcinoma to human mammary carcinoma. The former tumour involves young animals, while the latter appears most commonly at the end of fertile life or after the menopause. According to Furth (1972) a major difference is that the former tumour tends to be alveolar in structure, while the latter is predominantly ductal. Nevertheless, there is a strong likelihood that both prolactin and oestradiol play major roles in maintaining tumour growth in both cases (see Chapter 12).

## OVARIAN STEROIDS AND CANCER REGRESSION

'High dosage' oestrogen or progestin therapy of advanced cancer involves the administration of a dosage which is at least ten times that used generally in the treatment of gynaecological disorders. Regression of breast cancer after such therapy is generally assumed to involve an indirect effect which deprives the tumour of steroid or pituitary hormones which are promoting its growth (Pearson, 1957; Martin and Cunningham, 1960; Stewart, Skinner and O'Connor, 1965; Curwen, 1970). On the other hand, the regression of endometrial cancer after high dosage progestin therapy is generally thought to involve a local effect by the steroid on the tumour (Kistner, 1959; Kelley and Baker, 1960; Sherman, 1966; Kaiser, 1970).

In the light of recently acquired knowledge, such assumptions are open to question, and it is timely to re-examine the mechanisms whereby high dosage of ovarian steroids causes regression in hormone responsive cancer. This has been done elsewhere for mammary, endometrial, prostatic and kidney cancers in the human (Stoll, 1972, 1973). In this chapter, the evidence will be set out which leads to a working hypothesis involving both oestrogen and prolactin, and both direct and indirect mechanisms, in the response of breast cancer to high dosage oestrogen therapy. An unstable equilibrium between stimulation and inhibition of tumour growth may result.

Before developing such a hypothesis, it is necessary to set out certain assumptions made concerning the control of mammary growth. The first is that there are not separate growth promoting and secretory hormones in the stimulation of normal mammary tissue. It is assumed that prolactin has a double function—stimulating the growth of mammary epithelium, and promoting its secretory function also (Furth, 1972)—and on this basis 'lactogenesis may be considered as the final stage in mammogenesis' (see Chapter 1). It is likely too that mitotic activity in the cell will tend to be decreased when the biochemical activity of the cell is directed towards secretory goals (Hilf, Bell and Michel, 1967).

The second assumption is that the prolonged administration of oestrogen by itself to post-menopausal women can stimulate the development of lobulo-alveolar growth in normal mammary tissue (Huseby and Thomas, 1954). It may depend on the presence and level of progesterone secretion which may arise either from the post-menopausal ovary or adrenal cortex (Novak, 1970). The stimulating effect of oestrogen on the growth of the mammary gland in animals is thought to be mediated partly by stimulating the release of prolactin from the anterior pituitary gland, and partly by sensitizing the mammary parenchyma to the effect of prolactin (Nagasawa and Yanai, 1971).

There is considerable species variation in the need for ovarian steroids relative to prolactin in causing the change from ductal growth to lobulo-alveolar differentiation (see Chapter 1). In the case of the human, prolactin has only recently been identified as a separate hormone, and information is therefore very limited. Nevertheless, it may not be too simplistic to suggest that in the human, both normal mammary growth and its differentiation are controlled *mainly* by the synergistic action of oestrogen and prolactin, while progesterone probably potentiates oestrogen effects. High blood levels of the hormones (such as are found in pregnancy) would favour lobulo-alveolar differentiation or secretory activity, while the effect of oestrogen and prolactin at lower concentrations is probably to favour cell proliferation or mitotic activity.

Finally, although one cannot assume that breast cancer which retains hormonal sensitivity has a similar enzymatic activity to its parent tissue, it is not unreasonable to assume that it will respond *in the same direction* to specific hormonal stimuli. This has been shown to apply both in the case of thyroid cancer and endometrial cancer (Crile, 1972; Kistner, 1972).

Given these assumptions, it is suggested that the mitotic activity of hormone-responsive breast cancer under high dosage oestrogen therapy depends on the absolute and relative concentration of prolactin and oestrogen actively available at the target site. This working hypothesis is compatible with observations described later in this chapter on experimental mammary carcinoma treated by high dosage of oestrogen (see p. 65). It is supported by the clinical observation that evidence of tumour stimulation under oestrogen therapy may be reversed by increasing the dosage rapidly (Stoll, 1969a). The hypothesis is also able to explain several anomalies or paradoxes discussed later both in the clinical and in the morphological responses of human mammary cancer to high dosage oestrogen therapy.

Support for the hypothesis is provided also, in my opinion, by the observation of a carcinostatic effect, in addition to a carcinocidal effect, in the response of mammary carcinoma to high dosage oestrogen therapy. As the terms are used by the author, a 'carcinostatic' effect is associated with decrease in the rate of cell mitosis, such a change being temporary and reversible. A 'carcinocidal' effect, on the other hand, implies an increase in the rate of cell loss by the tumour, an effect which is irreversible and which leads ultimately to necrobiosis.

## OESTROGEN MECHANISMS IN MAMMARY CANCER

To clarify the distinction between carcinocidal and carcinostatic effects, it may be useful to review briefly some recent developments in our knowledge of oestrogen mechanisms in the cell. Oestradiol or its metabolites have been shown to be concentrated from the serum in a proportion of breast cancers (Crowley et al., 1962; Braunsberg, Irvine and James, 1967). It is assumed that oestradiol (Jensen and Jacobson, 1962), and probably progesterone also (O'Malley, Sherman and Toft, 1970), must bind to separate cytoplasmic and nuclear receptors before they can exert a stimulatory effect upon the activity of the target cell.

Binding leads to the development of a hormone receptor complex which then stimulates specific hormone-dependent processes in the cell. Biochemically, this involves stimulation of RNA and protein synthesis, and changes in specific enzyme activity. It is important to note that the nature and extent of these changes is not constant but varies from clone to clone, depending on the degree of cell differentiation, its state of activation at the time of hormone binding and the response of the cell to other environmental stimuli (Turkington, 1972). As result of these factors, hormonal stimulation of mammary tissue may be directed more into mitotic activity or more into secretory activity, and considerable confusion has arisen in the literature because the two types of activity are not always clearly distinguished (Cowie and Tindal, 1971).

On the other hand, in the case of mammary cancer responding to high dosage of oestrogen, it is inhibition of activity which is usually noted and not stimulation. The visible morphological and biochemical changes are usually those which lead to necrobiosis, and the rate of cell loss is increased. While the mechanism is uncertain, it is assumed to involve an effect on plasma membranes or on lysosomal activity in the tumour. In contrast with this irreversible carcinocidal effect, there is another type of oestrogen effect which is clearly seen in several types of experimental mammary carcinoma, and is suggested in human mammary carcinoma. It is a reversible carcinostatic effect probably involving a modification of nuclear gene transcription, and leading to changes in protein and RNA synthesis in the cell.

Evidence adduced later in this chapter suggests that while administration of low dosage of oestrogen stimulates mitotic activity of mammary cancer, high dosage may stimulate the tendency towards maturation or secretory activity in the tumour cells. This carcinostatic effect is more likely in the case of differentiated carcinoma. As noted above, increase in the secretory activity of tumour cells tends to be associated with decrease in their mitotic activity, ultimately manifesting as regression of the tumour when natural death occurs in the adult cells and they are not replaced. It is therefore suggested that one of the effects of high dosage oestrogen therapy in human mammary cancer may be a stimulation of enzymatic activity of a prosecretory type in the tissue. It is seen later in the case of experimental tumours that functional stimulation does not need to go as far as a secretory appearance for it to be associated with tumour regression.

The administration of oestrogen may also exert indirect effects on the tumour in addition to direct carcinocidal and carcinostatic effects. First, it is possible for an administered oestrogen to interfere with the binding of endogenous hormones in the target cell (Jensen, Desombre and Jungblut, 1967). It is not certain whether this explains the action of 'anti-oestrogens' such as oestriol (see Chapter 4), or non-physiological oestrogens such as diethyl stilboestrol. Secondly, high dosage of oestrogen has been shown to oppose the mitosis stimulating effect of prolactin on DMBA-induced rat mammary carcinoma (Meites, Cassell and Clark, 1971). Although specific binding sites for prolactin in the mammary gland are likely (Turkington, 1972), the prolactin opposing mechanism of oestrogen under these circumstances is unlikely to involve competitive binding.

A third and very important way in which high dosage oestrogen therapy may exert an indirect effect on the tumour is by feedback effects on the hypothalamus and pituitary hormone secretion. Although it used to be thought that high dosage of oestrogen depressed prolactin secretion (Kim, 1965), it has been recently reported that both high and low dosage stimulate the release of prolactin from the rat pituitary (Chen and Meites, 1970). The action is both on the hypothalamus and upon the pituitary gland itself. It may be relevant to our problem that oestrogen administration also stimulates the secretion of growth hormone, and it has been suggested that the latter may act synergistically with prolactin in promoting the growth of mammary carcinoma (Meites, 1972).

It is the multiplicity of oestrogen mechanisms which has led to confusion and difficulty in rationalizing therapy. If the effect of oestrogen therapy in breast cancer was mainly a local one, it is difficult to explain the clinical observation of 'withdrawal regression'—tumour regression in a proportion of patients after withdrawal of oestrogen therapy in breast cancer (Segaloff et al., 1954; Delarue, 1955). If, on the other hand, the effect of oestrogen was exerted mainly through feedback effects on the hypothalamus and pituitary hormone secretion, one would not expect a response after hypophysectomy. Yet there have been occasional reports of response by breast cancer to progestin–oestrogen combinations even after pituitary ablation (Kennedy, 1965; Landau, Ehrlich and Huggins, 1962), and this would suggest the mediation of a local mechanism.

In the inhibition of the DMBA-induced rat mammary carcinoma by high dosage of oestrogen it has been shown that more than one of these different mechanisms may be involved at the same time. Although high dosage of oestrogen stimulates release of pituitary prolactin, it is able at the same time to counteract the mitosis-stimulating effect of prolactin on the tumour. This is probably a local or peripheral effect because it can in turn be overcome by administering further prolactin (Meites, Cassell and Clark, 1971). These important observations suggest that the mitotic activity of experimental mammary carcinoma depends on the absolute and relative concentration of prolactin and oestrogen actively available at the target itself. A possible corollary to this hypothesis is that the mitotic activity could vary from time to time because of the double mechanism involving both local and indirect effects of oestrogen.

If the local and indirect effects of oestrogen were to predominate at different times, it could explain the biphasic temporal response—preliminary stimulation of tumour growth followed by inhibition—which has been observed following the administration of high dosage of oestrogen to rats bearing hormone sensitive mammary carcinoma (Kim, 1965; McSweeney and Fletcher, 1969; Kiang and Kennedy, 1971). A similar biphasic temporal response has been observed clinically in human mammary cancer (see p. 70), and it is possible that a similar double mechanism might characterize the effect of oestrogen therapy on human mammary cancer.

A hypothesis involving control of mitotic activity according to the absolute and relative concentration of oestrogen and prolactin actively available at each tumour site could also account for other anomalous clinical observations such as stimulation of tumour activity and 'withdrawal regression', both of which are occasionally noted in the course of high dosage oestrogen therapy in human mammary cancer. To explain these manifestations (and also the development of hormonal autonomy), it is usually postulated that breast cancer may, in the same individual, comprise a variety of mutant cell types including some whose growth is inhibited by oestrogen–prolactin and others whose growth is stimulated by oestrogen–prolactin (Furth, 1972). The mechanism of oestrogen–prolactin action which has been suggested in the above hypothesis provides an alternative explanation for these puzzling observations (see p. 68).

# MORPHOLOGICAL EFFECTS OF OESTROGEN ADMINISTRATION

Having discussed the possible mechanisms involved, it may now be possible to account for some of the morphological responses which have been observed in human mammary cancer following the administration of ovarian steroids.

## Carcinocidal effect

It has been shown that the addition of oestradiol in very high concentration—about 50–200 µg/ml—can decrease tissue survival in organ cultures of human mammary carcinoma (Kellner and Turcic, 1962; Stoll, 1969b; Wellings and Jentoft, 1972). This decrease in tissue survival is associated with inhibition of DNA synthesis in the tissue (Welsch and Rivera, 1972). The exact mechanism is uncertain but it is thought to be achieved at the cellular level by blockage of metaphase. Microscopically the tumour cells show granularity or shrinkage of the cytoplasm, and karyorrhexis or pyknosis of the nuclei. On the other hand, reports on the effects of near pharmacological concentrations of oestradiol on organ cultures of human mammary carcinoma are conflicting. Some observers have claimed stimulation of biosynthetic activity in the tumour (Chayen, Altmann and Bitensky, 1970; Salih et al., 1972), while others have found no effect on DNA synthesis (Welsch and Rivera, 1972).

## Carcinostatic effect

Stimulation of secretory activity has been reported in human mammary carcinoma following the addition of ovarian steroids or ovine prolactin to organ cultures (Mioduscewska, 1968), although the nature of the secretion was not confirmed. It may be relevant that in the case of endometrial carcinoma in the human, several authors have now reported that the addition of progesterone to organ cultures stimulates differentiation and maturation and a possible analogy is discussed later. This carcinostatic effect is seen at concentrations of about 10 µg/ml (Kohorn and Tchao, 1968; Bonte, Drochmans and Ide, 1970), although at higher concentrations, carcinocidal effects are visible in organ cultures of endometrial cancer as in the case of breast carcinoma (Nordquist, 1964, 1969).

## Stromal and immunological effects

In mammary specimens showing regression of breast carcinoma following high dosage oestrogen therapy it is common to see evidence of an immune response in the mammary stroma around the tumour. The stromal reaction used to be considered secondary to the tumour changes induced by the oestrogen therapy, but it is now believed to be evidence of a primary response in the stroma to the presence of the tumour. It is possible that this stromal response is intensified following stimulation by oestrogen.

Following high dosage oestrogen therapy in breast cancer, fibrillary loosening of the stroma and influx of lymphocytes and plasma cells has been noted to occur concurrently with degeneration of the malignant cells (Emerson et al., 1953; Emerson, Kennedy and Taft, 1960; Huseby and Thomas, 1954). A similar loosening of the fibrovascular stroma associated with marked round cell infiltration is found in some cases of *untreated* breast cancer (Alderson, Hamlin and Staunton, 1971). Both these observations may represent evidence of stimulation of the immune response (see Chapter 19).

It is possible that all three types of morphological response mentioned above may be involved in breast cancer under high dosage oestrogen therapy. The relative importance of each of the effects in the individual patient is probably determined by tumoral factors, by host factors and by hormonal factors.

With regard to tumoral factors, the response may depend on:

(1) The heterogeneity of the cell population in the individual mammary cancer, and the genetically determined sensitivity of each clone to the hormonal changes induced. This may be related to receptor site levels.

(2) The degree of cell differentiation existing in the tumour—the more differentiated, the more important the carcinostatic mechanism.

(3) The stage of tumour growth—the later phases of malignant growth appear to show a progression to autonomy in experimental animals.

With regard to host factors, the response may depend on:

(1) The hormonal environment—the response is different in the pre-menopausal woman from that in the post-menopausal woman.

(2) The stage of the disease—later stages appear to be associated with failure of the immune response mechanism in the host.

With regard to hormonal factors, the response may depend on:

(1) The biological profile of the hormone administered.

(2) Its route of administration, its metabolism in the body and the steroid concentration achieved at each site of the tumour.

(3) The absolute and relative concentration of oestrogen and prolactin actively available at each site of the tumour.

The effect of these factors in causing individual variations in hormonal sensitivity is discussed later in the chapter. It is proposed to discuss first their effect on the mechanism of response.

## THE CARCINOSTATIC MECHANISM IN OESTROGEN THERAPY

It has been assumed in the past that a carcinocidal effect with increase in the rate of cell loss is the major effect of high dosage oestrogen therapy in breast cancer, and that a decrease in the rate of cell mitosis is an unlikely mechanism (Lipsett, 1969). However, a carcinostatic effect is better able to explain some anomalous morphological observations in the oestrogen therapy of both experimental and human mammary carcinoma. In the case of experimental mammary carcinoma we have noted above that high dosage oestrogen therapy is able to counteract the mitosis-stimulating effect of prolactin on the tumour (Meites, Cassell and Clark, 1971). It suppresses prolactin induced DNA synthesis (Chapter 2). Furthermore, only a carcinostatic mechanism can explain the following puzzling morphological observations in the response to oestrogen of certain types of hormone responsive mammary carcinoma in rats.

Secretory change has been noted in the hormone-responsive transplanted R3230AC tumour in the Fischer rat after diethylstilboestrol administration, and this is enhanced by the addition of prolactin (Hilf, Bell and Michel, 1967). The secretion has been shown to contain casein and other whey protein, and, concomitant with the secretory response, there occurs inhibition of tumour growth. However, because this transplanted tumour does not regress after oophorectomy, it is regarded as hormone-responsive but not hormone-dependent, and therefore not strictly comparable in its endocrine-influenced behaviour to human mammary cancer.

It should therefore be noted that also in the case of the DMBA-induced mammary carcinoma in the rat, which is both hormone-dependent and hormone-responsive, milk-like secretion has been noted in the ductules of the tumour when it regresses after high dosage oestrogen administration (Hilf et al., 1969; Kiang and Kennedy, 1971). The latter author has noted the secretory change to be more marked in the case of well differentiated tumour. It has also been noted by Huggins that in the case of the DMBA-induced tumour, administration of oestrogen and progesterone in a suitable proportion may lead to regression of the tumour and directs the growth processes into the path of functional biochemical activity (Huggins, Moon and Morii, 1962).

In the case of the hormone-responsive transplanted 13672 rat mammary carcinoma, it is reported that increasing dosages of oestrogen causes increasing slowing of tumour growth, until with the highest dosage used, the tumour shows a secretory appearance (Segaloff, 1966). This last observation supports a suggestion made earlier that the carcinostatic effect represents a swing to functional stimulation at the expense of mitotic activity. Moreover, it is clearly noted first that it is dose dependent, and secondly that it *does not need to go as far as a secretory appearance for it to be associated with slowing of tumour growth.*

Hilf, Bell and Michel (1967) make the following comment on this type of response: 'the genetic apparatus of this tumour is still capable of the recognition of the hormonal stimulus which results in the lactation-like response in the neoplasm following oestrogen treatment . . . When the biochemical impetus is directed towards secretion, growth of the neoplasm is significantly reduced, implying that energy is being channeled into protein synthesis for purposes other than for cell multiplication.'

This hypothesis can be coupled with the observation (Welsch, 1972), that all hormonal treatment leading to lactation in the murine mammary gland will suppress the growth of co-existent hormone-responsive mammary carcinoma. Decrease in the rate of cell mitosis leads eventually to decrease in the size of a tumour if the rate of cell wastage exceeds new cell production.

It now becomes possible to explain an apparent paradox in the morphology of human mammary cancer regressing following high dosage oestrogen therapy. Concomitant with depression of tumour growth in such cases, there is nearly always associated evidence of proliferation of the normal mammary epithelium (Emerson et al., 1953; 1960; Huseby and Thomas, 1954). The latter authors noted evidence of ductal stimulation in all but 2 of 36 cases submitted to pathological examination and lobular stimulation in one-third of the cases. They comment on the apparent paradox that extensive proliferation of normal breast epithelium, even to the extent of lobules of pregnancy, should be seen after oestrogen therapy, at the same time that the tumour tissue is showing regression of growth. These changes are not seen in breast cancer regressing after major endocrine ablation in patients of a comparable age group. If it is recognized that epithelial stimulation of this type is the normal prelude to alveolar differentiation and secretory changes, then the response observed in the normal tissues to high dosage oestrogen therapy is no longer paradoxical.

The likely role of the carcinostatic effect in the regression of human mammary cancer under high dosage oestrogen therapy has been overlooked in the literature. The reason is that it is difficult to demonstrate decrease in the rate of cell mitosis as distinct from increase in the rate of cell death and, furthermore, the two often exist side by side. However, when the carcinostatic effect is associated with the induction of *full* secretory differentiation in the tumour, it is easily recognizable as the cause of tumour regression, and this is clearly seen in the case of endometrial cancer regressing under progestin therapy (Thiery and Willighagen, 1968; Bonte, Drochmans and Ide, 1966; Moe, 1972; Kistner, 1972).

The difference between human endometrial and mammary cancer in the degree of secretory differentiation associated with the carcinostatic response to ovarian steroid therapy, may reflect the different hormonal requirements of the tissues for the induction of advanced secretory change (Stoll, 1973). In the case of human endometrial tissue, the action of administered progestin on tissue previously primed with oestrogen is sufficient to lead to advanced functional stimulation. In the case of human mammary tissue, the effect of administered oestrogen (in the presence presumably of endogenous progesterone), is enough to induce only early functional stimulation. The presence of prolactin or placental lactogen at *very high* levels (and possibly glucocorticoids also) is probably necessary for full secretory development of mammary tissue. Whether this is the case or not, it seems that the presence of full secretory development is not essential for the carcinostatic effect to cause reduction in mitotic activity, either in experimental or in human mammary carcinoma.

## CLINICAL ANOMALIES IN THE RESPONSE TO OESTROGEN THERAPY

It is sometimes overlooked that high dosage oestrogen therapy is the most effective of all methods of endocrine therapy in the older post-menopausal patients with advanced breast cancer. In large series, objective evidence of tumour regression has been noted overall in 31–37 per cent of post-menopausal cases (Stoll, 1969a). A prominent but so far unexplained feature of the response is that the likelihood of tumour regression following high dosage oestrogen therapy increases considerably with increasing number of years past the menopause (Table 3.1). It rises as high as 49 per cent in patients over 70 years of age, if oestrogen is persisted with for two months or longer (Stoll and Ackland, 1970).

TABLE 3.1

Regression of Breast Cancer after High Dosage Oestrogen Therapy in Relation to Menopausal Age Group (Stoll, 1969a)

| Years since menopause | Percentage with tumour regression |
|---|---|
| 0–5 | 9 |
| 6–9 | 28 |
| 10 + | 36 |

Another common but anomalous observation in the oestrogen therapy of breast cancer is that of differential site sensitivity—regression of the tumour lesion under observation while new manifestations of active growth appear in another system in the same patient. Thus, for example, metastatic liver enlargement or pleural effusion may manifest clinically even while skin nodules on the chest wall are decreasing in size. What is more surprising, nodular lesions may even disappear in the skin of one part of the chest wall, while new nodules grow in another part.

There are also two major clinical paradoxes in the therapy of breast cancer by high dosage of oestrogen. The first is 'withdrawal regression', in which, by stopping therapy after a temporary response to oestrogen therapy has been lost, there follows in a proportion of cases a second temporary regression of tumour (Segaloff et al., 1954; Delarue, 1955). A similar withdrawal regression has been noted in breast cancer patients treated by progestin therapy (Stoll, 1966).

Equally puzzling is the 'biphasic temporal' response—apparent stimulation of growth activity sometimes seen in a lesion before it begins to undergo regression following high dosage oestrogen therapy. Probably related to this paradox is the observation that although about 30–40 per cent of post-menopausal patients with breast cancer show tumour regression after oestrogen therapy, in approximately a further 10 per cent of patients, treatment with oestrogens has to be discontinued after the first few days because of so called tumour stimulation (Stoll and Ackland, 1970). It has been found difficult to explain why the same dosage of oestrogen should cause complete regression of the tumour in some patients, but stimulation of growth activity in others.

In passing, it should be emphasized that in order to provide objective evidence of tumour stimulation, one must compare serial measurements of tumour volume during therapy with similar serial measurements before therapy, in order to show that the rate of growth has altered. Many patients whose treatment is suspended because of so-called tumour stimulation are found to have a rapidly growing tumour whose rate of growth has not been affected in any way by oestrogen administration, but it is the development of symptoms of drug intolerance or idiosyncrasy which has caused suspension of treatment. Typical symptoms include nausea, malaise or the onset of fever which disappear when treatment is discontinued.

Subjective manifestations which are often quoted as evidence of tumour stimulation also include increase in pain at the site of bone metastases and increased itching in areas of skin infiltrated by tumour. These symptoms may well be caused by stimulation of tumour growth, but they can also represent a temporary stimulation of immune mechanisms in the region of the tumour.

Having described such anomalies and paradoxes in clinical oestrogen therapy as withdrawal regression, differential site sensitivity, biphasic temporal response and stimulation of tumour activity, an attempt will be made to explain them on the basis of the hypothesis which has been postulated at the beginning of this chapter. This suggests that the effect of high dosage oestrogen treatment in breast cancer depends critically on the absolute and relative concentration of prolactin and oestrogen actively available at the target site.

## Dose dependence and tumour stimulation

It has been noted in the DMBA-induced rat mammary carcinoma that both the tumour and the normal mammary epithelium show a response which varies with the dose of oestrogen administered. Smaller doses cause stimulation of growth while large doses cause inhibition of activity (Huggins, Moon and Morii, 1962; Dao, 1964). Dose dependence has been shown in the oestrogen therapy of mammary cancer in the human also, but is not so clearly defined. In pre-menopausal patients, 15 mg stilboestrol daily (or 1·5 mg ethinyl oestradiol) will usually cause stimulation of tumour growth (Haddow et al., 1944; Nathanson, 1947), but a *massive* dose of up to 1 g stilboestrol daily can cause regression of tumour in a proportion of such patients (Nathanson, 1952; Kennedy, 1962). In post-menopausal patients, 15 mg stilboestrol daily will cause regression of tumour in about one-third of cases, but (especially in the early years after the menopause), it may also cause tumour stimulation in a small proportion. With increasing number of years past the menopause the likelihood of tumour regression increases, and the risk of tumour stimulation becomes less from this dose (Stoll, 1969a). Thus, the level of oestrogen dosage at which tumour stimulation is replaced by inhibition seems to decrease with increasing age of the patient.

It is well established that the effect of oestrogen on the release of both gonadotrophin and thyrotrophin is dose dependent—low doses stimulate, while high doses inhibit, release of these hormones. Although assumed for many years (Kim, 1965), there is no evidence of a similar dose-dependent effect by oestrogen on the release of prolactin from the pituitary gland. Both low and high doses *stimulate* prolactin release in the experimental animal (Chen and Meites, 1970). However, the observation of dose dependence in the tumour growth may be explained by the hypothesis that the tumour activity depends on the relative and absolute concentration of oestrogen and prolactin actively available at the target. In experimental animals, oestrogen administration at low dosage levels stimulates release of prolactin from the anterior pituitary gland, and this is associated with growth stimulation of hormone-responsive rat mammary carcinoma (Chen and Meites, 1970). Oestrogen at high dosage also stimulates prolactin release, but at these levels oestrogen is able to oppose the mitosis-stimulating effect of prolactin by a peripheral mechanism and thus causes inhibition of tumour growth (Meites, Cassell and Clark, 1971).

In the human too, it has recently been shown that high dosage of oestrogen stimulates the release of prolactin from the pituitary gland in post-menopausal women (L'Hermite and Heuson, 1973), yet the effect of such therapy is often to inhibit the growth of breast cancer. The mechanism may be similar to that which has been suggested in experimental mammary cancer and depends, as in that case, on an adequate level of oestrogen administration. Oestrogen at high dosage probably counteracts, by some peripheral mechanism, the mitosis-stimulating effect of prolactin. On this basis, the appearance of stimulation of tumour growth following oestrogen administration, at whatever age it occurs, suggests that the level of oestrogen at the target is inadequate for that particular tumour. This suggestion is confirmed by the observation that a rapid increase in dosage in such cases may occasionally lead to tumour regression (Stoll, 1969a).

With increasing age of the patient, a smaller dose of oestrogen is required to inhibit tumour activity in breast cancer and this may possibly reflect a lower prolactin level at the target. Because of decreasing hypothalamic sensitivity with increasing age (see Chapter 10), the same dose of oestrogen may stimulate the release of a relatively lower level of prolactin from the anterior pituitary gland. In a similar way, variations in the absolute and relative concentration of oestrogen and prolactin at the tumour, possibly associated with variations in receptor site levels, could explain differences in the degree of tumour response to oestrogen therapy from patient to patient, from site to site and even from time to time.


## Biphasic temporal response

In the high dosage oestrogen therapy of post-menopausal women with breast cancer, it is not uncommon to see evidence of a biphasic temporal response–temporary stimulation of tumour growth followed by prolonged inhibition of growth. Such a biphasic temporal response is most easily recognized clinically in the case of metastases in bone. Thus, hypercalcaemia occurring in the first week of oestrogen therapy is commonly accepted as evidence of tumour stimulation (Hall, Dederick and Nevinny, 1963; Moore et al., 1967), yet in the majority of such cases, objective evidence of tumour regression occurs if oestrogen therapy is persisted with in spite of the hypercalcaemia (Hall, Dederick and Nevinny, 1963).

A biphasic temporal response has been demonstrated in hormone-responsive mammary carcinoma in rats, being reported following oestrogen therapy of the transplanted MT tumour (Kim, 1965), and of the DMBA-induced tumour (Kiang and Kennedy, 1971). It has also been noted following oestrogen–progestin therapy of the DMBA-induced tumour in rats (McSweeney and Fletcher, 1969). In all these cases, initial stimulation of tumour growth is followed by evidence of tumour regression. Kiang and Kennedy (1971) reported that the biphasic response is more likely to occur in well differentiated tumours, while poorly differentiated tumours are more likely to show continuous stimulation of growth from the beginning.

In the case of soft tissue lesions in human mammary cancer, it has been suggested above that evidence of initial stimulation of tumour growth from high dosage oestrogen therapy may be followed by tumour regression if oestrogen therapy is continued at increased dosage. However, there is also indirect evidence of spontaneous subclinical biphasic response in human mammary cancer. Attempts have been made to establish objective parameters of tumour activity, and measurements of tumour temperature have been used for this purpose by the author and others during therapy by steroids of different types. It has been noted that tumour regression is predicted either by *increase* in tumour temperature within five days of instituting hormonal therapy

(Gillespie, Burrows and Edelstyn, 1971) or by *decrease* in skin nodule temperature after two weeks of hormonal therapy (Stoll, 1971). These observations are difficult to explain except on the basis of a subclinical biphasic temporal response to hormonal therapy in a hormone-responsive breast cancer.

Oestrogen is known to demonstrate a biphasic effect on the activity of hormone responsive mammary carcinoma in rats as noted above. The mechanism of a biphasic temporal response in breast cancer is not clear but could result from the action of two distinct oestrogen mechanisms if they manifested consecutively. Thus, in the case of experimental mammary carcinoma, it has been mentioned earlier that high dosage of oestrogen stimulates prolactin release from the anterior pituitary gland, but in addition it is able to counteract peripherally the mitosis-stimulating effect of prolactin on the tumour (Meites, Cassell and Clark, 1971). If this peripheral effect should be delayed, a biphasic response would be apparent.

The biphasic response observed after high dosage oestrogen therapy in mammary cancer could also result indirectly from a biphasic effect upon the release of gonadotrophin. It has been mentioned above that inhibition of gonadotrophin release may follow high dosage of oestrogen, but recent reports suggest that the direction of response may become reversed in post-menopausal women given continuous high dosage of oestrogen (Callantine, Humphrey and Nesset, 1966; Yen and Tsai, 1971). Thus 400 µg ethinyl oestradiol daily causes initial suppression of both FSH and LH by negative feedback, but if continued after three days this is followed by rebound stimulation of the LH level. The 'flare' in the LH level is even more marked when oestrogen administration is stopped and shifts in gonadotrophin might account also for the withdrawal regression sometimes seen in breast cancer after stopping oestrogen therapy. There is evidence of antagonism between gonadotrophin and prolactin secretion by the anterior pituitary both in animals and man (Ben-David, Danon and Sulman, 1971; Besser and Edwards 1972), and a rise in the gonadotrophin level may be associated with a fall in prolactin secretion (see Chapter 16).

Whatever the mechanism for the biphasic response to oestrogen therapy in breast cancer, it is important to make use of the evidence of hormonal sensitivity provided by the initial manifestation of tumour stimulation. Because of our ignorance of hormonal mechanisms in breast cancer, it has been the general practice in such a case to stop oestrogen administration immediately on the appearance of tumour stimulation and to take refuge in cytotoxic agents or corticosteroid therapy. As pointed out above, however, it is more rational to persist in therapy with oestrogens after the appearance of tumour stimulation, and also to increase dosage very considerably in order to achieve high concentration at the tumour as quickly as possible. The author has shown tumour regression to occur within six weeks in some such cases, while corticosteroids or symptomatic therapy can still be given concomitantly to relieve the subjective complaints of tumour aggravation.

## Site sensitivity

Differences in site sensitivity are often encountered in the endocrine therapy of breast cancer. Differences in the degree of tumour response from organ to organ, e.g. liver and lung, are usually ascribed to biochemical differences between the tissues. Differences in the degree of tumour regression from area to area in the same tissue are often ascribed to differences in vascularity. However, the regression of one group of lesions under endocrine therapy while similar lesions elsewhere are showing evidence of active growth, is usually explained on the basis of genetic differences existing in the tumour. It is assumed that in the same individual, mammary carcinoma may be composed of several clones of cells differing in their hormonal sensitivity—some are stimulated by prolactin or oestrogen, some are inhibited by prolactin or oestrogen and some are unaffected by either (Furth, 1972). It is possible, however, that a difference in response between lesions represents differences in the absolute and relative concentrations of prolactin and oestrogen achieved at each target site, possibly associated with variations in binding characteristics.

Laboratory studies may assist in elucidating the cause of these site differences in sensitivity. Thus a specimen of the tumour may be examined for its level of specific binding receptor for oestradiol (Jensen et al., 1972) and possibly also for prolactin. Its ability to synthesize or conjugate oestradiol may be significant in relation to its hormonal sensitivity (Adams and Wong, 1969; Dao and Libby, 1969). The effect of oestradiol or prolactin in enhancing pentose shunt activity in an organ culture of the tumour can also be investigated (Salih et al., 1972). The last technique may be particularly useful as it may also reflect the level of oestradiol and prolactin binding receptors in the specimen examined.

## ROLE OF PROGESTINS IN THERAPY

After high dosage oestrogen therapy has failed to control tumour growth, breast cancer may regress after high dosage progestin therapy (Stoll, 1966), or after oestrogen and progestin in combination (Stoll, 1965; Crowley and MacDonald, 1965; Berndt, 1970). There are also reports suggesting that a combination of oestrogen and progestin causes tumour regression in a higher proportion of breast cancers than does oestrogen alone (Muggia et al., 1967; Berndt et al., 1971), and it therefore seems likely that the presence of progestin favours a response by breast cancer to oestrogen therapy. Furthermore, it has been suggested that the presence of endogenous oestrogen increases the likelihood of response by breast cancer to progestin therapy, because tumour response after such therapy is found to be much more frequent in the presence of an initially oestrogenic vaginal smear (Stoll, 1967b). The presence of *both* steroids thus appears to increase the likelihood of tumour response, and it is interesting that vaginal smear observation made in the progestin therapy of endometrial cancer also suggests a similar conclusion (Bonte, Drochmans and Ide, 1970).

The mechanism by which progestins at high dosage assist in causing regression of breast cancer is not clear, but as in the case of oestrogen, it is likely that both direct and indirect mechanisms play a part. Thus progestins undoubtedly have an effect on gonadotrophin secretion in the human, but the evidence is conflicting because of crossover in the immunoassay of FSH and LH. It is likely that a decrease in the luteinizing component is the effect common to all members of the group (Diczfalusy, 1965; Dufau et al., 1970). Like oestrogen, progesterone administration at high dosage stimulates prolactin release from the pituitary in rats (Chen and Meites, 1970), but it may also interfere at the target site with the effect of prolactin. Thus it has been shown that high levels of progesterone will prevent the mammary gland of the pregnant rat from responding to the prolactin–adrenal complex which triggers off lactation in that animal (Kuhn, 1969).

Because of their similar mechanism it could be expected that the effect of high dosage progestin would be synergistic to or potentiate high dosage oestrogen effects at the target site. This has indeed been demonstrated both in lactation and in experimental mammary cancer. Blocking lactogenesis in the ovariectomized lactating rat normally requires the administration of 1 mg oestradiol (a very high dose), but if combined with 2 mg progesterone, only 10 µg of oestradiol is required (Cowie, 1972). Similarly, a combination of oestrogen and progesterone is much more effective in blocking lactogenesis in the rabbit than either steroid separately (Meites and Sgouris, 1953). This observation has been confirmed in the case of human lactation also (Toaff and Jewelowicz, 1963).

In the case of DMBA-induced mammary carcinoma in rats, it has been reported that progesterone potentiates the effect of high dosage oestrogen in retarding the growth of the tumour in the intact animal (Huggins, Moon and Morii, 1962). After oophorectomy, it has been reported that administration of progesterone potentiates the effect of oestrogen in reactivating the growth of the tumour (Young, Cowan and Sutherland, 1963). All these examples of oestrogen–progestin synergism lead to the suggestion that in mammary cancer the addition of progestin to oestrogen potentiates its peripheral action (Stoll, 1973).

This may apply also to the treatment of human mammary cancer. Oestrogen and progestin when used separately in the treatment of breast cancer need to be given at a very much higher dosage than that used in the treatment of gynaecological disorders. However, when given in combination at the relatively low dose found in oral contraceptives, they cause regression in over 20 per cent of breast cancers (Stoll, 1965). It is interesting that a similar observation has been made in the treatment of endometrial cancer by an oral contraceptive combination of oestrogen and progestin (Stoll, 1967a).

The therapy of breast cancer with high dosage oestrogen–progestin combinations has been reported frequently in the past ten years (Landau, Ehrlich and Huggins, 1962; Stoll, 1965, 1967a; Crowley and MacDonald, 1965; Kennedy, 1965; Notter, 1966; Landau, 1967; Muggia et al., 1967; Talley et al., 1970; Berndt, 1970). The basis of such treatment being empirical, a variety of agents and ratios of progestin to oestrogen have been utilized in these trials. The majority of trials have been in post-menopausal women, but evidence of tumour regression has been seen in pre-menopausal women also from comparable dosage (see Chapter 13). This is important in relation to current speculation as to the possible effect of oestrogen–progestin oral contraceptives on the development of breast cancer.

The reports mentioned above have noted tumour regression from the hormone combination in about 25 per cent of breast cancer patients in whom either oestrogen alone or progestin alone has yielded no response. Response to the combination has been reported even after hypophysectomy (Landau, Ehrlich and Huggins, 1962; Kennedy, 1965), a stage at which response to oestrogens alone has never been recorded. Although it has not been proven that the administration of the two hormones together in the first place is more effective than either alone (Ahmann, Hahn and Bisel, 1972), this would probably occur if the optimal progestin–oestrogen ratio could be assessed for each individual. Unfortunately, we have no certain method of determining this.

## FACTORS IN HORMONAL SENSITIVITY

One conclusion to be derived from this review is that there is unlikely to be a single hormonal relationship or unitary hypothesis capable of explaining the response by human mammary cancer to all methods of endocrine therapy including high dosage oestrogen therapy. On the assumption that both prolactin and oestrogen are required for maintaining the growth of hormone-sensitive breast cancer, it is here suggested that there are two ways by which the same tumour can be made to regress—one by depriving it of both prolactin and oestrogen as far as is possible by endocrine ablation, and the other by increasing the level of the two hormones at the target as a result of high dosage oestrogen therapy. The morphological reaction seen in breast ductal tissue after high dosage oestrogen therapy is quite different from that seen associated with tumour response to major endocrine ablation in patients of a similar age group. Our hypothesis can explain response to oestrogen therapy followed by response to oophorectomy (Kennedy, 1962), response to oestrogen therapy followed by response to hypophysectomy (Stoll, 1969a), and response to hypophysectomy followed by response to oestrogen–progestin combination therapy (Landau, Ehrlich and Huggins, 1962). There is no need to postulate the existence of genetically distinct prolactin–oestrogen dependent clones, and prolactin–oestrogen responsive clones in such cases.

There is not even clear evidence in the human of two genetically distinct types of breast cancer—hormone sensitive and hormone insensitive. An apparent clinical distinction may reflect the criteria of regression set by the clinician, and it is equally possible that some degree of hormonal sensitivity is present in all tissues. However, if this is so, some explanation must be found for the high proportion of apparently null responses to hormonal administration in breast cancer. Autonomy may develop so rapidly in a tumour that a very temporary regression may not be recognized clinically. Again, even if cell division is considerably slowed up by a carcinostatic effect, death of existing adult cells may be so delayed that obvious reduction in the size of the tumour does not manifest. Again, evidence of hormone response may be limited by defective reactivity in the stroma and failure of local immune response mechanisms. It is therefore obvious that hormonal sensitivity is not synonymous with measurable tumour regression after steroid administration.

The criteria for a 'significant' clinical response to hormonal therapy in breast cancer are not universally agreed, but are widely accepted as a 50 per cent reduction in volume of *all* measurable tumour lesions for a minimum period of six months with no new lesions appearing. The selection of such criteria is not arbitrary—it is one which is usually found to be associated with worthwhile palliation and prolongation of life (Stoll, 1969a). On this definition, it is generally accepted that only 25 per cent of patients show significant response to steroid therapy.

In most reported series of breast cancer patients treated by hormonal methods, a further 25 per cent of patients show undoubted regression of tumour, but to less than the degree specified above, and of the residual 50 per cent of patients, a proportion will be, of necessity, categorized as failures of response only because they do not survive eight months after initiating therapy. (This will effectively exclude them from the possibility of significant response, because it takes at least two months to show the first sign of tumour regression, and it must persist for six months to qualify as 'significant'.) Thus, although it is authoritatively stated that 75 per cent of breast cancers fail to respond to hormonal therapy (Hall, 1969), this does not deny the likelihood of genetically determined hormonal sensitivity in some or all of these cases. This point is important if we are suggesting the possibility of increasing tumour sensitivity to endocrine manipulation.

## CONCLUSION

The hormonal mechanisms involved in the regression of breast cancer under high dosage oestrogen therapy are analysed with the aim of developing a working hypothesis which can be used to improve the results of such therapy. The findings suggest a distinction between an irreversible carcinocidal effect and a reversible carcinostatic effect, and the effect of high dosage oestrogen therapy probably involves also indirect effects including stimulation of the immune response mechanism.

The relative importance of each of these mechanisms in the regression of breast cancer following high dosage oestrogen therapy depends on tumoral factors, host factors and hormonal factors. Tumoral factors include the heterogeneity of the cell population, the genetically determined responsiveness of the cell clones (possibly related to receptor site levels), the degree of tumour differentiation and the stage tumour growth has reached. Host factors include the hormonal environment before treatment and the immunosurveillance mechanism. Hormonal factors include the biological profile of the administered hormone, its route of administration and metabolism in the body, and the oestrogen concentration achieved at each tumour site in relation to that of prolactin. Only the last of these factors can be controlled in treatment and, even then, only to the extent permitted by the local receptor site levels.

It is likely that *both* oestradiol and prolactin normally stimulate both mitotic activity and secretory activity in normal mammary tissue. It is suggested that in the case of hormonally responsive mammary carcinoma, the absolute and relative concentration of prolactin and oestrogen actively available at the target site will determine its mitotic activity. A dose-related response of this type (in addition to tumoral factors) may explain the following clinical anomalies in the response of human mammary cancer to oestrogen therapy: stimulation of tumour activity in some cases, differences in site response, the biphasic temporal response and the withdrawal response. An important conclusion is that evidence of stimulation of tumour growth following oestrogen administration suggests hormone sensitivity and the need to increase considerably the level of oestrogen dosage.

The administration of a combination of oestrogen and progestin in an optimal ratio may lead to a higher proportion of regressing tumours than either agent alone in the treatment of breast cancer. Progestin appears to potentiate or facilitate the action of oestrogen in this respect.

## REFERENCES

Adams, J. B. and Wong, M. S. F. (1968'. 'Paraendocrine behaviour of human breast carcinoma. In vitro transformation of steroids to physiologically active hormones.' *J. Endocr.* **41**, 41.

## REFERENCES

Ahmann, D. L., Hahn, R. G. and Bisel, H. F. (1972). 'Disseminated breast cancer—evaluation of hormonal therapy utilising stilbestrol and medrogestone singly and in combination.' *Cancer (Phil.)* **30**, 651.

Alderson, M. R., Hamlin, I. and Staunton, M. D. (1971). 'Prognostic factors in breast carcinoma.' *Br. J. Cancer* **25**, 646.

Ben-David, M., Danon, A. and Sulman, F. G. (1971). 'Evidence of antagonism between prolactin and gonadotrophin secretion.' *J. Endocr.* **51**, 719.

Berndt, G. (1970). 'Management of metastasising mammary carcinoma with oestrogen–gestagen combination therapy by SH 834.' *Dt. Med. Wochenschrift* **95**, 2399.

— Eckel, H., Notter, G. and Stender, H. S. (1971). 'The action of oestrogen–gestagen combination therapy in advanced breast cancer with special reference to lung metastases.' *Strahlentherapie* **141**, 540.

Besser, G. M. and Edwards, C. R. W. (1972). 'Galactorrhoea.' *Br. med. J.* **2**, 280.

Bonte, J. B., Drochmans, A. and Ide, P. (1966). '6a-methyl-17a-hydroxyprogesterone acetate as a chemotherapeutic agent in adenocarcinoma of the uterus.' *Acta obstet. gynaec. scand.* **45**, 121.

— — — (1970). 'Cytologic evaluation of exclusive medroxyprogesterone acetate treatment for vaginal recurrence of endometrial adenocarcinoma.' *Acta cytol. (Baltimore)* **14**, 353.

Braunsberg, H., Irvine, W. T. and James, V. H. T. (1967). 'A comparison of steroid hormone concentrations in human tissue including breast cancer.' *Br. J. Cancer* **21**, 714.

— James, V. H. T., Irvine, W. T., James, F., Jamieson, C. W., Sellwood, R. A., Carter, A. E. and Hulbert, M. (1973). 'Prognostic significance of oestrogen uptake by human breast cancer tissue.' *Lancet* **1**, 163.

Callantine, M. R., Humphrey, R. R. and Nesset, B. C. (1966). 'LH release by 17 β estradiol in the rat.' *Endocrinology* **79**, 455.

Chayen, P., Altmann, F. P. and Bitensky, L. (1970). 'Response of human breast cancer to steroid hormones in vitro.' *Lancet,* **1**, 869.

Chen, C. L. and Meites, I. (1970). 'Effects of estrogen and progesterone on serum and pituitary prolactin levels in ovariectomised rats.' *Endocrinology* **86**, 503.

Cowie, A. T. (1972). Personal communication.

— and Tindal, J. S. (1971). In *The Physiology of Lactation,* p. 361. London; Edward Arnold.

Crile, G. (1972). In *Endocrine Therapy in Malignant Disease,* p. 369, Ed. by B. A. Stoll. London: Saunders.

Crowley, L. G., Demetriou, J., Macdonald, T., Kotin, P., Kashinsky, S. and Donovan, A. J. (1962). 'Levels of exogenous estrogens in tissues in human mammary carcinoma.' *Surg. Forum* **13**, 103

— and MacDonald, I. (1965). 'Delalutin and estrogens for the treatment of advanced mammary carcinoma in postmenopausal women.' *Cancer (Phil.)* **18**, 346.

Curwen, S. (1970). 'The treatment of advanced carcinoma of the breast with SH 420.' *Clin. Radiol.* **21**, 221.

Dao, T. L. (1964). 'Carcinogenesis of mammary gland in the rat.' *Progr. Expl Tumor Res.* **5**, 157.

Dao, T. L. and Libby, P. R. (1969). 'Conjugation of hormones by breast cancer tissue and selection of patients for adrenalectomy.' *Surgery (Baltimore)* **66**, 162.

Delarue, N. C. (1955). 'Fundamental concepts determining a philosophy of treatment in mammary carcinoma.' *Canad. med. Ass. J.* **73**, 597.

Diczfalusy, E. (1965). 'Probable modes of action of oral contraceptives.' *Br. med. J.* **2**, 394.

Dufau, M., Catt, K. J., Dulmanis, A., Fullerton, M., Hudson, B. and Burger, H. G. (1970). 'Suppression of oestradiol secretion and luteinising hormone release during oestrogen–progestogen oral contraceptive therapy.' *Lancet* **1**, 271.

Emerson, W. J., Kennedy, B. J., Graham, J. R. and Nathanson, I. T. (1953). 'Pathology of primary and recurrent carcinoma of the human breast after administration of steroid hormones.' *Cancer (Phil.)* **6**, 641:

— — and Taft, E. B. (1960). 'Correlation of histological alterations in breast cancer with response to hormonal therapy.' *Cancer (Phil.)* **13**, 1047.

Folca, P. J., Glascock, R. F. and Irvine, W. T. (1961). 'Studies with tritium labelled hexoestrol in advanced breast cancer.' *Lancet* **2**, 796.

Furth, J. (1972). In *Prolactin and Carcinogenesis* (4th Tenovus Workshops), p. 137, Ed. by A. R. Boyns and K. Griffiths. Cardiff; Alpha Omega Alpha.

Gillespie, P. J., Burrows, B. D. and Edelstyn, G. A. (1971). 'Possible clinical implications of therapeutically induced temperature changes in a continuously monitored tumour mass.' *Br. J. Cancer* **25**, 85.

Haddow, A., Watkinson, J. M., Paterson, E. and Kunkler, P. (1944). 'Influence of synthetic oestrogens upon advanced malignant disease.' *Br. med. J.* **2**, 393.

Hall, T. C. (1969). 'Endocrinologic factors in the design of more selective antitumor agents.' *Cancer Res.* **29**, 2412.

— Dederick, M. M. and Nevinny, H. B. (1963). 'Prognostic value of hormonally induced hypercalcemia in breast cancer.' *Cancer Chemother. Rep.* **30**, 21.

Hilf, R., Bell, C. and Michel, I. (1967). 'Biochemical responses of normal and neoplastic mammary tissue to hormonal treatment.' *Recent Progr Hormone Res.* **23**, 229.

— Goldenberg, H., Michel, I., Carrington, M. J., Bell, C., Greenstein, M., Merauze, D. R. and Shimkin, M. B. (1969). 'Biochemical characteristics of mammary glands and mammary tumours of rats induced by 3 MCA and 7,12 DMBA.' *Cancer Res.* **29**, 977.

Huggins, C. and Hodges, C. V. (1941). 'Studies on prostatic cancer. Effect of castration, estrogen and androgen injections on serum phosphatases in metastatic carcinoma of the prostate.' *Cancer Res.* **1**, 293.

— Moon, R. C. and Morii, S. (1962). 'Extinction of experimental mammary cancer. 1. Estradiol 17β and progesterone.' *Proc. natn Acad. Sci.* **48**, 379.

Huseby, R. A. and Thomas, L. B. (1954). 'Histological and histochemical alterations in the normal breast tissue of patients with advanced breast cancer being treated with estrogenic hormones.' *Cancer (Phil.)* **7**, 54.

Jensen, E. V., Block, G. E., Smith, S., Kyser, K. and Desombre, E. R. (1972). In *Oestrogen Target Tissue and Neoplasia*, p. 23, Ed. by T. L. Dao. University of Chicago Press.

— Desombre, E. R. and Jungblut, P. W. (1967). In *Endogenous Factors Influencing*

*Host–Tumor Balance,* Ed. by R. W. Wissler, T. Dao and S. Wood. University of Chicago Press.

Jensen, E. V. and Jacobson, H. I. (1962). 'Basic guides in the mechanism of estrogen action.' *Recent Progr Hormone Res.* **18**, 387.

Kaiser, H. (1970). 'Endocrine mechanisms offering protection against endometrial and mammary cancer.' *German Med. Monthly* **15**, 309.

Kellner, G. and Turcic, G. (1962). 'The importance of tissue culture for hormonal therapy of mammary carcinoma.' *Klin. Med. (Wien)* **17**, 83.

Kennedy, B. J. (1962). 'Massive oestrogen administration in premenopausal women with metastatic breast cancer.' *Cancer (Phil.)* **15**, 641.

— (1965). 'Hormone therapy for advanced breast cancer.' *Cancer (Phil.)* **18**, 1551.

Kelley, R. M. and Baker, W. H. (1960). 'Progestational agents in the treatment of carcinoma of the endometrium.' *New Engl. J. Med.* **264**, 216.

Kiang, D. T. and Kennedy, B. J. (1971). 'Combination of cyclophosphamide and estrogen therapy in DMBA induced rat mammary cancer.' *Cancer (Phil.)* **28**, 1202.

Kim, U. (1965). 'Pituitary function and hormonal therapy of experimental mammary cancer.' *Cancer Res.* **25**, 1146.

Kistner, R. W. (1959). 'Histological effects of progestins on hyperplasia and carcinoma in situ of the endometrium.' *Cancer (Phil.)* **12**, 1106.

— (1972). In *Endocrine Therapy in Malignant Disease,* p. 322, Ed. by B. A. Stoll. London; Saunders.

Kohorn, E. I. and Tchao, R. (1968). 'The effect of hormones on endometrial carcinoma in organ culture.' *J. Obstet. Gynaec. Br. Commnw.* **75**, 1262.

Kuhn, N. J. (1969). 'Progesterone withdrawal as the lactogenic trigger in the rat.' *J. Endocr.* **44**, 39.

Landau, R. L. (1967). 'Can endocrine therapy be expected to replace the surgical treatment of advanced breast cancer?' In *Cancer of the Breast,* Ed., by M. Dargent and C. Romieu. Lyon; Simep.

— Ehrlich, E. N. and Huggins, C. (1962). 'Estradiol benzoate and progesterone in advanced human mammary cancer.' *J. Am. med. Ass.* **182**, 632.

L'Hermite, M. and Heuson, J. C. (1973). 'Stimulation of basal serum prolactin levels by oral ethinyl oestradiol'. In Press.

Lipsett, M. B. (1969). 'Prospects in endocrinology for chemotherapy.' *Cancer Res.* **29**, 2408.

McSweeney, E. D., Jnr., and Fletcher, W. S. (1969). 'Synthetic estrogen, progestin combination effect on hormone sensitive breast cancer in the rat.' *Archs Surg.* **99**, 652.

Martin, L. and Cunningham, K. (1960). 'Suppression of pituitary gonadotrophins by 17a ethinyl 19 nortestosterone in patients with metastatic carcinoma of the breast.' *J. clin. Endocr.* **20**, 529.

Meites, J. (1972). In *Prolactin and Carcinogenesis* (4th Tenovus Workshop), p. 54, Ed. by A. R. Boyns and K. Griffiths. Cardiff; Alpha Omega Alpha.

— Cassell, E. and Clark, J. (1971). 'Estrogen inhibition of mammary tumor growth in rats. Counteraction by prolactin.' *Proc. Soc. expl Biol. Med.* **137**, 1225.

— and Sgouris, J. T. (1953). 'Can ovarian hormones inhibit mammary response to prolactin?' *Endocrinology* **53**, 17.

Mioduscewska, O. (1968). In *Prognostic Factors in Breast Cancer*, p. 347, Ed. by A. P. M. Forrest and P. B. Kunkler. Edinburgh; Livingstone.

Moe, N. (1972). 'Short term progestogen treatment of endometrial carcinoma.' *Acta obstet. gynec. scand.* **51**, 55.

Moore, F. D., Woodrow, S. I., Aliopoulios, M. R. and Wilson, R. E. (1967). 'Carcinoma of the breast. A decade of new results and old concepts.' *New Engl. J. Med.* **277**, 460.

Muggia, F. M., Cassileth, P. A., Flatow, F. A., Gellhorn, A. A., Hyman, G. A. and Ochoa, M. (1967). 'Treatment for breast cancer with medroxyprogesterone.' *Ann. intern. Med.,* **66**, 1066.

Nagasawa, H. and Yanai, R. (1971). 'Increased mammary gland response to pituitary mammotropic hormone by estrogen in rats.' *Endoc. jap.* **18**, 53.

Nathanson, I. T. (1947). 'Hormonal alteration of advanced cancer of the breast.' *Surg. Clins N. Am.* **27**, 1144.

— (1952). 'Clinical investigative experience with steroid hormones in breast cancer.' *Cancer (Phil.)* **5**, 754.

Nordquist, R. S. (1964). 'Hormone effects on carcinoma of the uterine body studied in organ culture. A preliminary report.' *Acta obstet. gynec. scand.* **43**, 296.

— (1969). 'Hormonal effects on endometrial carcinoma in vitro.' *Acta obstet. gynec. scand.* **48**, 118.

Notter, G. (1966). 'Toxic effects of progestogens and estrogen in breast cancer.' *Cancer Chemother. Abst.* **7**, 408.

Novak, E. R. (1970). 'Ovulation after fifty.' *Obstet. Gynaec.* **36**, 903.

O'Malley, B. W., Sherman, M. R. and Toft, D. O. (1970). 'Progesterone receptors in the cytoplasm and nucleus of chick oviduct target tissue. 'Proc. natn Acad. Sci.* **67**, 501.

Papaionnaou, A. N. (1972). 'Prolactin, levodopa and immune response in breast cancer.' *Lancet* **2**, 226.

Pearson, O. H. (1957). 'Observations on the role of androgens and estrogen in body balance.' *Ann. intern. Med.* **100**, 724.

Salih, H., Flax, H., Brander, W. and Hobbs, J. R. (1972). 'Prolactin dependence in human breast cancers.' *Lancet* **2**, 1103.

Segaloff, A. (1966). 'Hormones and breast cancer.' *Recent Progr. hormone Res.* **22**, 351.

— Gordon, D., Carabasi, R. H., Horwitt, B. N., Schlosser, J. V. and Murison, P. J. (1954). 'Hormonal therapy in cancer of the breast. 7. Effect of conjugated estrogen (equine) on clinical course and hormonal excretion.' *Cancer (Phil.)* **7**, 758.

Sherman, A. I. (1966). 'Progesterone caproate in the treatment of endometrial cancer.' *Obstet. Gynaec.* **28**, 309.

Stewart, J. G., Skinner, L. G. and O'Connor, P. J. (1965). 'Hormonal therapy in metastatic breast cancer, clinical response and urinary gonadotrophins.' *Acta endoc. (Kobn)* **50**, 345.

Stoll, B. A. (1965). In *Recent Advances in Ovarian and Synthetic Steroids,* Ed. by R. Shearman. Sydney; Globe.

— (1966). 'Therapy by progestational agents in advanced breast cancer.' *Med. J. Aust.* **1**, 331.

Stoll, B. A. (1967a). 'Effect of Lyndiol, an oral contraceptive, on breast cancer.' *Br. med. J.* **1**, 150.

— (1967b). 'Vaginal cytology as an aid to hormone therapy in postmenopausal breast cancer.' *Cancer (Phil.)* **20**, 1807.

— (1969a). In *Hormonal Management in Breast Cancer*. London; Pitman.

— (1969b). 'Investigation of organ culture as an aid to the hormonal management of breast cancer.' *Cancer (Phil.)* **25**, 1228.

— (1971). 'The thermoprofile as an early indicator of breast cancer response to hormonal therapy.' *Cancer (Phil.)* **27**, 1379.

— (1972). In *Endocrine Therapy in Malignant Disease*. London; Saunders.

— (1973). 'Hormonal therapy of gynecologic malignancy.' *Clin. Obstet. Gynec.*

— and Ackland, T. H. (1970). 'Management of breast cancer in old age.' *Br. med. J.* **4**, 201.

Talley, R. W., O'Bryan, R. M., Burrows, J. H., and SanDiego, E. L. (1970). 'Comparison of testololactone and an estrogen–progestin combination in the treatment of metastatic breast cancer.' *Cancer Chemother. Rep.* **54**, 249.

Thiery, M. and Willighagen, R. G. J. (1968). 'The influence of progesterone caproate on the enzyme profile of endometrial carcinoma.' *Bull. Soc. Roy. Belg. Gynec. Obstet.* **38**, 1.

Toaff, R. and Jewelowicz, R. (1963). 'Inhibition of lactogenesis by combined oral progestogens and oestrogen.' *Lancet* **2**, 322.

Turkington, R. W. (1972). In *Prolactin and Carcinogenesis* (4th Tenovus Workshop), p. 39, Ed. by A. R. Boyns and K. Griffiths. Cardiff; Alpha Omega Alpha.

Wellings, S. R. and Jentoft, V. L. (1972). 'Organ cultures of normal, dysplastic, hyperplastic and neoplastic human mammary tissue.' *J. natn Cancer Inst.* **4**, 329.

Welsch, C. W. (1972). Personal communication.

— and Rivera, E. M. (1972). 'Differential effects of estrogen and prolactin on DNA synthesis in organ cultures of DMBA induced rat mammary carcinoma.' *Proc. Soc. expl. Biol. Med.* **139**, 623.

Yen, S. S. C. and Tsai, C. C. (1971). 'The biphasic pattern in the feedback action of ethynyl estradiol on the release of pituitary FSH and LH.' *J. clin. Endocr.* **33**, 882.

Young, S., Cowan, D. M. and Sutherland, L. E. (1963). 'The histology of induced mammary carcinoma in rats.' *J. Path. Bact.* **85**, 337.

# 4

# Anti-oestrogens and Their Role in Mammary Cancer

## L. Terenius

Before discussing the role of anti-oestrogens in the treatment of breast cancer, it may be useful to review very briefly some recent developments in our knowledge of hormone receptors in mammary carcinoma. Although our knowledge is very incomplete, an understanding of hormone receptor mechanisms may be very important in the management of hormone-sensitive breast cancer.

## HORMONE RECEPTORS AND TUMOUR SENSITIVITY TO HORMONES

During the 1960s it was found that target tissues for hormonal steroids have specific binding proteins for the hormones. These proteins have a 'functional' specificity so that, for example, oestrogen receptors will bind only oestrogens and competitive anti-oestrogens, but not androgens or progestogens. They have very high dissociation constants—about $10^{-11}$ to $10^{-10}$ M—and occur only in hormone-sensitive cells, and have therefore been named 'receptors' (Hechter, 1971). Their high specificity and high affinity, and the high stability of steroid hormone receptor complexes (a half life *in vivo* of several hours), have suggested their importance in mediating steroid effects on the target cell (Jensen and DeSombre, 1972).

A number of investigators have confirmed that oestrogen receptors are present not only in ovary-dependent DMBA-induced rat mammary carcinoma, but also in between 30 and 50 per cent of biopsies from human mammary carcinoma (see below). Progestogen receptors seem to be present in a somewhat lower proportion of biopsies from human mammary carcinoma, and it is interesting that the levels of oestrogen and progestogen receptors do not bear a constant relationship to each other (Terenius, 1973). Work on prolactin receptors has so far provided less conclusive evidence of their identity.

It would seem likely that tumours which have a particular type of receptor are also *sensitive* to that particular hormone. However, this does not necessarily mean that the tumour is *dependent* on the hormone or that a clinical response will be observed following a treatment which causes a change in the stimulation of that particular receptor. The kind and degree of response may vary according to the types and number of receptors involved, and where several kinds of receptors exist, on the relative level of each receptor. It should also be remembered that the effect of a hormone on a target depends greatly on its *local* concentration, and this can be affected by alterations in the turnover of the hormone and in the regional blood flow.

Experimental data and clinical experience suggest that oestrogen, progesterone and prolactin are all necessary for the development of mammary tissue, and these hormones are presumed to be important also in the growth of mammary carcinoma. Assuming that a tumour may be responsive to none or any one of these hormones, or to any combination of hormones, it is theoretically possible for eight different kinds of hormone sensitivity to exist (Jull, 1958).

However, for the sake of simplicity let us consider a tumour with oestrogen receptors only and presumably oestrogen dependent. Castration of the host will reduce the secretion of oestrogen, as will also adrenalectomy or pharmacological suppression of adrenal secretion of oestrogen. Provided such treatment reduces the local oestrogen concentration at the target, less oestrogen will occupy the receptors and, having lost this stimulus for growth, the tumour may regress. Alternatively one could advocate treatment with an anti-oestrogen in which case the oestrogen receptors will be occupied, but not very much stimulated, by the agent (see below).

High dose therapy with oestrogens can lead to a local concentration of such magnitude that the receptors may be saturated, which does not appear to occur physiologically. It is possible that such strong stimulation of receptors is responsible for the therapeutic effect but other processes in hormone-responsive cells may be affected as well. Such effects may involve an action on plasma membranes, capillary permeability in the tumour or stimulation of lysosomal activity. All these effects are known to occur in the normal cells of the target tissue in response to oestrogens and it is uncertain whether they involve a different kind of receptor.

It is obvious that in order to define the role of tumoral receptors in the clinical response to any of the three methods of treatment described above, attempts must be made to relate the clinical response to the measurement of receptor levels. There is already some limited information available of a convincing relation between oestrogen receptor level and response to adrenalectomy (Folca, Glascock and Irvine, 1961; Jensen et al., 1971). Similar investigations are necessary of progestogen and prolactin receptor levels in relation to therapy.

## TUMOUR BIOLOGY AND HORMONE RECEPTORS

The concept of tumour progression (Foulds, 1954) involves an irreversible transition from a pre-malignant stage to true malignant growth and then towards autonomy. In tumours originating from endocrine responsive tissue, autonomy involves hormone insensitivity. The stages in such a process are exemplified in the virus-induced mammary tumours in mice (Foulds, 1959). During the pre-malignant stage, the presence of a hormonal stimulus is essential for progression to the malignant phase, and this may be necessary to overcome immunosurveillance mechanisms. The mechanism for further progression to the autonomous stage probably involves the loss of hormone receptors in these tumours. It has been shown in the case of mammary tumours of GR mice with the Mühlbock virus, that hormone-dependent tumours possess oestrogen receptors while actively growing tumours in the later stages have not (Terenius, 1972).

It is possible that a mammary tumour may be composed of cells arising from different cell lines or clones, each with a different hormonal sensitivity. Suppression of a sensitive cell line may lead to overgrowth of lines with a different sensitivity spectrum or of non-sensitive lines which were previously restrained. It is difficult to distinguish this, as a cause of the development of autonomy, from a progression of a cell line from hormone sensitivity to autonomy. It is well known that the synthesis of hormone receptors is stimulated by hormones, and the administration of oestrogens may increase synthesis of new oestrogen and progestogen receptors. It seems desirable, therefore, in order to postpone progression to autonomy, to maintain the synthesis of new hormone receptors.

One might be permitted to speculate that in the hormonal therapy of breast cancer, one should aim at the stimulation of the receptors without stimulation of tumour growth. In the case of oestrogen receptors, this might be brought about by therapy with high dosage of oestrogens or with anti-oestrogens.

## DEFINITION AND SCOPE OF ANTI-OESTROGENS

In about one-third of women with metastatic breast cancer, remission of the disease can be brought about by endocrine-ablative procedures (Dao, 1972). There is evidence that such treatment does not completely eliminate endogenous production of oestrogens (Bulbrook and Greenwood, 1957; Bulbrook et al., 1958; Scowen, 1958). For this reason, compounds which antagonize the actions of oestrogens (anti-oestrogens) have been studied as potential therapeutic agents in the disease.

The term anti-oestrogen is used to describe an agent which counteracts the activity of oestrogens. Since the potencies of oestrogens depend on the experimental situation and the test used, the term anti-oestrogen has little meaning unless the test system and the oestrogen are specified.

In the broadest sense any compound which reduces the response to an oestrogen is an anti-oestrogen, irrespective of whether the mechanism involves reduction of biosynthesis or increase in metabolism or excretion of the oestrogen, or involves specific events at the target organ level. Conventionally, compounds which influence oestrogen kinetics outside the target tissues such as stimulators of liver microsomal enzymes (Levin, Welch and Conney, 1968), or inhibitors of protein synthesis, are not considered anti-oestrogenic. On the other hand, substances with androgenic or progestogenic activity often are included among the anti-oestrogens by some authors (Emmens and Miller, 1969). In this communication a narrower definition will be followed: the anti-oestrogens described are agents which reduce the response of target tissues to oestrogen, but themselves have a specific effect on oestrogen-sensitive target tissue. A number of such compounds are known and they fulfil a second criterion: they have an affinity for oestrogen receptors (see below).

These anti-oestrogens antagonize the actions of endogenous or administered oestrogens on uterine growth, vaginal cornification or pituitary secretion. They *also* have more or less oestrogen-like activity in several tests. A subdivision of receptor-blocking anti-oestrogens has been proposed (Terenius, 1970, 1971a). It is based on the anti-oestrogenic as well as on the oestrogenic profile of an agent. A first category includes those agents which are more or less antagonistically active after systemic administration. A second category comprises compounds which are antagonistic only under certain circumstances and which give ano-malous dose-response curves for uterotrophic activity (the so-called impeded response). Compounds in the first category seem to be retained by the oestrogen receptor while those in the latter category manifest a transient occupation.

*Figure 4.1a* shows the differences in dose–response behaviour recorded for *oestrogenic* (uterotrophic) activity. *Figure 4.1b* shows that because of the inherent oestrogenic activity of the anti-oestrogens only partial antagonism may be obtained (Terenius, 1971a).

Compounds in the first category which have been studied in relation to breast cancer are MER-25, *cis*- and *trans*-clomiphene, EMD 16–795,* nafoxidine (U-11, 100A), ICI-46, 474, PD C1-628,* CN-55, 945 and in the second category oestriol, dimethyl stilboestrol (DMS) and erythro-MEA.

Although dependent on species and test it can be generalized that compounds in the first of the categories noted have higher anti-oestrogenic–oestrogenic ratio than those in the second category. It should also

---

* Tentative identification only.

85

be noted that most available data on this ratio for these compounds come from studies on the uterus and vagina and it is by no means certain that such data

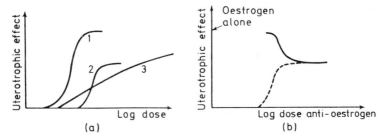

*Figure 4.1(a). Typical dose-response curves for uterotrophic activity in rodents. Curve 1, oestrogen; curve 2, anti-oestrogen of category 1; and curve 3, anti-oestrogen of category 2. (b) typical dose–response curve for anti-uterotrophic activity (anti-oestrogen of category 1). The dotted line indicates uterotrophic activity of the anti-oestrogen alone. The antagonism is therefore only partial*

can be extrapolated to activity on breast cancer. These problems will be discussed below.

A third category of compounds includes the receptor directed cytotoxics. One of these, estramustine phosphate, has been tried in advanced mammary carcinoma in women. Structurally it is a combination of a nitrogen mustard and oestradiol-17-phosphate via a carbamate linkage. Since it is anti-oestrogenic in mice, albeit only at high doses (Müntzing, 1972), it is included here.

Those compounds which have been tested therapeutically against breast cancer either in experimental animals or in women are shown in *Figure 4.2*.

## ANTI-OESTROGENS AND THE INITIATION OF BREAST CANCER

The female sex hormones probably contribute to the induction of breast cancer and induction has never been reported to occur in undeveloped breast tissue (Mühlbock, 1972). It has therefore been suggested that excessive exposure during the reproductive years to female hormones, notably oestrogens, may be one important factor in the genesis of the disease.

Oestriol, if injected, is known to be anti-oestrogenic on the uterus and vagina of experimental animals. Since it is produced and excreted in large amounts, the hypothesis has been advanced that oestriol could be a physiological anti-oestrogen protecting the receptors in breast tissue from excessive stimulation (Lemon et al., 1966; Lemon, 1970; MacMahon et al., 1971). In addition to 'oestriol', it is possible that its epimers and other weak oestrogens oxidized at C2 and C6 could play a similar role. Lemon, Miller

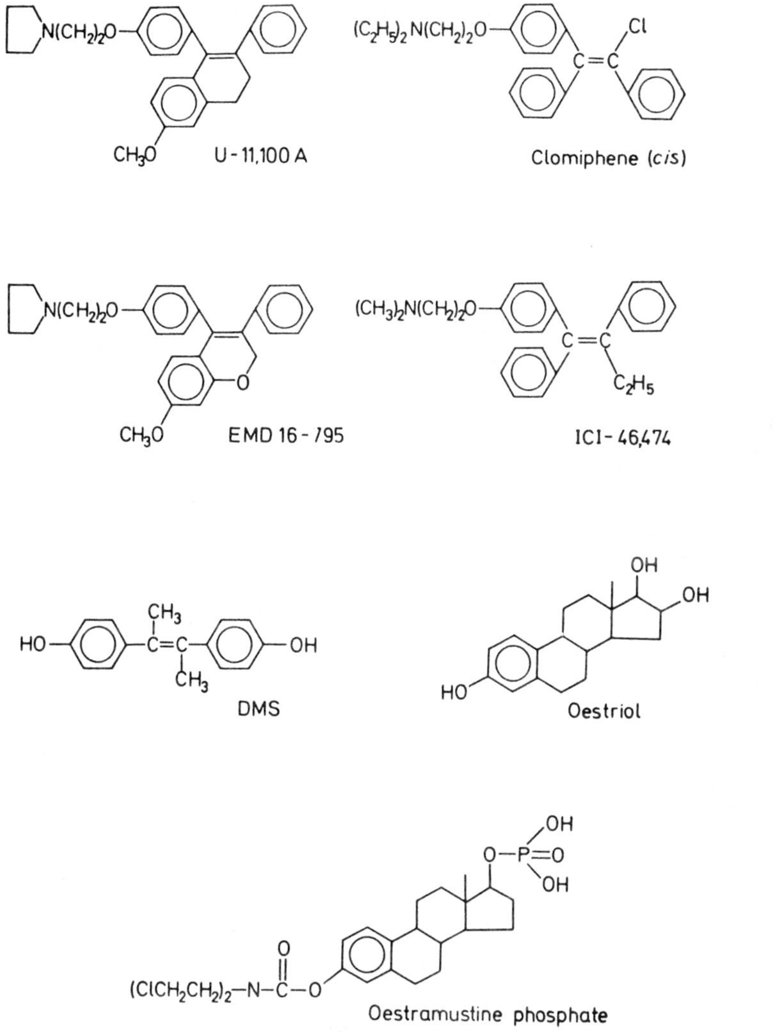

*Figure 4.2. Formula chart*

and Foley (1971) have recently summarized the clinical support for this hypothesis.

Some experimental work in rats has shown that anti-oestrogens have indeed a protective role during the induction of breast cancer in rats by 7,12-dimethylbenzanthracene (DMBA). Terenius (1971b) induced mammary tumours by repeated injection of DMBA. During a period slightly overlapping the induction period, different groups of rats were treated with MER-25 or oestriol at doses which induced dioestrus. It was found that MER-25 and, to a lesser extent, oestriol delayed and reduced the tumour incidence. (No significant effect was seen after treatment with progesterone or testosterone, although such treatment also led to vaginal dioestrus.) When oestriol was given in a polymerized form which releases the active compound slowly, neither vaginal dioestrus nor protection of the mammary glands was demonstrated.

The conclusions drawn by the author were that only receptor-blocking anti-oestrogens were protective under the test conditions. Furthermore, it seemed as if oestriol had to be given intermittently in order to be an antagonist and this would fit in with observations made by Miller (1969) on the uterus and vagina of mice. However, the anti-carcinogenic role of oestriol under conditions of continuous release, as occurs physiologically, remains undetermined and should preferably be studied at various dose levels.

In similar experiments, Lemon, Miller and Foley (1971) found that implanting oestriol pellets within 24–48 hours of a single administration of DMBA reduced the incidence of breast cancer significantly. A similar effect was also seen after implantation of oestriol-17β. Since no information is given on the concomitant effects of the two different hormones on oestrus cycles it is not possible to determine whether the oestriol-induced inhibition of tumour growth was a result of anti-oestrogenic or oestrogenic activity.

Lemon, Miller and Foley (1971) also report an unsuccessful attempt to induce breast cancer in Sprague–Dawley rats by implantation of about 1 mg of oestriol every two months. No breast tumours were developed after 120–500 days of observation. When given to spayed, DMBA-treated rats, however, oestriol alone or in combination with oestradiol-17β or oestrone, induced tumours in a few rats (doses are not stated). Spayed rats which received only DMBA developed no tumours and thus oestriol seemed to have a synergistic effect in promoting tumour development.

Very recently, Heuson et al. report that nafoxidine protects the mammary gland in the DMBA-treated rat from the development of carcinoma (EORTC Breast Cancer Group, 1972).

## ANTI-OESTROGENS IN THE TREATMENT OF EXPERIMENTAL BREAST CANCER

The only model system which seems to have been used for the study of anti-oestrogens is the 7,12-dimethylbenzanthracene (DMBA)-induced mammary cancer in rats. Injection of the carcinogen into 50–56-day-old female rats produces breast tumours within 30 to 90 days in almost every rat (Huggins, Grand and Brillantes, 1961). The tumour is strongly dependent on ovarian and pituitary function and cannot be induced in castrated or hypophysectomized animals. Although much used as a model for the human disease, it differs in some respects as, for example, it does not undergo metastatic spread (Dao, 1969). This tumour is also dependent on caloric intake (Gropper and Shimkin, 1967) and insulin (Heuson, Legros and Heimann, 1972).

Early reports that clomiphene (Schulz, Haselmeier and Hölzel, 1969) and nafoxidine (Terenius, 1970) reduced the growth of the DMBA tumour were later substantiated. Schulz et al. have studied the two anti-oestrogens clomiphene and EMD 16–795 in the DMBA tumour system. Clomiphene exists in two geometric isomers: the cis-isomer with both anti-oestrogenic and oestrogenic properties, while the trans-isomer is only oestrogenic. Schulz, Haselmeier and Hölzel (1971) used both isomers separately in treatment. Tumours of 1–2 cm in diameter were observed. The clomiphene isomers were given either subcutaneously or orally for 30 days. The cis-isomer of clomiphene significantly inhibited tumour growth as compared with untreated controls, while the trans-isomer was inactive or even seemed to stimulate tumour growth. Unfortunately no information is given on the effect of the treatment on the body weight of the rats or the effect on oestrus cycles.

Schulz, Haselmeier and Hölzel (1971) also report on the incorporation of labelled clomiphene in the mammary tumours, uterus and skeletal muscle. An isomer mixture labelled with $^{14}C$ was used. Since the specific activity of the compound was as low as $22 \cdot 5$ µCi/µg and the binding affinities of the clomiphene isomers are rather low (Terenius, 1971a), practically no receptor labelling can occur. The information obtained in these experiments therefore gives no indication on receptor occupation.

Treatment with EMD 16–795 similarly reduced or inhibited tumour growth (Schulz and Wüstenburg, 1971), and reduction in tumour growth occurred even at doses which did not influence body growth. The tumour inhibitory activity of the agent was reversible since tumour growth recurred after cessation of treatment. Again, no information is given on the effect on the oestrus cycle.

Terenius (1971c) observed that nafoxidine was effective in reducing tumour growth in DMBA-treated rats. The anti-oestrogen was given when the rats had one or more tumours of about $0 \cdot 8$ cm in diameter and treatment was continued for three weeks. The animals were kept for 5–7 weeks after cessation of the treatment. Nafoxidine treatment markedly reduced tumour growth in comparison with control animals, both the number and volume of tumours being less at the end of the treatment period than at the beginning. After the end of the treatment several tumours started to grow immediately but a majority remained static for at least two or three weeks. A few of these regressed tumours started to grow again later, while others remained in permanent remission. The complex growth pattern showing the individuality in response is shown in *Figures 4.3* and *4.4*.

At the dose level used, nafoxidine only slightly affected the increase in body

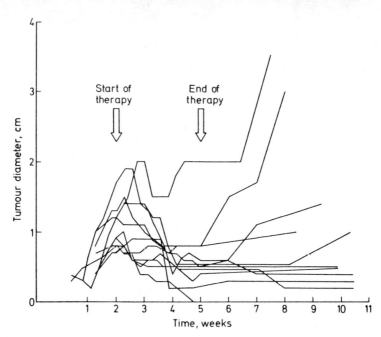

*Figure 4.3. Response of the DMBA-induced tumour to anti-oestrogen (nafoxidine) treatment. Large tumours (0·8 cm in diameter or larger during observation period) occurring singly in each rat are shown*

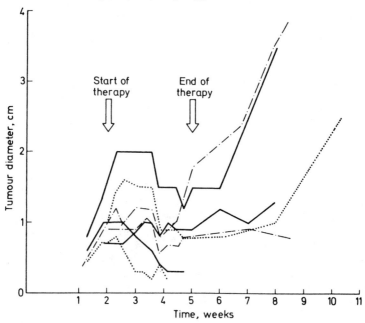

*Figure 4.4. As in Figure 4.3 but animals with multiple large tumours. The symbols refer to individual rats*

[Reproduced from Terenius (1971c) by courtesy of Pergamon Press]

weight in these growing animals (an increase in the treated groups of $5 \pm 5$ g as compared with $15 \pm 10$ g for the controls). Since a comparison of the body-weight changes in tumour-bearing animals is difficult, the effect of nafoxidine on the growth of normal animals of the same age was studied. Nafoxidine had a small effect on weight (an increase in the treated group of $12 \pm 2$ g against $22 \pm 4$ g in controls). It is unlikely, however, that these small differences are responsible for the dramatic reduction in tumour number and volume. Nafoxidine changed the normal vaginal cyclic pattern to an acyclic pattern, but the vaginal smears could be classified as mainly dioestrus since they contained leucocytes and less than 50 per cent nucleated cells.

Very little has been published on the anti-tumour effects of anti-oestrogens of category 2. Lemon, Miller and Foley (1971), who have been investigating the effects of oestriol in carcinogenesis (see above), state, however, that 'estriol administration has not visibly affected the growth rate of established (DMBA) tumours in our rats'.

## CLINICAL TRIALS WITH ANTI-OESTROGENS

To date, very few patients with breast cancer have been treated with anti-oestrogens. An early trial with MER-25 was apparently not followed up because of severe side effects (Callantine, 1967). It should be noted that although this anti-oestrogen is considered to be almost devoid of oestrogenic activity it has to be given in massive doses because of its low potency.

The largest and most complete reported trial is that carried out with ICI-46,474* by Cole, Jones and Todd (1971). A series of 46 patients at an advanced stage of the disease were treated for at least three months. Good response according to objective and subjective criteria was seen in 10 patients, 19 failed to respond while 17 demonstrated an intermediate degree of response. Side reactions were usually mild, although treatment had to be discontinued in 2 cases because of hot flushes and gastro-intestinal intolerance.

In the final evaluation a comparison was made with a similarly conducted trial with an oestrogen (stilboestrol 5 mg × 3 per day orally) or with an androgen (methylandrostenediol 50 mg × 4 per day sublingually). Thirty-one of these patients later participated in the series treated with ICI-46,474. The rate of remission was similar for all drugs although somewhat lower for androgen treatment. No correlation between sensitivity to androgen and ICI-46,474 seemed to exist. The incidence of severe side effects was lower with ICI-46,474 than with the other drugs, particularly when compared with oestrogen treatment. Very little information is given on the hormonal effects of ICI-46,474 and it is only stated that it gave no virilizing effects, whereas these were troublesome with the androgen. Furthermore, it is reported that 'vaginal smears showed no characteristic pattern'.

* Recently named Tamoxifen.

Very recently a short report on a co-operative multi-hospital trial of nafoxidine in human breast cancer was published (EORTC Breast Cancer Group, 1972). Of 24 treated patients, 8 demonstrated objective remissions in a three month observation period. In one case, hypercalcaemia developed and treatment was discontinued. In the other cases only mild side effects were observed but marked skin photosensitivity (erythema) was seen in 13 of the 23 evaluated cases. Vaginal cytology was recorded in 14 patients at the beginning and at the end of the treatment and transformation from atrophy to oestrogen-like stimulation was seen in 11 cases.

Two anti-oestrogens of category 2, DMS and oestriol, have been used for limited clinical trials. Dimethylstilboestrol (DMS) has been tested by the Co-operative Breast Cancer Group (Segaloff, 1966). Of 22 patients only 13 per cent (3) showed objective regressions. No more details are given. In mice, DMS has been found to be anti-oestrogenic when applied locally, but only weakly active when given systemically (Emmens, Cox and Martin, 1962).

Lemon, Miller and Foley (1971) give some data on the initial phase of a study of oestriol (2·5–10 mg/day) in advanced breast cancer. No remissions were seen in two patients who tolerated 2·5–5 mg oestriol per day for two months. In contrast, a rapid exacerbation of bone pain was observed in two other patients. These initial results are clearly not encouraging.

According to the hypothesis advanced by Lemon (1970) oestriol plays an anti-carcinogenic role, protecting the breast tissue from neoplastic transformation (see above). If this is true one might expect endocrine-induced remission in patients secreting subnormal amounts of oestriol. However, in trials described by Jull, Shucksmith and Bonser (1963) and Lemon et al. (1966) no statistical correlation was seen between oestriol quotient* and remission subsequent to various types of ablative endocrine therapy.

A trial with oestramustine phosphate has been carried out by the EORTC Breast Cancer Group (1969). Criteria for the selection of patients and the evaluation of results were similar to those followed by the same Group in the nafoxidine trial. A total of 34 post-menopausal patients were treated with oestramustine phosphate for at least three months. Only 2 objective remissions were observed, both being in patients with cutaneous metastases. Vaginal smears from 6 patients were indicative of hormonal stimulation—in 3 cases the smears were typically cornified. Although these results are not encouraging and further trials were not recommended, it might be profitable to explore other compounds based on the same principles. Incidentally, the drug is said to manifest a favourable effect in advanced prostatic cancer (Jönsson and Högberg, 1971).

---

* Excretion in urine: $\dfrac{\text{oestriol, } \mu g/24 \text{ hours}}{\text{oestrone} + \text{oestradiol-}17\beta, \mu g/24 \text{ hours}}$

## ANTI-OESTROGENS AND OESTROGEN RECEPTORS

Oestrogen receptors are present in the ovarian dependent but to a lesser extent in the independent DMBA-tumour (King, Cowan and Inman, 1965; Mobbs 1966), as well as in some human breast tumours (references given below). Both oestrogens and some anti-oestrogens bind to these receptors. All anti-oestrogens dealt with in this review are competitive inhibitors of oestrogen binding to the receptors, and the current concept is that they act by receptor blockade.

It has been demonstrated that anti-oestrogens inhibit oestrogen binding to experimental and human breast tumours. Thus, nafoxidine (Jensen, DeSombre and Jungblut, 1967; Terenius, 1968, 1971c; James et al., 1971) inhibits oestrogen binding in the DMBA-tumour and human breast cancer. Jensen, DeSombre and Jungblut (1971) used the inhibition caused by another anti-oestrogen, PD CI-628, as a criterion of binding specificity, i.e. the presence of receptors in a tumour sample, while Görlich and Heise (1971), Hähnel and Twaddle (1971) and Maass et al. (1971) used nafoxidine for the same purpose. This application is illustrated in *Figure 4.5*.

Korenman and Dukes (1970) determined the competitive binding capacity of the anti-oestrogens epi-oestriol, oestriol, erythro-MEA, DMS, cis-clomiphene and CN-55,945, in 15 breast cancer specimens. It was found that every anti-oestrogen tested was inhibitory in the 7 cases where specific (i.e. saturable) binding occurred. These authors suggest that such tests with several anti-oestrogens might reveal some binding selectivity for the *tumour* receptors. A possible general selectivity in tumour receptors or an individuality of the tumour receptors might give important information for therapy, but so far there seems to be no experimental support for this possibility.

## DISCUSSION

There is considerable vagueness in the current use of the term 'anti-oestrogen' and also an apparent ignorance of the fact that at antagonistic doses all anti-oestrogens are also at least minimally oestrogenic when given alone. Even MER-25, which is inactive as an oestrogen in several tests (Lerner, Holthaus and Thompson, 1958; Emmens, Cox and Martin, 1962; Terenius, 1971a) gave oestrogen-like effects on enzyme levels in rat uterus (Harris, Lerner and Hilf, 1968) as well as oestrogen-like ultrastructural changes in rat endometrium (Terenius and Ljungkvist, 1972).

Clinical documentation of multiple trials is available for only one anti-oestrogen, clomiphene. Charles et al. (1969) compared the activity of both isomers in various gynaecological disorders. The *cis*-isomer was the more potent antagonist as judged from studies of changes in cervical mucus and vaginal smears. Other examples of the antagonistic activity of clomiphene are

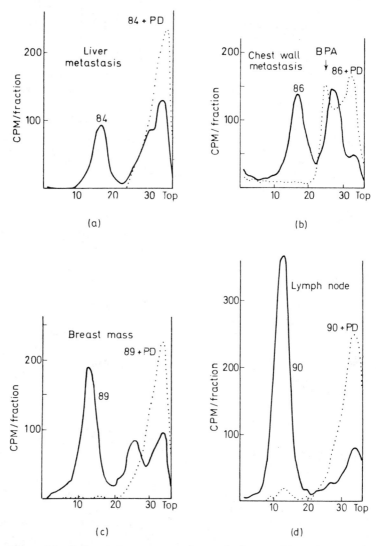

*Figure 4.5. Sedimentation patterns of cytosols from positive primary and metastatic tumours by use of 0·5 nM oestradiol-6,7-³H and 0·2 μM Parke-Davis (PD) CI-628. Centrifugation: No. 84, 12 hours at 308,000 × g; No. 86 and No. 90, 12 hours at 300,000 × g; No. 89, 13 hours at 300,000 × g. in 10–30 per cent sucrose. In No. 86, BPA indicates position of bovine plasma albumin marker* [Reproduced from Jensen *et al.* (1971) by courtesy of the National Cancer Institute]

inhibition of oestrogen effects on ovulation in regularly menstruating women (Roy et al., 1963) and inhibition of oestrogen effects on pituitary secretion (Vaitukaitis et al., 1971).

Induction of ovulation (indicative of anti-oestrogenic activity) has also been demonstrated after treatment with ICI-46,474 (Klopper and Hall, 1971). These and other studies indicate that these compounds act as anti-oestrogens in women *before the ordinary menopausal age*. The situation may be quite different in the woman with advanced breast cancer who is several years past the menopause. In the post-menopausal women, the observed effect of an anti-oestrogen may be more oestrogenic than anti-oestrogenic. Observations in a trial of nafoxidine in post-menopausal women with breast cancer indicated that the treatment actually stimulated the vagina in most studied patients (EORTC Breast Cancer Group, 1972).

It could then be argued that the anti-oestrogens affect mammary cancer by virtue of their oestrogenic activity in the same way as large amounts of oestrogens do. However, this seems unlikely. Oestrogens like ethinyloestradiol or stilboestrol are given in very high doses in mammary cancer compared with those for gynaecological disorders, whereas the dose of ICI-46,474 used in the mammary cancer trial was 10 milligrams once or twice daily (Cole, Jones and Todd, 1971), a dose also used for the induction of ovulation (Klopper and Hall, 1971). To control the DMBA-induced rat mammary tumour huge doses of oestradiol are necessary, about 20 times the dose giving maximum oestrogenic effect in the rat (Huggins, Moon and Morii, 1962). The anti-oestrogens, on the other hand, reduce growth of this tumour at a dose where they are only weakly oestrogenic. It should also be noted that anti-oestrogens never induce a full oestrogenic response (see *Figure 4.2*, and Terenius, 1971a).

If the anti-oestrogens do not act by antagonizing the endogenous production of oestrogens or by being oestrogens, what else remains? One hypothesis that can be advanced is that these compounds act as anti-metabolites causing lethal synthesis. Thus, although some oestrogen-like stimulation may be observed with nafoxidine in post-menopausal women (EORTC Breast Cancer Group, 1972) this does not necessarily mean that the cancer tissue receives the proper stimulus which an 'oestrogen' would give. Some support for this hypothesis of an anomalous response has been found by studying the effects of these compounds on the luminal epithelium of rat uterus (Terenius and Ljungkvist, 1972).

Another possibility is that the anti-oestrogens act by influencing the release of prolactin as the triad, oestrogen, progesterone and prolactin is probably responsible for some breast cancer growth. Studies on prolactin levels in plasma before and during anti-oestrogen treatment are highly desirable. A different line of research would be to give antibodies to one or several of these hormones to define their role in mammary tumour growth. Such antibodies would of course be much purer 'anti-hormones' than those described here.

It should be pointed out that the DMBA-induced mammary cancer suffers from several disadvantages as a model for the human disease. This cancer grows very rapidly as compared with the human cancer and requires intense hormonal support for growth. Hormonal conditions similar to those in the woman past the menopause are therefore not present.

The evaluation of clinical trials with hormones in breast cancer is complicated by the fact that more than 50 per cent of the patients do not respond irrespective of the treatment chosen. Whether the resistant cases are really hormone-independent or whether the hormone treatment is inadequate is never known. It seems clear, however, that breast cancer in women cannot be considered as a uniform disease. Some tumours may be independent of every hormone, while other tumours may depend on hormones but of different kinds. One indication of this is the finding (Terenius, 1973) that human breast cancer tissue occasionally contains progesterone receptors which usually (but not always) occur together with oestrogen receptors. Furthermore, there is no evidence of a correlation between the levels of one receptor with those of the other.

Support for the considerations expressed above may come from the clinical observation by Cole, Jones and Todd (1971) that there is no observed correlation between sensitivity to androgen (methylandrostenediol) and anti-oestrogen (ICI-46,474). This suggests that combinations of hormones, for instance androgens and anti-oestrogens, might give further improvement in remission rates. There is clearly need for more investigations of this kind. Combination therapy may also, in view of the fair success noted for combination cytotoxic therapy in other tumours, be valuable *per se*. If breast cancer is a composite disease, it is possible that different parts of a tumour or different metastases in one patient may depend on hormonal stimulation of different kinds.

Because of differences in hormone dependency, a method of patient selection is highly desirable. Considerable interest has therefore been focused on studies such as those of Folca, Glascock and Irvine (1961) and Jensen et al. (1971), indicating that tumours with oestrogen receptors may be caused to go into remission by ablative surgery. Measurements of receptor levels may therefore be the long sought tool for selecting patients for hormonal intervention, besides giving fundamental knowledge of what hormonal sensitivity means. Studies are then needed to investigate whether the presence of oestrogen receptors in human breast cancer also implies sensitivity to anti-oestrogen treatment. Such studies are being initiated here.

Also for the purpose of selecting suitable therapy, other investigators have studied the effects of hormones on tumours in organ culture (Stoll, 1970; Burstein et al., 1971). An *in vitro* response is taken as evidence of sensitivity to that particular hormone. Dao and Libby (1969) showed that tumour slices from patients who responded to adrenalectomy had a different capacity to conjugate steroids (oestradiol and dehydroepiandrosterone) than non-responders. Again it would be helpful to know the relation between these two parameters and tumour sensitivity to treatment by anti-oestrogens. Should a clear-cut relationship exist between one or more of the parameters described above and tumour sensitivity to anti-oestrogens, then a powerful tool for selecting patients and treatment of the disease may follow.

Finally, mention should be made of such studies as that of Bulbrook and his colleagues (Bulbrook, 1971) who are attempting to establish a relationship between urinary levels of steroid hormone metabolites and subsequent risk of developing breast cancer. If, by such methods a high-risk category can be found, preventive therapy with anti-oestrogens may be considered. The time interval between primary treatment of a cancer and recurrence might also be lengthened by preventive therapy, and to select suitable cases for such treatment one or more of the selection methods outlined above might be helpful.

## ACKNOWLEDGMENT

Work by the author was supported by the Swedish Cancer Society.

## REFERENCES

Bulbrook, R. D. (1971). 'Some basic difficulties in attempting to predict response to therapy by endocrine assays.' *Natn Cancer Inst. Monogr.* **34**, 39.

— and Greenwood, F. C. (1957). 'Persistence of urinary oestrogen excretion after oophorectomy and adrenalectomy.' *Br. med. J.* **1**, 662.

— — Hadfield, G. J. and Scowen, E. F. (1958). 'Hypophysectomy in breast cancer. An attempt to correlate clinical results with oestrogen production.' *Br. med. J.* **2**, 15.

Burstein, N. A., Kjellberg, R. N., Raker, J. W. and Schmidek, H. H. (1971). 'Human carcinoma of the breast in vitro: the effect of hormones.' *Cancer* **27**, 1112.

Callantine, M. R. (1967). 'Nonsteroidal estrogen antagonists.' *Clin. Obstet. Gynec.* **10**, 74.

Charles, D., Klein, T., Lunn, S. F. and Loraine, J. A. (1969). 'Clinical and endocrinological studies with the isomeric components of clomiphene citrate.' *J. Obstet. Gynaec. Br. Cwlth.* **76**, 1100.

Cole, M. P., Jones, C. T. A. and Todd, I. D. H. (1971). 'A new anti-oestrogenic agent in late breast cancer. An early clinical appraisal of ICI46474.' *Br. J. Cancer* **25**, 270.

Dao, T. L. (1969). 'Studies on mechanism of carcinogenesis in the mammary gland.' *Progr. expl. Tumor Res.* **11**, 235.

— (1972). 'Ablation therapy for hormone-dependent tumors.' *Ann. Rev. Med.* **23**, 1.

— and Libby, P. R. (1969). 'Conjugation of steroid hormones by breast cancer tissue and selection of patients for adrenalectomy.' *Surgery* **66**, 162.

Emmens, C. W., Cox, R. I. and Martin, L. (1962). 'Antiestrogens.' *Recent Progr. Hormone Res.* **18**, 415.

— and Miller, B. G. (1969). 'Estrogens, proestrogens and antiestrogens.' *Steroids* **13**, 725.

EORTC Breast Cancer Group (1969). 'Essai clinique du phénol bis (2-chloroéthyl) carbamate d'oestradiol dans le cancer mammaire en phase avancée.' *Europ. J. Cancer* **5**, 1.

— (1972). 'Clinical trial of nafoxidine, an oestrogen antagonist in advanced breast cancer.' *Europ. J. Cancer* **8**, 387.

Folca, P. J., Glascock, R. F. and Irvine, W. T. (1961). 'Studies with tritium-labelled hexoestrol in advanced breast cancer.' *Lancet* **2**, 796.

Foulds, L. (1954). 'The experimental study of tumor progression: a review.' *Cancer Res.* **14**, 327.

— (1959). *Neoplastic Development.* London and New York: Academic Press.

Gropper, L. and Shimkin, M. B. (1967). 'Combination therapy of 3-methylcholanthrene-induced mammary carcinoma in rats: effect of chemotherapy, ovariectomy, and food restriction.' *Cancer Res.* **27**, 26.

Görlich, M. and Heise, E. (1971). 'Die Bestimmung der Östradiolrezeptoren in menschlichen Mammakarzinomen.' *Arch Geschwulzforsch.* **38**, 139.

Harris, D. N., Lerner, L. J. and Hilf, R. (1968). 'The effects of progesterone and ethamoxytriphetol on estradiol-induced changes in the immature rat uterus.' *Trans. N. Y. Acad. Sci.* **30**, 774.

Hechter, O. (1971). 'Reflections concerning steroid hormone receptors.' *Adv. Biosci.* **7**, 395.

Heuson, J.-C., Legros, N. and Heimann, R. (1972). 'Influence of insulin administration on growth of the 7,12-dimethylbenz(a)anthracene-induced mammary carcinoma in intact, oophorectomized, and hypophysectomized rats.' *Cancer Res.* **32**, 233.

Huggins, C., Grand, L. C. and Brillantes, F. P. (1961). 'Mammary cancer induced by a single feeding of polynuclear hydrocarbons and its suppression.' *Nature, Lond.* **189**, 204.

— Moon, R. C., and Morii, S. (1962). 'Extinction of experimental cancer. I. Estradiol-17β and progesterone.' *Proc. Natn. Acad. Sci. U.S.* **48**, 379.

Hähnel, R. and Twaddle, E. (1971). 'Estrogen receptors in human breast cancer. 1. Methodology and characterization of receptors.' *Steroids* **18**, 653.

James, F., James, V. H. T., Carter, A. E. and Irvine, W. T. (1971). 'A comparison of *in vivo* and *in vitro* uptake of estradiol by human breast tumors and the relationship to steroid excretion.' *Cancer Res.* **31**, 1268.

Jensen, E. V. and DeSombre, E. R. (1972). 'Mechanism of action of the female sex hormones.' *Ann. Rev. Biochem.* **41**, 203.

— — and Jungblut, P. W. (1967). 'Estrogen receptors in hormone responsive tissues and tumours.' In *Endogenous Factors Influencing Host–Tumor Balance,* p. 15, Ed. by R. W. Wissler, T. L. Dao and S. Wood, Jnr. Chicago University Press.

— Block, G. E., Smith, S., Kyser, K. and DeSombre, E. R. (1971). 'Estrogen receptors and breast cancer response to adrenalectomy.' *Natn. Cancer Inst. Monogr.* **34**, 55.

Jull, J. W. (1958). 'Hormonal mechanisms in mammary carcinogenesis.' In *Endo-*

*crine Aspects of Breast Cancer*, p. 305, Ed. by A. R. Currie. Edinburgh; Livingstone.

Jull, J. W., Shucksmith, H. S. and Bonser, G. M. (1963). *J. clin. Endocr.* **23**, 433.

Jönsson, G. and Högberg, B. (1971). 'Treatment of advanced prostatic carcinoma with estracyt.' *Scand. J. Urol. Nephrol.* **5**, 103.

King, R. J. B., Cowan, D. M. and Inman, D. R. (1965). 'The uptake of 6,7-$^3$H oestradiol by dimethylbenzanthracene-induced rat mammary tumours.' *J. Endocr.* **32**, 83.

Klopper, A. and Hall, M. (1971). 'New synthetic agent for the induction of ovulation: preliminary trials in women.' *Br. med. J.* **1**, 152.

Korenman, S. G. and Dukes, B. A. (1970). 'Specific estrogen binding by the cytoplasm of human breast carcinoma.' *J. clin. Endocr.* **30**, 639.

Lemon, H. M. (1970). 'Abnormal estrogen metabolism and tissue estrogen receptor proteins in breast cancer.' *Cancer* **25**, 423.

— Wotiz, H. H., Parsons, L. and Mozden, P. J. (1966). 'Reduced estriol excretion in patients with breast cancer prior to endocrine therapy.' *J. Am. med. Ass.* **196**, 1128.

— Miller, D. M. and Foley, J. F. (1971). 'Competition between steroids for hormonal receptor.' *Natn Cancer Inst. Monogr.* **34**, 77.

Lerner, L. J., Holthaus, F. J. Jnr. and Thompson, C. R. (1958). 'A non-steroidal estrogen antagonist 1-(*p*-2-diethylaminoethoxyphenyl)-1-phenyl-2-*p*-methoxyphenyl ethanol.' *Endocrinology* **63**, 295.

Levin, W., Welch, R. M. and Conney, A. H. (1968). 'Effect of phenobarbital and other drugs on the metabolism and uterotropic action of estradiol-17β and estrone.' *J. Pharmac. expl Therap.* **159**, 362.

Maass, H., Engel, B., Hohmeister, H. and Trams, G. (1971). 'Bindung von 17β-Östradiol in Mammacarcinomgewebe und Uterus des Menschen.' *Acta endocr. (Kbh.)*, suppl. 152, 58.

MacMahon, B., Cole, P., Brown, J. B., Aoki, K., Lin, T. M., Morgan, R. W. and Woo, N. C. (1971). 'Oestrogen profiles of Asian and North American women.' *Lancet* **2**, 900.

Miller, B. G. (1969). 'The relative potencies of oestriol, oestradiol and oestrone on the uterus and vagina of the mouse.' *J. Endocr.* **43**, 563.

Mobbs, B. G. (1966). 'The uptake of tritiated oestradiol by dimethylbenzanthracene-induced mammary tumours of the rat.' *J. Endocr.* **36**, 409.

Mühlbock, O. (1972). 'Role of hormones in the etiology of breast cancer.' *J. Natn Cancer Inst.* **48**, 1213.

Müntzing, J. (1972). Personal communication.

Roy, S., Greenblatt, R. B., Mahesh, V. B. and Jungck, E. C. (1963). 'Clomiphene citrate: further observations on its use in induction of ovulation in the human and on its mode of action.' *Fertil. Steril.* **14**, 575.

Schulz, K.-D., Haselmeier, B. and Hölzel, F. (1969). 'The influence of clomid and its isomers upon dimethylbenzanthracene-induced rat mammary tumours.' *Acta endocr. (Kbh.)* Suppl. 138, 236.

— — — (1971). 'The influence of clomid and its isomers on dimethylbenzanthracene-induced rat mammary tumours.' In *Basic Actions of Sex Steroids on Target Organs*, p. 274. Basel; Karger.

— and Wüstenberg, B. (1971). 'Growth inhibition of estrogen-dependent rat

99

mammary cancer by EMD 16-795, a new synthetic anti-estrogen.' *Hormone Metab. Res.* **3**, 295.

Scowen, E. F. (1958). Oestrogen excretion after hypophysectomy in breast cancer.' In *Endocrine Aspects of Breast Cancer*, p. 208, Ed. by A. R. Currie. Edinburgh; Livingstone.

Segaloff, A. (1966). 'Hormones and breast cancer.' *Recent Progr. Hormone Res.* **22**, 351.

Stoll, B. A. (1970). 'Investigation of organ culture as an aid to the hormonal management of breast cancer.' *Cancer* **25**, 1228.

Terenius, L. (1968). 'Selective retention of estrogen isomers in estrogen-dependent breast tumors of rats demonstrated by *in vitro* methods.' *Cancer Res.* **28**, 328.

— (1970). 'Two modes of interaction between oestrogen and anti-oestrogen.' *Acta endocr. (Kbh.)* **64**, 47.

— (1971a). 'Structure–activity relationships of anti-oestrogens with regard to interaction with 17β-oestradiol in the mouse uterus and vagina.' *Acta endocr. (Kbh.)* **66**, 431.

— (1971b). 'Effect of anti-oestrogens on initiation of mammary cancer in the female rat.' *Europ. J. Cancer* **7**, 65.

— (1971c). 'Anti-oestrogens and breast cancer.' *Europ. J. Cancer* **7**, 57.

— (1972). 'Parallelism between estrogen binding capacity and hormone responsiveness of mammary tumours in GR/A mice.' *Europ. J. Cancer* **8**, 55.

— (1973). 'Estrogen and progestogen binders in human mammary carcinoma.' *Europ. J. Cancer* **9**, 291.

— and Ljungkvist, I. (1972). 'Aspects on the mode of action of anti-estrogens and antiprogestogens.' *Gynec. Invest.* **3**, 96.

Vaitukaitis, J. L., Bermudez, J. A., Cargille, C M., Lipsett, M. B. and Ross, G. T. (1971). 'New evidence for an anti-estrogenic action of clomiphene citrate in women.' *J. clin. Endocr.* **32, 503.**

# 5

# Corticotrophin Secretion in Relation to Breast Cancer

Simone Saez

The relationship between adrenocorticotrophic hormone (ACTH) and breast cancer can be considered from two aspects. The first is, the way in which ACTH is able to modify the progression of breast cancer, and the second is the way in which the progression of breast cancer can modify the secretion of ACTH, which in turn will have its own consequences.

Both situations require to be studied from two points of view—the evolution of neoplastic disease in general and of those characteristics that are specific to breast cancer.

## ACTION OF CORTICOTROPHIN ON BREAST CANCER

At the present time it is considered that ACTH does not exert a general anti-neoplastic action, but that it modifies the growth of certain tumours on account of particular biological characteristics. In such cases it is thought that ACTH acts indirectly by stimulating hormone secretion from the adrenal glands. It can be readily appreciated, therefore, that the consequences will differ according to whether stimulation of the glycogenic steroids or of the CI8 or CI9 steroids is being considered.

### Corticotrophin in relation to glycogenic steroids

The effect of ACTH on the growth of experimental tumours is variable. Corticoid stimulation, as by the administration of prednisolone, enhances pulmonary dissemination of the Lewis sarcoma T241 grafted in C57 BL mice

(Arons et al., 1962). In this case it is acting on a grafted and non-hormone-dependent tumour, whose conditions of development depend on factors very different to those in mammary cancer. On the other hand, the effect of ACTH on experimental mammary tumours is to slow the growth of mammary adenocarcinoma in C3H mice, proportionally to the dose administered (Glenn et al., 1960).

With regard to normal tissue, ACTH or corticoids can stimulate mammary growth and induce lactation in the rat (Cowie and Folley, 1957). In the differentiation of such mammary tissue, corticoids have been clearly demonstrated to act in conjunction with steroids and polypeptide hormones (Turkington, 1971).

In women suffering from breast cancer, the effects of prolonged treatment by ACTH or by cortisone acetate have been compared (Segaloff et al., 1954). The results of the two agents were similar—both induce a feeling of well being, but there was no objective regression of the tumours. For some considerable time, therefore, the administration of prolonged courses of ACTH has been replaced by large doses of hydrocortisone or prednisolone, which apparently yield comparable results (Dao, Tan and Brooks, 1961; Stoll, 1960; Gardner, Thomas and Gordon, 1962). The similarity of response to prednisolone and to ACTH may appear to be contradictory at first sight as prednisolone is an inhibitor of ACTH secretion but, to the contrary, it demonstrates that the action of ACTH depends on the hypersecretion of corticosteroids that it induces.

The agents that are most active in controlling the growth of a malignant tumour are those which have the greatest anti-inflammatory effect. It is accepted that this action is a general one against any neoplastic process and is not specific for mammary cancer (Dao, Tan and Brooks, 1961).

## Corticotrophin in relation to oestrogens

Since the first attempt at radical suppression of the hormone cycle in a reproductively active woman (Beatson, 1896), it has been acknowledged that oestrogens provide a stimulus for the progression of breast cancer, even though the mechanisms involved in this process are unknown. The radical suppression of oestrogen production has proved to be very complex, and ovariectomized women usually continue to excrete oestrogens in the urine. This has been shown in earliest reports by biological assay (Dao and Huggins, 1955), more precisely by biochemical assays (Brown et al., 1957; Brown, Bulbrook and Greenwood, 1957; Strong et al., 1956; Jull, Shucksmith and Bonser, 1963), and confirmed by the presence in vaginal smears of cells showing oestrogenic stimulation (Zarate et al., 1970).

Menopausal women with or without breast cancer may show evidence of oestrogen-induced differentiation of vaginal cells (Struthers, 1956; Stoll, 1967; De Waard and Thijssen, 1970; Nissen-Meyer and Sanner, 1963; Castellanos et al., 1963), and an irregular excretion of oestrogens (Brown, Bulbrook and Greenwood, 1957; Strong et al., 1956).

Histopathological signs of ovarian activity after the menopause have been described to be more common in women with breast cancer (Sommers and Teloh, 1952). The possibility of post-menopausal ovarian oestrogen production cannot, therefore, be ruled out, especially as it has been shown that oestrogen excretion is reduced by ovariectomy or irradiation of the ovaries (Lemon, 1959; Nissen-Meyer and Sanner, 1963; Persson and Risholm, 1964). Undoubtedly, however, this is not the most important source of oestrogen.

On the other hand, the administration of ACTH to ovariectomized women increases the secretion of the three fractions—oestrone, oestradiol and oestriol (Strong et al., 1956; West, Damast and Pearson, 1958) which suggests their adrenal origin. Recently, it has been demonstrated, using more precise methods (Barlow, Emerson and Saxena, 1969), that the administration of ACTH increases the production of oestrogens in post-menopausal women and this increase is not modified by ovariectomy, indicating its adrenal origin. This effect involves a true production of oestrogens and not the transformation of cortisone and hydrocortisone into oestrogens oxygenated at C11 which was thought to be produced in adrenalectomized patients given 50 mg cortisone daily (Chang and Dao, 1961). Subsequently this was not confirmed and is no longer held to be correct. It should be added that the production of oestrogens of adrenal origin is not peculiar to women suffering from breast cancer, but in these women it is liable to have more serious consequences than in normal women.

With the aim of suppressing adrenal oestrogen production in breast cancer patients, prolonged treatment with cortisone or prednisolone has been proposed at the dosage usually used to inhibit ACTH secretion. This treatment, when associated with bilateral ovariectomy, should theoretically produce the same suppression of oestrogen production as does bilateral adrenalectomy. In the opinion of several authors (Lemon, 1959; Persson and Risholm, 1964) such treatment is of particular interest as it causes little side effects and, started immediately after ovariectomy, it might inhibit the adrenals taking over the production of oestrogens. However, it has been shown that oestrogen excretion in patients treated in this way is not completely stopped (Nissen-Meyer and Sanner, 1963).

It can be asked if the administration of classical ACTH inhibitors is equally effective at all stages in the development of breast cancer. This question is discussed later in the chapter.

## MODIFICATION OF CORTICOTROPHIN SECRETION IN THE PRESENCE OF CANCER

The idea that oestrogens of adrenal origin support the growth of breast cancer after ovariectomy has focused attention on the activities of corticosteroids as a whole, during the natural history of breast cancer. However, interpretation of the results obtained from such investigations requires:

(1) Distinction between the elements that contribute to the growth of the cancer and those that are a consequence of the cancer.

(2) Identification of those changes that are related to the progression of malignant disease in general and those that are peculiar to breast cancer.

(3) Investigation of the mechanism whereby, under these conditions, the secretion of corticosteroids is altered.


## Paraneoplastic hypercorticism

Cushing's syndrome has been frequently described to be associated with the growth of non-endocrine tumours (Meador and Liddle, 1962; Lipsett et al., 1964). It is induced by the primary tumour or its metastases secreting a substance similar to ACTH which causes hyperstimulation of the adrenal cortex independent of the normal hypothalamo-hypophyseal regulation.

This syndrome is only one among other so-called 'paraneoplastic' endocrine syndromes, where there is inappropriate secretion by tumour tissue of a protein substance that mimics the action of a hormone protein. Hypercorticism (Goodall, 1969) is the most frequent syndrome after erythraemia (their incidence being respectively 25 and 34 per cent) and is more frequent than hypoglycaemia, hypercalcaemia and the syndromes arising from inappropriate secretion of serotonin, anti-diuretic hormone, gonadotrophin and thyrostimulin.

Cushing's syndrome in association with breast cancer occurs much less often than with oat cell carcinoma of the bronchus (Lipsett et al., 1964). The clinical signs of Cushing's syndrome in such cases are pronounced, rapidly become worse and may finally predominate over the symptoms arising from the cancer *per se* (Allott and Skelton, 1960). Corticosteroid secretion in these patients has certain special features—the level of plasma cortisol is higher than that usually found in Cushing's syndrome, and varies from day to day. When the secretion of cortisol is very high, it is not modified by large doses of dexamethasone (8 mg/24 hours), although this lowers the cortisol level by more than 50 per cent in Cushing's syndrome not associated with tumours (Liddle et al., 1969; Liddle, 1960). The urinary 17-hydroxy-corticosteroids (17-OHCS) are not increased in response to metopirone (Lipsett et al., 1964).

These two tests show that the ACTH secretion in these patients is independent of its normal regulatory system.

In patients with paraneoplastic hypercorticism, the clinical signs are in proportion to the extent of the disturbance of the endocrine system. However, several authors have shown that during the growth of certain types of cancer (Noble, 1964; Marks, Anderson and Lieberman, 1961; Deshpande, Hayward and Bulbrook, 1965) the plasma 17-OHCS may be considerably raised, without any clinical signs of hypercorticism or disturbance of the plasma electrolytes (Werk and Sholiton, 1960; Borkowski et al., 1966).

Logically this suggests a change in either: *(a)* transport or catabolism of steroids; or *(b)* production or regulation of their secretion. This problem has been investigated in our laboratories by different methods and under various biological conditions:

(1) The plasma 17-OHCS levels and their response to stimulation by exogeneous ACTH.

(2) The hypothalamo-hypophyseal response to stress and to metopirone.

(3) Cortisol response to suppression by dexamethasone.

## Changes in the regulation of corticotrophin secretion

*Plasma 17-OHCS levels and their response to stimulation by exogeneous ACTH*

Hymes and Doe (1962) have clearly demonstrated that patients with advanced lung cancer, three weeks to three months before death, had plasma 17-OHCS levels considerably higher than the normal resting value and an increased response to ACTH stimulation. These changes were less pronounced than in Cushing's syndrome due to ectopic ACTH secretion, and were accompanied by an alteration of circadian rhythm. These patients presented absolutely no other clinical signs of hormone imbalance. Patients with other forms of tumour when given the same test showed the same response as normal controls (Hymes and Doe, 1962; McNamara, Aron and Paulson, 1968).

We have used the ACTH test in two groups of patients with cancer. Twenty-five i.u. of ACTH were given according to the method of EikNess et al. (1955) as a six-hour intravenous perfusion in normal glucose. The baseline plasma 17-OHCS was measured between 8 and 9 a.m., then at two-hourly intervals. The patients were aged 25–70 years and had not received any chemotherapy, radiotherapy or hormone therapy.

Group (a) comprised 37 patients with a variety of different histological types of cancer including bronchial carcinoma, sarcoma, melanoblastoma, carcinoma of the cervix and adenocarcinoma of the endometrium (cerebral tumours were not included). All the cancers were growing actively. The plasma 17-OHCS, non-conjugated, were measured according to the method of Samuels and Nelson and expressed in µg/100 ml plasma (Table 5.1).

It can be seen that the values are significantly increased compared to normal controls. The ACTH stimulation induces a rapid increase of the plasma 17-OHCS. The level reached at the end of the perfusion was not related to the extent that the level was raised at the beginning of the test. Overall the curve appeared to be set about 10 µg above that in normal controls. None of the patients had any evidence of hypercorticism either clinically or in laboratory tests.

TABLE 5.1

Variation of Plasma Non-conjugated 17-OHCS (μg/100 ml ± SD) during Stimulation by 25 i.u. ACTH i.v. in 37 Patients with Various Tumours (Group a)

| | Basal level | 2 Hours | 4 Hours | 6 Hours |
|---|---|---|---|---|
| Normal | 14·6 ± 2·5 | 31·3 ± 3·9 | 39·3 ± 4·2 | 44·6 ± 4·3 |
| Various tumours | 25·96 ± 4·25 | 46·46 ± 8·78 | 54·35 ± 8·72 | 56·06 ± 9·19 |

Group (b) consisted of 66 women with breast cancer in various stages of the disease given the same ACTH test. The mean values for the group were comparable to those in group (a) and higher than in normal controls (Table 5.2).

TABLE 5.2

Variation of Plasma Non-conjugated 17-OHCS (μg/100 ml ± SD) during Stimulation by 25 i.u. ACTH i.v. in 37 Patients with Various Tumours and 66 Cases of Advanced Breast Cancer

| | Basal level | 2 Hours | 4 Hours | 6 Hours |
|---|---|---|---|---|
| Various tumours 37 | 25·96 ± 4·25 | 46·43 ± 8·78 | 54·35 ± 8·72 | 56·06 ± 9·19 |
| Breast tumours 66 | 24·86 ± 5·72 | 39·88 ± 6·5 | 48·21 ± 6·22 | 51·05 ± 12·86 |

It is known that patients with advanced breast cancer have a 30 per cent incidence of adrenal metastasis (Karsner, 1941; Saphir and Parker, 1941; Saez-Poulain et al., 1965). They are nearly always silent although theoretically one would expect the existence of these metastases to disturb the secretion of corticosteroids. Anatomically these metastases nearly always present as nodules of varying size and number that do not destroy the adrenal cortical parenchyma. However, one patient (not included in this series given the ACTH test) presented with an Addisonian syndrome and histological examination of the adrenal gland showed that the tumour cells infiltrated the paryenchymal cords isolating them from one another. This is à rare phenomenon (Hill and Wheeler, 1965).

The patients with breast cancer given the ACTH test were treated by ablative endocrine surgery two weeks after the test and the state of their adrenals was assessed. Anatomo-pathological examination confirmed that in 25 patients one or both adrenals contained metastatic cancer nodules of varying number and size (Table 5.3). The level of plasma 17-OHCS during the ACTH perfusion was not significantly different in the patients with adrenal metastases from those with histologically normal adrenals.

TABLE 5.3

Concentration of Plasma Non-conjugated 17-OHCS ($\mu$g/100 ml $\pm$ SD) during the Perfusion of ACTH in Women with Breast Cancer, with or without Adrenal Metastases

| | Basal level | 2 Hours | 4 Hours | 6 Hours |
|---|---|---|---|---|
| 66 cases | $24 \cdot 86 \pm 5 \cdot 72$ | $39 \cdot 88 \pm 6 \cdot 5$ | $48 \cdot 21 \pm 6 \cdot 22$ | $51 \cdot 05 \pm 6 \cdot 41$ |
| With adrenal metastases (25 cases) | $26 \cdot 73 \pm 6 \cdot 41$ | $41 \cdot 18 \pm 8 \cdot 11$ | $51 \cdot 49 \pm 8 \cdot 8$ | $54 \cdot 52 \pm 7 \cdot 22$ |
| Without adrenal metastases (41 cases) | $23 \cdot 63 \pm 5 \cdot 18$ | $38 \cdot 71 \pm 5 \cdot 25$ | $46 \cdot 11 \pm 4 \cdot 49$ | $48 \cdot 77 \pm 5 \cdot 64$ |
| P | N S | N S | N S | N S |

Finally, the patients with breast cancer were sub-divided according to Taylor's staging and the results analysed according to this sub-division (Taylor and Perlia, 1960):

*Stage I:* Local tumours with local recurrence and pleural metastases.

*Stage II:* Bone metastases with or without local recurrence.

*Stage III:* Visceral metastases including hepatic, pulmonary and choroid metastases.

It should be noted that in staging the cases, no account was taken of adrenal metastases which otherwise would all have been entered into group III by definition. Nevertheless, analysis of the results shows that the frequency of adrenal metastasis increased with other visceral involvement. Table 5.4 shows that the baseline mean plasma 17-OHCS level increased between group I and group III, but there was a wide variation of the values within each group, and therefore no significant difference between the groups. In each of the groups, as for all the tumours studied previously, the 17-OHCS level before the test and at six hours were above the normal level.

Wang and Bulbrook (1969) have shown in breast cancer that the capacity for the binding of steroids to plasma proteins is the same at all stages in the evolution of the cancer as in normal subjects (Wang and Bulbrook, 1969; Sandberg, Slaunwhite and Carter, 1960; Bell, Bulbrook and Deshpande, 1967) and that there is no alteration in the metabolic clearance of cortisol (Jensen et al., 1968a, b). We must therefore conclude that:

(1) The elevation of the plasma 17-OHCS is not related to any abnormality in the transport and degradation of cortisol.

(2) It is independent of any secondary involvement of the adrenal cortex and tends to increase with the general advance of the cancer.

(3) It is not related to the extent of metastatic spread.

## TABLE 5.4

Variation of the Plasma 17-OHCS Non-conjugated (μg/100 ml ± SD) during the Course of Stimulation by 25 i.u. ACTH i.v. in 66 Patients with Breast Tumour

| Extent of tumour (stage) | Number of cases | Number of cases with adrenal metastases | Non-conjugated 17-OHCS | | | |
|---|---|---|---|---|---|---|
| | | | Basal level | 2 Hours | 4 Hours | 6 Hours |
| I | 12 | 2 | 19·90 ± 3·22 | 36·10 ± 5·01 | 43·27 ± 5·42 | 52·45 ± 5·85 |
| II | 34 | 10 | 23·75 ± 4·74 | 41·65 ± 5·80 | 48·73 ± 6·14 | 51·56 ± 6·5 |
| III | 20 | 13 | 29·86 ± 7·53 | 39·41 ± 8·28 | 49·05 ± 6·95 | 49·25 ± 6·75 |

(4) The modifications which have been reported are not unique to breast tumours but also feature in various other tumours with metastatic spread.

(5) If the raised initial value of plasma 17-OHCS is taken into account, the increase in response to ACTH is normal.

## Hypothalamo-hypophyseal response to stress and metopirone

At present it is thought that there are two regulatory systems in the hypothalamus which will contribute under different conditions to the stimulation of the adrenal cortex (Estep et al., 1963; McCarthy et al., 1964). One determines the response to stress, and is independent of the second, which regulates ACTH secretion in response to the circulating cortisol level. Their action can be observed during insulin-induced hypoglycaemia which acts as a stressor, or after the administration of metopirone which reduces cortisol secretion by blocking 11 β-hydroxylation.

In women suffering from breast cancer at an operable stage, Greenwood et al. (1968) have studied the variations of plasma cortisol after the administration of insulin. The resting cortisol levels were elevated in these women but the rise following hypoglycaemia was no different to that in the controls.

A paradoxical response was, however, observed in similar patients after the administration of glucose (Greenwood et al., 1968; Pearson et al., 1968). More than half the patients studied produced an abnormal increase of cortisol during the first or second hour after starting the test. The plasma growth hormone concentration undergoes the same variation (Pearson et al., 1968), whilst in normal subjects a fall is seen after starting the glucose infusion. In breast cancer the blood glucose curve was of the para-diabetic type.

These alterations suggest a disturbance of the hypothalamus comparable to that following stress. It manifests as an increased secretion of growth hormone and cortisol which escapes the normal regulation, and therefore is not reduced by the administration of glucose.

Cole and Mannheimer (1965) studied the response to metopirone in patients with advanced breast tumours and compared them with treated patients who had been disease free for five years. Both groups were found to have a normal urinary output of 17-OHCS.

We carried out the same test in two groups of patients with advanced cancer. One group comprised 34 patients with breast cancer, the other 27 patients of both sexes with various malignant tumours excluding cerebral tumours. Metopirone was given at a dose of 500 mg three-hourly for 24 hours, to a total dose of 4 g (Cleveland, Nikezic and Migeon, 1962; Kaplan, 1963). The urinary 17-OHCS were measured by the method of Porter and Silber for two days preceding the test, the day of the test, and the day after.

To assess the relation of changes in the regulation of ACTH secretion to the progress of the cancer, the patients were subdivided into those who survived in good health for six months after the test, and those in which their condition became worse during this period. The magnitude of the response to metopirone was judged from the percentage increase in the urinary 17-OHCS the day after administration of metopirone compared with the mean of the two days preceding the test.

In a series of normal subjects studied under the same conditions the 17-OHCS excretion was raised a little more than two fold. The increase was 6-7 mg and these results are in agreement with previous observations (Kaplan, 1963). In the two groups of cancer patients (breast tumours and various tumours), the mean urinary 17-OHCS output after metopirone was similar in both groups, and higher than in the controls (Table 5.5).

In the patients who remained in reasonable health for more than six months, the increase of urinary 17-OHCS was greater than three fold. It was close to four fold in the patients whose cancer progressed rapidly.

TABLE 5.5

Modification in the Urinary 17-OHCS (mg/24 hours $\pm$ SD) after Administration of Metopirone in 34 Cases of Breast Cancer and 27 Other Cancers

|  | Control days 1–2 | Metopirone day 3 | day 4 |
|---|---|---|---|
| Normal controls | $4 \cdot 85 \pm 1 \cdot 5$ | $8 \cdot 07 \pm 1 \cdot 9$ | $11 \cdot 82 \pm 2$ |
| *Breast tumours* | | | |
| > 6 months * 23 cases | $6 \cdot 40 \pm 1 \cdot 9$ | $10 \cdot 29 \pm 2 \cdot 02$ | $20 \cdot 07 \pm 5 \cdot 20$ |
| < 6 months 11 cases | $8 \cdot 06 \pm 2 \cdot 10$ | $13 \cdot 92 \pm 3 \cdot 75$ | $30 \cdot 27 \pm 8 \cdot 59$ |
| *Various tumours* | | | |
| > 6 months 14 cases | $5 \cdot 18 \pm 1 \cdot 30$ | $14 \cdot 41 \pm 3 \cdot 75$ | $21 \cdot 13 \pm 3 \cdot 5$ |
| < 6 months 13 cases | $6 \cdot 92 \pm 1 \cdot 9$ | $19 \cdot 65 \pm 4 \cdot 9$ | $30 \cdot 84 \pm 4 \cdot 65$ |

* For definition of < and > 6 months see the text.

It should be noted there was a great scatter in the results and some of them were very high, in particular in the two groups whose tumours became widespread rapidly. It is possible that the patients were in a more advanced state than those examined by Cole and Mannheimer (1965) and this would explain the apparent discordance between our results and theirs. These increased responses to metopirone suggest a change in the regulation by ACTH of cortisol secretion, as is suggested also by the disappearance of the circadian rhythm (Lichter and Sirett, 1968). This change seemed to be most pronounced when the tumour progressed rapidly despite treatment. This was observed in both breast cancer and other forms of cancer.

### Dexamethasone suppression of cortisol production

It is known that the level of cortisol production in patients with breast cancer is higher than in normal subjects, and is higher in advanced tumours than at an early stage (Jensen et al., 1968).

In a reasonably large series of patients (40 cases of breast cancer, 40 with other forms of cancer) we studied the effects of dexamethasone on cortisol production. The cortisol was measured by the isotope dilution technique (Kenny, Preeyasombat and Migeon, 1966; Kenny, Malvaux and Migeon, 1963; Bertrand et al., 1963). Two tests were made successively on each patient under resting conditions, then on the third day after giving dexamethasone (20 µg/kg/24 hours) (Liddle, 1960). Some of these patients were submitted subsequently to a third test on the third day after giving them 8 mg dexamethasone in 24 hours. The results are expressed in milligrammes of cortisol per square meter of body surface per 24 hours *(Figure 5.1)*, and are discussed later.

The patients were between 25 and 70 years old and were not receiving any hormonal or chemotherapeutic treatment at the time of the examination or recently prior to the examination. The women with breast cancer were at various stages of the disease, from an early operable local lesion to widespread metastatic disease—Taylor's stage III (Taylor and Perlia, 1960). The second group comprised both men and women with a variety of forms of cancer (Melanoblastoma, sarcoma, epithelioma of buccopharynx or bronchus and uterine adenocarcinoma in different stages of progress) (Table 5.6).

TABLE 5.6

Production of Cortisol (mg/m$^2$/24 hours $\pm$ SD) in 80 Patients with Malignant Tumours, Under Basal Conditions and during Adrenal Suppression with Dexamethasone (20 µg/kg/24 hours)

|  | Basal level | After adrenal suppression |
|---|---|---|
| Various tumours (40 cases) | $16 \cdot 08 \pm 4 \cdot 16$ | $9 \cdot 36 \pm 4 \cdot 23$ |
| Breast tumours (40 cases) | $14 \cdot 98 \pm 3 \cdot 19$ | $5 \cdot 39 \pm 2 \cdot 87$ |

There was no significant difference in the result of dexamethasone suppression between the two groups, but the production of cortisol in the two groups of cancer patients was greater than in normal controls, both under basal conditions and when suppressed with 20 μg/kg/24 hours dexamethasone (Saez, 1971). Analysis of the results showed that suppression was less marked when the basal level was higher.

Among the breast tumours, 7 patients were at an operable stage. Their production of cortisol was in all respects comparable to normal controls, both under basal conditions and during suppression by dexamethasone 20 μg/kg/24 hours, when it fell to 2 mg/m$^2$/24 hours. In stages I, II and III the values showed little difference but were significantly higher than in normal subjects. These results (Table 5.7) mirror those described for plasma 17-OHCS.

TABLE 5.7

Production of Cortisol (mg/m$^2$/24 hours ± SD) in 40 Patients with Breast Cancer in Relation to the Stage of the Disease

| Stage of breast cancer | Number of cases | Basal level | After adrenal suppression |
|---|---|---|---|
| Operable | 7 | 11·34 ± 1·46 | 2·20 ± 0·67 |
| I | 8 | 14·37 ± 3·17 | 3·83 ± 1·80 |
| II | 15 | 16·41 ± 3·22 | 6·05 ± 3·6 |
| III | 10 | 15·11 ± 3·11 | 7·37 ± 3·48 |

When results are classified according to the Taylor staging (which corresponds to the extent of the cancer) cases with *different eventual outcome* tend to be grouped together. For this reason we have re-grouped the patients according to their clinical fate during the six months after the test. The first group comprises women with breast cancer who had not relapsed or were improved for at least six months, and the second group those who relapsed rapidly or did not obtain any improvement during the same period. Patients with early operable cancer were excluded from this analysis (Table 5.8).

The patients with breast cancer whose prognosis was worse had the highest basal level of cortisol production, and the least degree of suppression by dexamethasone. Tumours at other sites studied in the same way gave similar responses. It is interesting that, in some patients, an elevated plasma cortisol that was difficult to suppress preceded clinical deterioration and enabled a poor response to therapy to be predicted. Conversely, if surgery or chemotherapy led to a good remission there was a tendency for the cortisol production and the degree of suppression to become closer to normal. The study of plasma 17-OHCS during the progress of lung cancer has given comparable results (Van Hove and Vermeulen, 1970; Bishop and Ross, 1970).

In 33 of our breast cancer patients, the production of cortisol was calculated after administration of 8 mg of dexamethasone per 24 hours (Liddle, 1960; Liddle et al., 1969). Under these conditions cortisol production was suppressed

TABLE 5.8

Production of Cortisol (mg/m²/24 hours ± SD) in 73 Patients with Progressive Cancer in
Relation to the Eventual Outcome

| | Breast tumours (stages I–II–III) | | Various tumours | |
|---|---|---|---|---|
| | Basal conditions | Suppression | Basal conditions | Suppression |
| > 6 months | 15·27 ± 3·33 22 cases | 4·04 ± 2·08 | 12·65 ± 3 19 cases | 4·50 ± 2·67 |
| < 6 months | 17·22 ± 3·07 11 cases | 9·69 ± 3·53 | 19·66 ± 4·72 21 cases | 13·75 ± 4·28 |
| p | N S | <0·01 | <0·01 | <0·001 |

by more than 50 per cent in all cases *(Figure 5.1)*. This confirms that the
hypercorticism is not due to the production of ectopic ACTH, but rather to a
change in the central regulatory system for the secretion of ACTH.

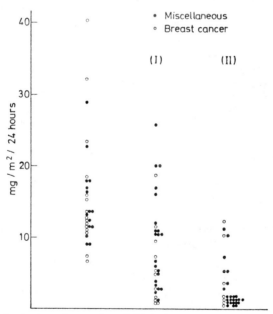

*Figure 5.1. Production of cortisol (mg/m²/24 hours) in 33 cancer patients in basal
conditions, after adrenal suppression by dexamethasone 20 μg/kg/24 hours (I) and
after adrenal suppression by dexamethasone 8 mg/day (II)*

113

Our results can be summarized as follows:

(1) The paraneoplastic hypercorticism syndrome caused by ectopic ACTH secretion occurs only rarely in the course of breast cancer.

(2) The level of plasma 17-OHCS is nevertheless frequently higher than normal under basal conditions, without any evidence of anatomical change in the adrenals or alteration in the degradation of the steroids.

(3) The metopirone test suggests that the regulation of ACTH secretion by the level of cortisol persists, but with a higher threshold than normal in patients with rapidly advancing cancer. The response to insulin stress is modified in the same direction and suggests a pre-existing condition of non-specific stress.

(4) Suppression with small doses of dexamethasone (20 μg/kg/24 hours) allowed the production of cortisol to persist at a higher level than in normal subjects under the same conditions.

The different tests for examining the regulation of ACTH secretion tend to support the same hypothesis: that there is in patients with breast cancer *an abnormally high threshold in the hypothalamo–hypophyseal mechanism regulating the secretion of the adrenal steroids.* In patients with other forms of cancer showing similar progression, comparable changes in the mechanism were observed. They are not specific for breast cancer, but related to the general evolution of neoplasms which act as a non-specific somatic stress (Wilson and Moore, 1968; Beisel and Rapoport, 1969).

Mackay et al. (1971) have demonstrated changes in steroid level associated with variations of the immune reaction during the progress of breast cancer. They have shown that in patients in whom the 17-OHCS were raised, immune reactions were depressed and these were generally found among the more advanced tumours. It is possible that when the immune defences against cancer have been overcome, changes in the regulation of steroid secretion characteristics of stress will appear, at the same time as other hypothalamic reactions.

This might explain why these changes precede the clinical deterioration and are not accompanied by hypercorticism. It is compatible with the observation that when these changes are pronounced they indicate a bad prognosis, for they will be a sign that the disease has extended beyond the reach of therapy.

*Relationship between changes in the regulation of ACTH secretion and the secretion of adrenal oestrogens*

It has been shown that oestrogen production continues after ovariectomy (Barlow, Emerson and Saxena, 1969; Hellman and Fishman, 1970) and also after the natural menopause (Editorial, 1967, 1969; Rogers, 1969; Kase and Cohn, 1967; Baird and Guevara (1969). The fact that it responds to stimulation by exogenous ACTH suggests that its origin is adrenal, arising either directly or indirectly via intermediary precursors (Poliak et al., 1971; Procope, 1969).

Oestrogen production varies with modification of ACTH secretion (Schmidt and Christiaans, 1964; Zarate et al., 1970). It has been shown that in ovariectomized women the oestrogenic index of the vaginal smear is increased as a result of a psychological or somatic stress. A similar reaction has been reproduced experimentally in animals (Schmidt and Christiaans, 1964), and can be suppressed by adrenalectomy or hypophysectomy (Schmidt and Christiaans, 1964).

On the other hand, adrenal suppression reduces the urinary oestrogen excretion to very low levels and lowers the karyopyknotic index of the vaginal smear (De Waard and Thÿssen, 1970). However, it does not seem that adrenal suppression can completely suppress the adrenal secretion of corticoids and oestrogens. This is in agreement with the histological appearances of the adrenal cortex (Jantet et al., 1963), which show that atrophy is more complete after hypophysectomy than after prolonged treatment with corticosteroids.

Direct measurements of the level of oestrogens in the adrenal venous blood compared with that in the peripheral circulation, show that there is adrenal production of oestrone (Baird, Uno and Melby, 1969), and that it is increased by ACTH (Saez et al., 1972). Plasma levels of oestrone and oestradiol have been measured in parallel to the production of cortisol (Saez et al., 1972) under basal conditions and after three days' suppression with dexamethasone (20 $\mu g/kg/24$ hours). The plasma concentration of oestrone was significantly reduced, even when the initial value was low. The percentage reductions were $55 \pm 16$ per cent for oestrone, $84 \pm 9 \cdot 5$ per cent for cortisol but only $2 \pm 18$ per cent for oestradiol. In ovariectomized and adrenalectomized women the plasma oestrone and oestradiol levels are equivalent to the theoretical 'blank' of the method of estimation, that is less than 15 pg per specimen.

*Figure 5.2* shows the plasma oestrone and oestradiol levels and production of cortisol, measured simultaneously under basal conditions and during adrenal suppression, in 13 ovariectomized or post-menopausal women with miscellaneous tumours at various stages of evolution. According to these preliminary findings the adrenal production of oestrone seems to vary with that of cortisol. This is said to apply to circadian rhythm also (Tulshinsky and Korenman, 1970). It should be noted that in 2 patients (cases 1 and 2) the production of cortisol was only slightly lowered by the suppression, and at the same time the level of plasma oestrone was almost unchanged.

It has been reported that in lung cancer also, both the urinary oestrogen and 17-OHCS excretion may be raised together (McNamara, Aron and Paulson, 1968). In the majority of cancers these changes in hormone production do not have any profound effect on the progress of the cancer—cortisol increases as the disease becomes more widespread. In breast cancer, on the other hand, the effect of this process may be very different. Patients whose condition is deteriorating are those in whom there is the greatest risk from adrenal stimulation. If the formation of oestrogens rises parallel with corticosteroid

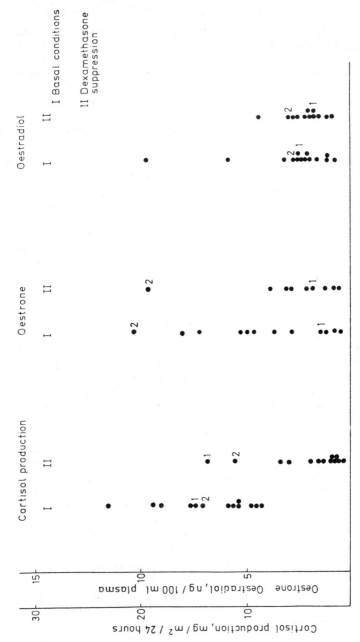

Figure 5.2. Production of cortisol (mg/m²/24 hours) and plasma oestrone and oestradiol (ng/100 ml) in 13 post-menopausal or castrated female cancer patients in basal conditions (I) and after adrenal suppression by dexamethasone 20 μg/kg/24 hours (II).

production, the growth of a hormone-dependent tumour could be enhanced. The vicious circle can only be broken by hypophysectomy or bilateral adrenalectomy.

In summary, what begins as a non-specific reaction to the presence of the tumour can result in stimulating the growth of breast cancer.

## SUMMARY

The different tests for the investigation of the hypothalamic regulation of ACTH secretion have provided evidence that in patients with breast cancer the hypothalamic regulatory mechanism controlling the secretion of cortisol is set at a higher threshold than normal. Similar changes have been described in the progression of cancers at other sites and they are not related specifically to breast cancer or to hormone dependency. High levels of adrenal steroids in the plasma indicate a bad prognosis and appear to be a reflection of somatic stress caused by the cancer. This process is not specific for breast cancer, but it must be accepted that if the adrenal secretion of oestrogen rises at the same time as that of corticosteroids, then the growth of a hormone dependent breast cancer could be stimulated by this mechanism.

## ACKNOWLEDGMENTS

We are indebted to A. Gerson who carried out the statistical calculations and to Dr. J. M. Saez for the determination of plasma oestrogens in our patients.

## REFERENCES

Allott, E. N. and Skelton, M. O. (1960). 'Increased adrenocortical activity with malignant disease.' *Lancet* 2, 278.

Arons, M. S., Wexler, H., Sabesin, S. and Mantel, N. (1962). 'Effect of cortisone and amputation on metastases.' *Cancer* 15, 227.

Baird, D. T. and Guevara, A. (1969). 'Concentration of unconjugated estrone and estradiol in peripheral plasma in non-pregnant women throughout the menstrual cycle, castrated and post-menopausal women, and in men.' *J. clin. Endocr.* 29, 149.

— Uno, A. and Melby, J. D. (1969). 'Adrenal secretion of androgen and oestrogens.' *J. Endocr.* 45, 135.

Barlow, J. J., Emerson, K. and Saxena, B. N. (1969). 'Estradiol production after ovariectomy for carcinoma of the breast.' *New Engl. J. Med.* 280, 633.

Beatson, G. T. (1896). 'On the treatment of inoperable cases of carcinoma of the mamma: Suggestions for a new method of treatment with illustrative cases.' *Lancet* 2, 104.

Beisel, W. R. and Rapoport, M. I. (1969). 'Inter-relation between adrenocortical functions and infectious illness.' *New Engl. J. Med.* 280, 541.

Bell, E., Bulbrook, R. D. and Deshpande, N. (1967). 'Transcortin in plasma of patients with breast cancer.' *Lancet* 2, 395.

Bertrand, J., Loras, B., Gilly, R. and Cauthenet, B. (1963). 'Contribution à l'étude de la secrétion et du metabolisme du cortisol chez le nouveau né et le nourrisson.' *Path. Biol.* **11**, 997.

Bishop, M. C. and Ross, E. J. (1970). 'Adrenocortical activity in disseminated malignant disease in relation to prognosis.' *Br. J. Cancer* **24**, 719.

Borkowski, A., Levin, S., Mahler, A. and Verhas, V. (1066). 'A study of adrenal function in seventy-six consecutive cases of bronchial carcinoma.' *Europ. J. Cancer* **2**, 263.

Brown, J. B., Bulbrook, R. D. and Greenwood, F. C. (1957). 'An evaluation of a chemical method for the estimation of oestriol, estrone and estradiol 17 β in human urine.' *J. Endocr.* **16**, 41.

— Bruce, J., Douglas, M., Klopper, A., Loraine, J. A. and Strong, J. A. (1957). 'The excretion of pituitary gonadotrophines, oestrogens, pregnanediol and neutral 17 ketosteroids in the urine of patients with metastatic and recurrent mammary carcinoma.' *Acta endocr.* Suppl. **31**, 273.

Butler, P. W. P. and Besser, G. M. (1968). 'Pituitary adrenal function in severe depressive illness.' *Lancet* **1**, 1234.

Castellanos, H., Fairgrieve, J., O'Morchoe, P. J. and Moore, F. D. (1963). 'Corticotropin stimulation of urethral cornification. A measure of adrenal oestrogen capacity in carcinoma of the breast.' *J. Am. med. Ass.* **184**, 295.

Chang, R. and Dao, T. L. (1961). 'Adrenal estrogens—conversion of 4 C 14 cortisone acetate to 11 oxygenated estrogens in women.' *J. clin. Endocr.* **21**, 624.

Cleveland, W. W., Nikezic, M. and Migeon, Cl. J. (1962). 'Response to an 11 β hydroxylase inhibitor (Su-4885) in males with adrenal hyperplasia and their parents.' *J. clin. Endocr.* **22**, 281.

Cole, W. and Mannheimer, I. (1965). 'Urinary Porter–Silber chromogens following I.V. metopyron and ACTH in patients with breast cancer.' *Cancer* **18**, 313.

Cowie, A. T. and Folley, S. J. (1957). 'Endocrine aspects of mammary growth and function particularly in relation to pituitary hormones.' In *Endocrine Aspects of Breast Cancer*, p. 266, Ed. by A. R. Currie. Edinburgh; Livingstone.

Dao, T. and Huggins, C. (1955). 'Estrogen excretion in women with mammary cancer before and after adrenalectomy.' *Archs Surg.* **71**, 645.

— Tan, E. and Brooks, V. (1961). 'A comparative evaluation of adrenalectomy and cortisone in the treatment of advanced mammary carcinoma.' *Cancer* **14**, 1259.

Deshpande, N., Hayward, J. L. and Bulbrook, R. D. (1965). 'Plasma 17 OHCS and oxosteroids in patients with breast cancer and in normal women.' *J. Endocr.* **32**, 167.

De Waard, F. and Thijssen, J. H. H. (1970). 'Relationship between hormonal cytology and steroid excretion in post menopausal women.' *J. Endocr.* **48**, XXXVI.

— Pot, H., Tonckens-Nanninga, N. E., Baanders, J. Van., Halewijn, E. A. and Thijssen, J. H. H. (1972). 'Longitudinal studies on the phenomenon of post ménopausal estrogen production.' *Acta cytol.* **16**, 273.

Editorial (1967). 'Extragonadal estrogen production.' *New Engl. J. Med.* **276**, 57.

— (1969). 'Goodbye to the menopausal ovary.' *New Engl. J. Med.* **280**, 667.

Eik-Ness, T., Sandberg, A. A., Migeon, Cl. J., Tyler, F. and Samuels, L. T. (1955). 'Changes in plasma levels of 17 OHCS during the intravenous administration of ACTH.' *J. clin. Endocr.* **15**, 15.

Estep, H., Island, D., Ney, R. and Liddle, G. (1963). 'Pituitary adrenal dynamics during surgical stress.' *J. clin. Endocr.* **23**, 419.

Gardner, B., Thomas, A. N. and Gordon, G. S. (1962). 'Antitumor efficacy of prednisolone and sodium liothyronine in advanced breast cancer.' *Cancer* **15**, 334.

Glenn, E. M., Richardson, S. L., Bowman, B. J. and Lyster, S. C. (1960). 'Steroids and experimental mammary cancer.' In *Biological Activities of Steroids in Relation to Cancer*, p. 257, Ed. by G. Pincus and E. P. Wollmer. New York; Academic Press.

Goodall, G. M. (1969). 'On para-endocrine cancer syndromes.' *Int. J. Cancer* **4**, 1.

Greenwood, F. C., James, V. H. T., Meggitt, B. F., Miller, J. D. and Taylor, P. H. (1968). 'Pituitary function in breast cancer.' In *Prognostic Factors in Breast Cancer*, p. 409, Ed. by A. P. M. Forrest and P. B. Kunkler. Edinburgh; Livingstone.

Hellman, L. and Fishman, J. (1970). 'Oestradiol production rates in man before and after orchiectomy for cancer.' *J. Endocr.* **46**, 113.

Hill, G. J. and Wheeler, H. B. (1965). 'Adrenal insufficiency due to metastatic cancer of the lung.' *Cancer* **18**, 1467.

Hymes, A. C. and Doe, R. P. (1962). 'Adrenal function in cancer of the lung, with and without Cushing's syndrome.' *Am. J. Med.* **33**, 398.

Jantet, G., Crocker, D. W., Shiraki, M. and Moore, F. D. (1963). 'Adrenal suppression in disseminated carcinoma of the breast.' *New Engl. J. Med.* **269**, 1.

Jensen, H. K. and Blichert-Toft, M. (1971a). 'Serum corticotrophin, plasma cortisol and urinary excretion of 17 Ketogenic steroids in the elderly.' *Acta endocr.* **66**, 25.

— — (1971b). 'Investigation of pituitary–adrenocortical function in the elderly during standardized operations and postoperative intravenous metyrapone test assessed by plasmacortisol, plasma compounds and eosinophil cell determinations.' *Acta endocr.* **67**, 495.

Jensen, V., Deshpande, N., Bulbrook, R. D. and Douss, T. W. (1968a). 'Adrenal function in breast cancer: the distribution of cortisol in patients with early or advanced breast cancer and in normal women.' *J. Endocr.* **42**, 433.

— — — — (1968b). 'Adrenal function in breast cancer: production and metabolic clearance rate of cortisol in patients with early or advanced breast cancer and in normal women.' *J. Endocr.* **42**, 425.

Jull, J. W., Shucksmith, H. S. and Bonser, G. M. (1963). 'A study of urinary estrogen excretion in relation to breast cancer.' *J. clin. Endocr.* **23**, 433.

Kaplan, N. M. (1963). 'Assessment of pituitary ACTH secretory capacity with metopirone: interpretation.' *J. clin. Endocr.* **23**, 945.

Karsner, H. T. (1941). 'Tumors of the Adrenal.' In *Atlas of Pathology*. Armed Forces Institute of Pathology.

Kase, N. and Cohn, G. L. (1967). 'Clinical implication of extragonadal estrogen production.' *New Engl. J. Med.* **276**, 28.

Kenny, F. M., Malvaux, P. and Migeon, Cl. J. (1963). 'Cortisol production rates in newborn babies, older infants and children.' *Pediatrics* **31**, 360.

— Preeyasombat, C. and Migeon, Cl. J. (1966). 'Cortisol production rate. 11 Normal infants, children and adults.' *Pediatrics* **37**, 34.

Lemon, H. M. (1959). 'Prednisone therapy of advanced mammary cancer.' *Cancer* **12**, 93.

Lichter, I. and Sirett, N. E. (1968). 'Plasma cortisol level in lung cancer.' *Br. med. J.* **2**, 154.

Liddle, G. W. (1960). 'Test of pituitary suppressibility in diagnosis of Cushing's syndrome.' *J. clin. Endocr.* **20**, 1530.

— Nicholson, W. E., Island, D. F., Orth, D. N., Abe, K. and Lowder, S. C. (1969). 'Clinical and laboratory studies of ectopic syndromes.' *Recent Progr. Hormone Res.* **25**, 283.

Lipsett, M. B., Odell, X. D., Rosenberg, L. E. and Waldmann, T. A. (1964). 'Hormonal syndromes associated with non endocrine tumors.' *Ann. intern. Med.* **61**, 633.

McCarthy, C. F., Wills, M. R., Keane, P. M., Gough, K. R. and Read, A. E. (1964). 'Su—4885 response after head injury.' *J. clin. Endocr.* **24**, 121.

Mackay, W. D., Edwards, M. H., Bulbrook, R. D. and Wang, D. Y. (1971). 'Relation between plasma androgen sulphates and immune response in women with breast cancer.' *Lancet* **2**, 1001.

McNamara, J. J., Aron, H. H. and Paulson, D. L. (1968). 'Steroid hormone abnormalities in patients with carcinoma of the lung.' *J. thorac. cardiovasc. Surg.* **56**, 371.

Marks, L. J., Anderson, A. E. and Lieberman, H. (1961). 'Carcinoma of the lung associated with marked adrenocortical hyperplasia and adrenal hyper-responsivenes to ACTH in the absence of Cushing's syndrome.' *Ann. intern. Med.* **54**, 1243.

Meador, C. K. and Liddle, G. W. (1962). 'Cause of Cushing's syndrome in patients with tumors arising from "non-endocrine tissue".' *J. clin. Endocr.* **22**, 693.

Migeon, Cl. J., Kenny, F. M., Hung, W. and Voorhess, M. L. (1967). 'Study of adrenal function in children with meningitis.' *Pediatrics* **40**, 163.

Miller, M. and Moses, A. M. (1968). 'Effect of temperature and dexamethasone on the plasma 17 OHCS and G. H. response to pyrogen.' *J. clin. Endocr.* **28**, 1056.

Nissen-Meyer, R. and Sanner, T. (1963a). 'Excretion of oestrone, pregnanediol and pregnanetriol in breast cancer patients. I. Excretion after spontaneous menopause.' *Acta endocr.* **44**, 325.

— — (1963b). 'The excretion of estrone, pregnanediol and pregnanetriol in breast cancer patients. II. Effects of ovariectomy, ovarian irradiation and corticosteroids.' *Acta endocr.* **44**, 334.

Noble, R. L. (1964). 'Tumors and hormones.' In *The Hormone,* p. 559, Ed. by G. Pincus. New York; Academic Press.

Pearson, O. H., Llerena, O., Samaan, N. and Gonzalez, D. (1968). 'Serum growth hormone and insulin levels in patients with breast cancer.' In *Prognostic Factors in Breast Cancer,* p. 421, Ed. by A. P. M. Forrest and P. B. Kunkler. Edinburgh; Livingstone.

Persson, B. H. and Risholm, L. (1964). 'Oophorectomy and cortisone treatment as a method of eliminating oestrogen production in patients with breast cancer.' *Acta endocr.* **47**, 15.

Poliak, A., Smith, J. J., Friedlander, D. and Romney, S. (1971). 'Estrogen synthesis in castrated women: the action of human chorionic gonadotropin and corticotropin.' *Am. J. Obstet. Gynec.* **110**, 376.

Procope, B. J. (1969). 'Studies on the urinary excretion, biological effects and origin of oestrogens in post-menopausal women.' *Acta endocr.* Suppl. **135**, 110.

Rogers, J. (1969). 'Estrogen in the menopause and post menopause.' *New Engl. J. Med.* **280**, 364.

Saez, J. M., Morera, A. M., Dazord, A. and Bertrand, J. (1972). 'Adrenal and testicular contribution to plasma oestrogens.' *J. Endocr.* **55**, 41.

Saez, S. (1971). 'Adrenal function in cancer: relation to the evolution.' *Europ. J. Cancer* **7**, 381.

Saez-Poulain, S., Pommatau, E., Dargent, M. and Mayer, M. (1965). 'Modifications des 17 OHCS plasmatiques libres au cours d'une perfusion d'ACTH chez 62 malades atteintes d'un cancer mammaire evolué avec ou sans metastases surrénaliennes.' *Annls d'Endocr.* **26**, 513.

Sandberg, A. A., Slaunwhite, W. R. and Carter, A. (1960). 'Transcortin: a corticosteroid binding of plasma. III. Effects of various steroids.' *J. clin. Invest.* **39**, 1914.

Saphir, O. and Parker, M. L. (1941). 'Metastases of primary carcinoma of the breast with special reference to spleen, adrenal glands and ovaries.' *Archs Surg.* **42**, 1002.

Schmidt, A. L. C. and Christiaans, A. P. L. (1964). 'An estrogenic effect as a component of the stress syndrome.' *Acta endocr.* **46**, 421.

Segaloff, A., Carabasi, R., Horwitt, B. N., Schlosser, J. V. and Murison, P. J. (1954). 'Hormonal therapy in cancer of the breast. VI. Effect of ACTH and cortisone on clinical course and hormonal excretion.' *Cancer* **7**, 331.

Shuster, S. (1960). 'Adrenal function in chronic wasting disease.' *J. clin. Endocr.* **20**, 675.

Sommers, S. C. and Teloh, H. (1952). 'Ovarian stromal hyperplasia in breast cancer.' *Archs Path.* **53**, 160.

Stoll, B. A. (1960). 'Dexamethasone in advanced breast cancer.' *Cancer* **13**, 1074.

— (1967). 'Vaginal cytology as an aid to tumor therapy in post-menopausal cancer of the breast.' *Cancer* **20**, 1807.

Strong, J. A., Brown, J. B., Bruce, J., Douglas, M., Klopper, A. and Lorraine, J. A. (1956). 'Sex hormone excretion after bilateral adrenalectomy and oophorectomy in patients with mammary carcinoma.' *Lancet* **2**, 955.

Struthers, R. A. (1956). 'Oestrogen production after menopausis.' *Br. med. J.* **1**, 1331.

Sweppe, J. S., Junghman, R. A. and Lewin, I. (1967). 'Urine steroid excretion in post-menopausal breast cancer. Response to corticotropin stimulation and dexamethasone suppression.' *Cancer* **20**, 155.

Taylor, S., G. and Perlia, C. P. (1960). 'Evaluation of endocrine ablative surgery in the treatment of mammary carcinoma: a preliminary study on survival.' In *Biological Activities of Steroids in Relation to Cancer*, Ed. by G. Pincus and E. Wollmer. New York; Academic Press.

Tulshinsky, J. and Korenman, S. G. (1970). 'Aradio-ligand assay for plasma-estrone, normal values and variation during menstrual cycle.' *J. clin. Endocr.* **31**, 77.

Turkington, R. W. (1971). 'Hormonal regulation of mammary gland in vitro.' In *The Sex Steroids*, p. 383, Edited by W. McKerns. New York; AppletonCentury-Crofts.

Van Hove, W. and Vermeulen, A. (1970). 'Plasma cortisol levels in bronchial carcinoma. Influence of cytostatic treatment.' *Rev. Europ. Etudes Clin. Biol.* **15**, 96.

Wang, D. Y. and Bulbrook, R. D. (1969). 'The binding of steroids to plasma proteins in normal women and women with breast cancer.' *Europ. J. Cancer* **5**, 247.

Werk, E. E. and Sholiton, L. J. (1960). 'Adrenocortical function in carcinoma of the lung.' *Cancer* **13**, 469.

West, C. D., Damast, B. and Pearson, O. M. (1958). 'Adrenal estrogens in patients with breast cancer.' *J. clin. Invest.* **37**, 341.

Wilson, R. E. and Moore, F. D. (1968). 'Biochemical and clinical factors in the selection of patients for endocrine surgery.' In *Prognostic Factors in Breast Cancer*, p. 339, Ed. by A. P. M. Forrest and P. B. Kunkler. Edinburgh; Livingstone.

Zarate, A., Hernandez, J., Ayup, S., Canales, E., Mungia, H. and Franco, E. (1970). 'Effect of adrenocorticotrophin hormone on urinary estrogens and vaginal epithelium in ovariectomised patients.' *J. Obstet. Gynaec. Br. Commwlth.* **77**, 757.

# 6

# Pituitary Gonadotrophin Production and Breast Cancer

K. Fotherby

## INTRODUCTION

The estimation of urinary gonadotrophins achieved some prominence in the early investigations carried out on patients with mammary carcinoma for a number of reasons. Until fairly recently urinary gonadotrophin excretion provided the only direct means of estimating pituitary function (see Chapter 15), as distinct from measuring changes resulting from an effect of pituitary trophic hormones on their target organs (for example, [131]I uptake by the thyroid, adrenocortical hormone production). Hence it was considered that estimation of gonadotrophin excretion might be useful in determining the completeness of hypophysectomy. Interest was centred on gonadotrophins also because of their influence in controlling the production of sex hormones in the ovary, and the possible importance of oestrogenic hormones of the ovary in the carcinogenic process. Although in pre-menopausal women the small amounts of gonadotrophins produced are known to control ovarian steroidogenesis, it is not known whether they exert any control over the ovary in post-menopausal women, or on the adrenal cortex in women after ovariectomy, when gonadotrophins are produced in large amounts.

Most of the active steroids used in the early investigations of the treatment of breast cancer—for example, oestrogens and androgens—were known to suppress gonadotrophin production and it was therefore thought (Segaloff et al., 1951) that there was a relationship between the clinical efficacy of hormonal compounds and their ability to inhibit gonadotrophin production. However, this concept is no longer tenable because compounds are now known which are effective in the treatment of breast cancer, and yet have relatively minor effects on gonadotrophin production. It had been hoped that some of the studies to be mentioned below would establish that measurements of urinary gonadotrophin excretion were of aid in predicting the response of patients with breast cancer to various forms of treatment. This is referred to again later.

The procedures available for the estimation of gonadotrophins and their reliability have been extensively reviewed by Stevenson and Loraine (1971). Unfortunately, almost all of the measurements of gonadotrophin excretion in urine in the investigations of breast cancer patients have been carried out using the mouse uterus test, in which the increase in the weight of the uterus of intact immature mice is measured after injection of suitable extracts of urine. The increase in weight produced is compared with that produced by known amounts of a standard preparation of gonadotrophins. The method is non-specific and measures both follicle stimulating hormone (FSH) and luteinizing hormone (LH) activity. In addition, the bioassay is relatively imprecise unless carried out under very strictly controlled conditions and, therefore, in many of the early studies the value of the results obtained, which were often expressed in arbitrary mouse units, is questionable.

# CHANGES IN GONADOTROPHIN EXCRETION WITH TREATMENT

## Oestrogens in breast cancer

Oestrogen produced from the ovary is known to be one of the factors controlling pituitary gonadotrophin secretion (Fotherby and James, 1972b). Administration of natural oestrogens, particularly in high dosage, inhibits gonadotrophin secretion and this inhibitory property is shared by the synthetic oestrogens, such as stilboestrol and ethynyl oestradiol. The mechanism is of especial interest in the treatment of breast cancer because of the large proportion of tumours regressing after high dose oestrogen therapy in post-menopausal patients.

Loraine and Bell (1966) have reviewed the early studies showing that the naturally occurring oestrogens administered orally or by implantation decrease the urinary excretion of gonadotrophins. Using stilboestrol Heller, Chandler and Myers (1944) found that whereas a dose of 0·5 mg/day was without any effect, a higher dose (5 mg/day orally) suppressed the elevated gonadotrophin excretion found in ovariectomized subjects. Smith and Albert (1955) also showed that the effect was dose related; doses of 1 mg or more per day had a suppressive effect and complete suppression was obtained with 10 mg of stilboestrol administered for five days. This finding is also supported by the work of Loraine and Bell (1966). Brown (1956) obtained variable effects on FSH and LH excretion when 0·5 mg of stilboestrol was given orally for three to five days and he suggested that the effect was to increase LH rather than FSH production. It is of interest that Smith and Albert (1958) found a slight increase in gonadotrophin excretion after giving low doses (0·1 mg/day) of stilboestrol and that more recent work (see below) has confirmed that small doses of oestrogen may stimulate the pituitary production of gonadotrophins.

With regard to patients with mammary carcinoma, one of the first studies concerning the effect of oestrogens on gonadotrophin excretion in this condition was carried out by Loraine, Strong and Douglas (1957). They studied 47 post-menopausal women with mammary carcinoma and collected urine samples for eight days before starting treatment with stilboestrol, 5 mg orally per day. At the end of six weeks their response to treatment was assessed. The mean gonadotrophin excretion before starting treatment in those patients whose tumours failed to respond was significantly higher than that of patients who showed no progression of the disease or tumour regression. Gonadotrophin excretion by the two latter groups of subjects did not show a significant difference from that of a group of control subjects of similar age with diseases other than cancer.

Despite the significant difference in the mean values for gonadotrophin excretion between those who failed to respond to treatment and the others, the range of values showed a considerable degree of overlap. However, Loraine, Strong and Douglas were able to suggest that if the urinary gonadotrophin excretion was greater than 55 units per 24 hours, the patient was unlikely to benefit from stilboestrol treatment. These results were interpreted as showing that a particular group of patients with mammary carcinoma may show differences in hormonal production from other patients with the disease, and also that gonadotrophin assays may be of use for predicting the response of patients to treatment.

O'Connor and Skinner (1964) also studied gonadotrophin excretion in patients with mammary carcinoma treated with stilboestrol, but from their studies they were not able to deduce any clear-cut relationship between gonadotrophin excretion and response to treatment. All patients showed a significant depression of gonadotrophin excretion during treatment but after cessation of treatment gonadotrophin excretion increased for periods of six months or more, showing that the suppression of the pituitary produced by the treatment was reversible. Gonadotrophin excretion was reduced during the treatment period to 8–27 per cent of the pre-treatment values, showing that pituitary production of gonadotrophins was not completely suppressed by the dose of stilboestrol used (10–20 mg daily).

In a subsequent study Stewart, Skinner and O'Connor (1965) found that, in patients showing an objective remission, gonadotrophin excretion remained low throughout the remission period although a low level of gonadotrophin excretion was not indicative of clinical remission. Thus the only two major reports suggest that high pre-treatment gonadotrophin levels predict a lesser likelihood of response to oestrogen therapy, while the appearance of objective

125

response to such therapy was associated with suppression of gonadotrophin secretion.

## Progestogens in breast cancer

The usefulness of progestogens in the treatment of cancer of the breast has been reviewed by Briggs, Caldwell and Pitchford (1967). Although a number of synthetic progestins have been tried those most widely tested include norethisterone (or esters of this compound) and medroxyprogesterone acetate.

Moore et al. (1961) found no change in gonadotrophin excretion when progesterone was given orally in doses as high as 500 mg twice daily for 30–90 days, confirming the results obtained by Smith and Albert (1958) in post-menopausal and ovariectomized subjects. Norethisterone or its esters do depress gonadotrophin excretion of post-menopausal women but the possibility arises that this may be due to the conversion of the synthetic steroid to oestrogenic metabolites *in vivo* (Fotherby and James, 1972a). In pre-menopausal women administration of norethisterone or its acetate inhibits ovulation and was originally claimed not to affect gonadotrophin excretion (Brown, Fotherby and Loraine, 1962). However, under similar conditions Buchholz, Nocke and Nocke (1964) did show a decrease in the mid-cycle peak of gonadotrophin, and more recent studies involving estimation of gonadotrophins in blood show that administration of synthetic progestins suppresses the mid-cycle peak of LH.

Both Douglas, Loraine and Strong (1960) and Martin and Cunningham (1960) have measured gonadotrophin excretion in women with metastatic carcinoma of the breast treated with norethisterone oenanthate. This compound was administered intramuscularly in doses of 100–200 mg weekly. At this dose a progressive decrease in gonadotrophin excretion was seen, reaching a minimum value about four to six weeks after beginning of therapy, but even on prolonged treatment, gonadotrophin excretion was reduced only to pre-menopausal levels and not completely abolished. The number of patients used in these studies was too small to enable any conclusions to be drawn on the relationship between gonadotrophin excretion either prior to or during therapy, and subsequent clinical response.

From the studies of Martin and Cunningham (1960) and also those of Netter, Gorins and Thevenet (1969), it appears that administration of norethisterone acetate orally also decreases gonadotrophin excretion. Chow and Lederis (1969) measured the urinary excretion of FSH (using the ovarian augmentation assay) and luteinizing hormone (using the ovarian ascorbic acid depletion assay) in patients with breast cancer, both before and during 14 days of treatment with norethisterone acetate. They found that treatment led to a significant decrease in the excretion of FSH, but not apparently in the excretion of LH. In addition they claimed that tumour remissions were more frequent in patients with a higher pre-treatment gonadotrophin excretion (Curwen, 1970).

Thus although norethisterone acetate may have oestrogenic metabolites *in vivo*, the finding noted above is contrary to that of Loraine, Strong and Douglas (1957) for oestrogen therapy in breast cancer. The pituitary inhibitory activity of the related synthetic progestogen Norgestrel (17α-ethynyl-17β-hydroxy-13β-ethylgon-4-en-3-one) appears to be less than that of norethisterone since oral administration of 15 mg daily of Norgestrel for ten days did not reduce the urinary excretion of LH or total gonadotrophins (Svendsen, Fotherby and Fairweather, 1968).

## Androgens in breast cancer

Androgens appear to be less potent inhibitors of gonadotrophin production than oestrogens. Segaloff et al. (1951, 1953) found that long-term treatment of post-menopausal or ovariectomized patients with testosterone propionate or methyl testosterone in doses of 50–100 mg/day decreased, but did not abolish, gonadotrophin excretion. Over short periods of time (9–11 days) lower doses of methyl testosterone (50–100 mg/day) did not affect gonadotrophin excretion (Rosemberg and Engel, 1960). Loraine and Bell (1966) present observations in one patient who received testosterone phenylpropionate, 100 mg weekly. No decrease was found in gonadotrophin excretion although the same patient had shown suppression of gonadotrophin excretion when treated with stilboestrol. On the basis of these results, therefore, it seems unlikely that remission of the disease observed in patients treated with androgenic steroids can be ascribed to a reduction in the pituitary production of gonadotrophins.

## Adrenalectomy in breast cancer

Adrenalectomy appears to have a variable effect on gonadotrophin excretion. The most extensive study concerning changes in gonadotrophin excretion by patients with mammary carcinoma subjected to bilateral adrenalectomy and oophorectomy is that reported by Loraine et al. (1961). They studied 32 patients prior to adrenalectomy and ovariectomy, and found that there was no significant difference in gonadotrophin excretion between those patients who subsequently showed a remission from the treatment and those who showed no remission. Estimations were also performed on 37 patients, six weeks after the combined operation. In those patients who showed a remission of the disease it appeared that gonadotrophin excretion tended to increase or to remain high, whereas in those patients who showed no remission, gonadotrophin excretion decreased or remained at the previously low levels. The mean gonadotrophin excretion of those patients who showed a remission was significantly higher than those who showed no remission.

Pommatau et al. (1962) also studied gonadotrophin excretion in 90 post-menopausal or ovariectomized patients with advanced breast cancer and subjected to adrenalectomy. They found that in 29 of these subjects gonadotrophin excretion was low but increased post-operatively. An increase in gonadotrophin excretion after adrenalectomy was more frequent in patients who responded to operation, a similar observation to that noted above by Loraine et al. (1961).

## PLASMA LEVELS AND METABOLISM OF GONADOTROPHINS

All the estimates of gonadotrophin production in women with breast cancer treated with hormones or by surgery have been based on assay of urinary gonadotrophins. No studies have yet been reported in which the estimations of the gonadotrophins in serum have been made by radioimmunoassay procedures. Results obtained with the newer procedures may, however, help in the interpretation of the findings of some previous investigations and also in elucidating the relationship between sex hormone administration and gonadotrophin production.

The metabolic clearance rates and production rates of human LH and FSH have been determined by Kohler, Ross and Odell (1968) and Coble et al. (1969) using a constant infusion technique. They found that the metabolic clearance rates for the hormones were the same both in pre-menopausal and post-menopausal women and were not influenced by the presence or absence of the ovarian steroids. The metabolic clearance rate for LH was about twice that of FSH. The plasma level of LH in normal women was 32 mu/ml and very much higher values (99 mu/ml) were found in post-menopausal women. These values correspond to a production rate of LH in post-menopausal women of about 2,500 mu/min, a value about three times that of pre-menopausal women (734 mu/min). Thus, although the metabolic clearance rate does not change at the menopause or after ovariectomy, there is a large increase in the production rate. The endogenous FSH levels for pre-menopausal women were 10 mu/ml and for post-menopausal women 172 mu/ml, and the production rates were 146 mu/min and 3,141 mu/min respectively. In pre-menopausal women it has been suggested that the plasma concentrations of LH and FSH appear to be maintained by intermittent release of the hormones from the pituitary followed by periods of no secretion (Midgley and Jaffe, 1971). Whether this periodic release is maintained in post-menopausal women, or whether the increased production after the menopause is a result of continuous secretion, is not known. Ovariectomy appears to lead to a greater increase in FSH production than in that of LH (Yen and Tsai, 1971b). Gonadotrophin levels in plasma increase after ovariectomy, reaching a plateau by the end of the third week corresponding to a six- and eight-fold increase for LH and an eight- to twelve-fold increase for FSH.

LH appears to disappear rapidly from plasma (Yen et al. 1968) and, after surgical hypophysectomy, the initial half-life of LH is about 20 min, followed by a slower rate of disappearance with a half-life of about four hours. LH disappears more rapidly than FSH, which has an initial half-life of about three hours. Differences in the degree of suppressibility of the two gonadotrophins by various agents may be partly due to this difference in the rate of metabolism.

## OVARIAN STEROIDS AND THE REGULATION OF GONADOTROPHIN SECRETION

The role of the sex hormones in the regulation of gonadotrophin production by the pituitary, as assessed by urinary excretion of gonadotrophins, has been summarized by Stevens and Vorys (1967). More meaningful results have been obtained by use of radioimmunoassay methods for the separate estimation of FSH and LH in blood. The application of these methods to the study of the regulation of gonadotrophin production in humans has been extensively reviewed by Franchimont (1971a). The effects produced appear to depend on a number of factors, including the dose of the steroid, its duration and method of administration and, in pre-menopausal women, the time in the cycle when the steroid is administered.

### Pre-menopausal women

An interesting recent observation is that under certain conditions oestrogen administration can stimulate gonadotrophin release by positive feedback. Administration of low doses of the synthetic oestrogen mestranol (0·01 mg/day) throughout the menstrual cycle led to a stimulation of FSH excretion, but at higher doses (0·1 mg/day) excretion of FSH was depressed (Stevens and Vorys, 1967). The authors also suggest that administration of mestranol for short periods may lead to a biphasic response—first an elevation of the LH excretion, but on continued administration depression of LH excretion occurs. Small doses of the synthetic progestin ethynodiol diacetate (0·25 to 0·5 mg/day) were claimed to increase FSH excretion in pre-menopausal women, whereas large doses had no effect (Stevens and Vorys, 1967).

Tsai and Yen (1971) found that when oestradiol was infused into pre-menopausal women at doses greater than 50 μg/12 hours the serum levels of both FSH and LH were depressed, the depression of LH levels being greater than that of FSH.

### Post-menopausal women

Administration of oestrogens intravenously, intramuscularly or by infusion to post-menopausal subjects suppresses serum FSH and LH concentrations.

Odell and Swerdloff (1968) found gonadotrophin levels of post-menopausal women to fall to pre-menopausal levels within 10–15 days of administration of 500 µg daily of ethynyloestradiol or 15 mg/day of stilboestrol, the decrease in FSH being greater than that of LH. Similar findings were obtained by Yen and Tsai (1971a) who found that when ethynyloestradiol at a dose of 400 µg/day was given to post-menopausal women over a period of 5–8 days there was an initial decline in gonadotrophin levels, the fall in FSH being greater than that in LH. Surprisingly they further found that on about the third or fourth day there was an increase in the serum level of gonadotrophins, LH being stimulated more than FSH.

These findings were confirmed by Nillius and Wide (1971); they found that ethynyloestradiol administered orally at a dose of 100 µg/day suppressed gonadotrophin production and after four weeks the serum levels were similar to those found in pre-menopausal women. The relative decrease for FSH was greater than that for LH which is in contrast to their previous findings (Nillius and Wide, 1970), that a single intramuscular injection of 1 mg or 5 mg oestradiol benzoate or of oestradiol itself produced a greater decline of LH than of FSH levels. Although the same percentage decrease in LH was observed with both doses of oestrogen, for FSH levels the higher dose produced a more consistent decrease than the lower one.

Franchimont (1971b) found that low doses of oestrogen decreased FSH levels with little effect on LH until the plasma level of administered oestrogen decreased when there was a surge of LH secretion. With higher doses of oestradiol benzoate (5 mg intramuscularly) serum LH was depressed.

In post-menopausal women progestogens in low dosage appear to suppress LH but not FSH levels, whereas in high doses both gonadotrophins, particularly LH, are suppressed. Administration of progesterone (10–100 mg intramuscularly) to post-menopausal women does not change the serum concentration of gonadotrophins (Nillius and Wide, 1971; Franchimont, 1971b). However, progesterone does appear to have a positive feedback effect on the hypothalamus, and administration of small doses of progesterone intramuscularly to women in whom the serum levels of LH and FSH were depressed by oestrogen treatment, led to a sharp peak in LH concentration in plasma with a small increase in the FSH concentration (Nillius and Wide, 1971). When the dose of progesterone was increased to 100 mg, the peak in LH concentration was seen less consistently. These findings are similar to those reported by Odell and Swerdloff (1968).

## DISCUSSION AND CONCLUSIONS

It is obvious from what has been described above that no adequately designed extensive study has been carried out in women with breast cancer to determine the relationship of pituitary gonadotrophin production either to the disease process itself or to the effect of treatment. All studies so far have employed estimation of urinary gonadotrophins by relatively imprecise and insensitive bioassay procedures. No studies have been reported in which measurements have been carried out on blood, using more specific and sensitive radioimmunoassay procedures, and no adequate attempt has been made to assess the separate production of FSH and LH.

Investigation in these patients of blood levels of gonadotrophins and their response to treatment might give more meaningful results than urinary estimations. This is underlined by the findings of Kohler, Ross and Odell (1968) and Coble et al. (1969) that less than 5 per cent of the total amount of LH and FSH produced in humans is excreted in the urine in a biologically active form. In view of these facts one cannot expect to come to any useful conclusion regarding the relationship of the pituitary production of gonadotrophins to the various aspects of carcinoma of the breast.

Pre-treatment findings listed above of a higher excretion of gonadotrophins in patients responding to various types of treatment than in those who do not respond, are in agreement with those of Martin (1964). He studied 60 women subjected to various kinds of endocrine treatment, either surgical (including ovariectomy, adrenalectomy or hypophysectomy) or hormonal treatment (including the administration of androgens and corticosteroids). Martin suggested that there was a higher excretion of gonadotrophins in those patients whose clinical state was described as fair than those classified as poor. In addition, those patients who responded had a higher gonadotrophin excretion than those who did not. However, findings such as these may be merely related to the general clinical condition of the patient and it might be expected that those patients in a generally better clinical state respond better to treatment. It is possible therefore that changes in urinary gonadotrophin production may be merely a non-specific effect of the disease. Furthermore no studies have adequately taken into account the relationship of gonadotrophin excretion to the spread of metastases, and it is well known that some metastases may respond in a patient while others do not.

In attempting to relate changes in gonadotrophin production to the effect of treatment, the variety of treatment methods needs to be taken into account. Oestrogens, for example, will cause a marked decrease in gonadotrophin production to very low levels, whereas many of the androgens and progestogens used in the treatment cause a much less marked reduction in gonadotrophin production. The effect of surgical procedures is the converse of these, ovariectomy leading to a marked increase of gonadotrophin production and adrenalectomy producing variable effects but in general a slight increase. Thus as far as hormonal treatment is concerned, gonadotrophin excretion is not completely abolished but merely reduced by most agents while surgical removal or irradiation of the ovaries causes a marked rise in gonadotrophin excretion within one month, to within 10–20 times pre-operative values.

The factors regulating the production of gonadotrophins from the pituitary are still incompletely understood. The effect of the sex hormones in inhibiting the pituitary secretion of gonadotrophins by what has become known as the 'long-loop' feedback mechanism is now known to be due to a negative feedback action of the sex hormones on receptors in the hypothalamus leading to a decreased secretion of the gonadotrophin releasing factors and hence a decreased secretion of gonadotrophins from the pituitary. It has also been proposed that a 'short-loop' feedback mechanism exists, an increase in the blood level of the gonadotrophins themselves leading to an inhibition of the secretion of the releasing factors from the hypothalamus. In the case of the gonadotrophins it would appear that the 'long-loop' feedback mechanism is the dominant one since removal of the source of sex hormones by ovariectomy leads to an increased secretion of both FSH and LH, and the increased levels of these gonadotrophins in blood does not appear to inhibit their own secretion.

The increased secretion of gonadotrophins after ovariectomy (Yen and Tsai, 1971b) or ovarian irradiation (Loraine and Bell, 1966) occurs quickly. Loraine and Bell (1966) quote an example of a patient subjected to ovarian irradiation just after menstruation; an increased urinary excretion of gonadotrophin was apparent within 15 days and by 30 days after irradiation the excretion was 20 times higher than that observed during the preceding menstrual cycle. It is not known what function, if any, these large amounts of gonadotrophins perform. Once having increased either at the menopause or after ovariectomy, they seem to show only a slight decrease with advancing age (Loraine and Bell, 1966; Loraine, 1958). Further work is needed to determine the significance of these post-menopausal changes and this should preferably be done by the separate estimation of FSH and LH in blood.

In considering the relationship between gonadotrophin excretion and the response of patients with breast cancer to ovariectomy it must be borne in mind that the effect may be mediated not only by changes in gonadotrophin production but also by an effect on prolactin secretion. It has recently been shown that serum prolactin levels fall sharply after ovariectomy in rats, associated with a rise in serum gonadotrophin levels (Ben-David, Danon and Sulman, 1971). Suppression of gonadotrophin by methallibure administration caused a rise in the prolactin level. A reciprocal relationship between prolactin and gonadotrophin secretion by the pituitary is seen in patients with inappropriate lactation, and this relationship should be investigated in a wider group of patients now that assays of human prolactin are possible.

Similarly, in considering the relationship between gonadotrophin excretion and the response of breast cancer to oestrogen therapy, it is possible that the biphasic changes observed in gonadotrophin secretion may affect the secretion of other pituitary hormones. The observation by Yen and Tsai (1971a) that administration of high doses of ethynyloestradiol for more than three days caused an initial fall but later a rise in FSH and LH levels, may be relevant to this suggestion.

## REFERENCES

Ben-David, M., Danon, A. and Sulman, F. G. (1971). 'Evidence of antagonism between prolactin and gonadotrophin secretion.' *J. Endocr.* **51**, 719.

Boyland, E., Godsmark, B., Greening, W. P., Rigby-Jones, Stevenson, J. J. and Abdul-Fadl, M. A. M. (1958). 'The effect of irradiation of the pituitary on gonadotrophin excretion in women with advanced mammary cancer.' In *Endocrine Aspects of Breast Cancer* (Proceedings of a Conference at the University of Glasgow), p. 170, Ed. by A. R. Currie. Edinburgh; Livingstone.

Briggs, M. H., Caldwell, A. D. S. and Pitchford, A. G. (1967). 'The treatment of cancer by progestogens.' *Hosp. Med.* 63.

Brown, J. B., Fotherby, K. and Loraine, J. A. (1962). 'The effect of norethisterone and its acetate on ovarian and pituitary function during the menstrual cycle.' *J. Endocr.* **25**, 331.

Brown, P. S. (1956). 'Follicle stimulating and interstitial cell stimulating hormones in the urine of women with amenorrhoea.' *J. Endocr.* **14**, 129.

Buchholz, R., Nocke, L. and Nocke, W. (1964). 'The influence of gestagens on the urinary excretion of pituitary gonadotrophins, estrogens, and pregnanediol in women in the postmenopause and during the menstrual cycle.' *Int. J. Fertil.* **9**, 231.

Chow, Y. F. and Lederis, K. (1969). 'Urinary gonadotrophins in breast cancer patients: effects of treatment with norethisterone acetate.' *Acta endocr. (Kbh).* Suppl. **138**, 223.

Coble, Y. D., Kohler, P. O., Cargille, C. M. and Ross, G. T. (1969). 'Production rates and metabolic clearance rates of human follicle-stimulating hormone in premenopausal and postmenopausal women.' *J. clin. Invest.* **48**, 359.

Curwen, S. (1970). 'The treatment of advanced carcinoma of the breast with norethisterone acetate.' *Clin. Radiol.* **21**, 219.

Douglas, M., Loraine, J. A. and Strong, J. A. (1960). 'Studies with 19-norethisterone oenanthate in mammary carcinoma.' *Proc. R. Soc. Med.* **53**, 1.

Elstein, M. (1969). 'Urinary hormone excretion patterns in chlormadinone acetate treated patients and the associated cervical mucus changes.' In *Chlormadinone Acetate*, pp. 46–59, Ed. by G. A. Christie and M. Moore-Robinson. Maidenhead; Syntex Pharmaceuticals.

Fotherby, K. and James, F. (1972a). 'Metabolism of synthetic steroids.' *Adv. ster. Biochem.* **3**, 67.

— — (1972b). 'Biochemistry of steroids in normal subjects.' In *Endocrine Therapy in Malignant Disease*, pp. 3–23, Ed. by B. A. Stoll. London; Saunders.

Franchimont, P. (1971a). 'The regulation of FSH and LH secretion in humans.' In *Frontiers in Neuroendocrinology*, Ed. by L. Martini and W. F. Ganong. Oxford University Press.

— (1971b). 'Steroid feedback mechanisms on growth hormone and the gonadotropins in humans.' In *Proceedings of the Third International Congress on Hormonal*

*Steroids*, pp. 722–726, Ed. by V. H. T. James and L. Martini. Amsterdam; Excerpta Medica.

Heller, C. G., Chandler, R. E. and Myers, G. B. (1944). 'Effect of diethylstilboestrol on menopausal symptoms and urinary gonadotrophins in ovariectomized women.' *J. clin. Endocr.* **4**, 109.

Kohler, P. O., Ross, G. T. and Odell, W. D. (1968). 'Metabolic clearance and production rates of HLH in pre- and postmenopausal women.' *J. clin. Invest.* **47**, 38.

Loraine, J. A. (1958). 'The estimation of anterior pituitary hormones in patients with mammary carcinoma.' In *Endocrine Aspects of Breast Cancer* (Proceedings of a Conference, Glasgow), pp. 158–169, Ed. by A. R. Currie. Edinburgh; Livingstone.

— and Bell, E. T. (1965). 'The effect of various compounds on pituitary function in man as judged by urinary gonadotrophin assays.' In *Hormonal Steroids*, Vol. 2, pp. 281–291, Ed. by L. Martini and A. Pecile. New York; Academic Press.

— — (1969). *Hormone Assays and Their Clinical Application*. Edinburgh; Livingstone.

— Douglas, M., Falconer, C. W. A. and Strong, J. A. (1961). 'Urinary gonadotrophin excretion in relation to the treatment of mammary carcinoma by bilateral adrenalectomy and oophorectomy.' In *Progress in Endocrinology*, Part II, pp. 150–155, Ed. by K. Fotherby, J. A. Loraine, J. A. Strong and P. Eckstein. Cambridge University Press.

— Strong, J. A. and Douglas, M. (1957). 'The value of pituitary gonadotrophin assays in patients with mammary carcinoma.' *Lancet* **2**, 575.

Martin, F. I. R. (1964). 'Urinary gonadotrophins in postmenopausal women with breast cancer.' *Br. med. J.* **2**, 351.

Martin, L. and Cuningham, K. (1960). 'Suppression of pituitary gonadotrophins by 17-ethynyl-19-nortestosterone in patients with metastatic carcinoma of the breast.' *J. clin. Endocr.* **20**, 529.

Midgley, A. R and Jaffe, R. B. (1971). 'Regulation of human gonadotropins: X. Episodic fluctuation of LH during the menstrual cycle.' *J. clin. Endocr.* **33**, 962.

Moore, D. J., Roscoe, R. T., Heller, C. G. and Paulsen, C. A. (1961). 'Failure of progesterone to depress urinary gonadotropin excretion in normal menstruating women.' In *Human Pituitary Gonadotrophins*, p. 233, Ed. by A. Albert. Springfield; Thomas.

Netter, A., Gorins, A. and Thevenet, M. (1969). 'Étude des variations de l'élimination urinarie des oestrogèns biologiques, des gonadotrophines totales, des 17 cétostéroides et des 17 hydroxy-corticoïdes sous l'effet de l'acétate de noréthistérone administré a doses massives dans les cancers du sein métastiques.' *Ann. Endocr. Paris* **30**, 488.

Nillius, S. J. and Wide, L. (1970). 'Effects of oestrogen on serum levels of LH and FSH.' *Acta endocr. (Kbh.)* **65**, 583.

— — (1971). 'Effects of progesterone on the serum levels of FSH and LH in postmenopausal women treated with oestrogen.' *Acta endocr. (Kbh.)* **67**, 362.

O'Connor, P. J. and Skinner, L. G. (1964). 'The effect of chronic diethylstilboestrol administration and subsequent withdrawal on pituitary gonadotrophin excretion in patients with mammary carcinoma.' *Acta endocr. (Kbh.)* **45**, 623.

Odell, W. D. and Swerdloff, R. S. (1968). 'Progestogen-induced luteinizing and follicle-stimulating hormone surge in postmenopausal women; a simulated ovulatory peak.' *Proc. natn Acad. Sci.* **61**, 529.

Pommatau, E., Poulain, S., Dargent, M. and Mayer, M. (1962). 'FSH levels of menopausal or castrated women suffering from an advanced breast carcinoma.' *Ann. Endocr. Paris* **23**, 678.

Rosemberg, E. and Engel, I. (1960). 'The influence of steroids on urinary gonadotrophin excretion in a postmenopausal woman.' *J. clin. Endocr.* **20**, 1576.

Segaloff, A., Gordon, D., Horwitt, B. N., Schlosser, J. V. and Murison, P. J. (1951). 'Hormonal therapy in cancer of the breast. 1. The effect of testosterone proprionate therapy on clinical course and hormonal excretion.' *Cancer* **4**, 319.

— Horwitt, B. N., Carabasi, R. A., Murison, P. J. and Schlosser, J. V. (1953). 'Hormonal therapy in cancer of the breast. V. The effect of methyl-testosterone on clinical course and hormonal excretion.' *Cancer* **6**, 483.

Smith, R. A. and Albert, A. (1955). 'Effects of estrogen on urinary gonadotrophins.' *Proc. Mayo Clin.* **30**, 617.

— — (1958). 'The effects of intramuscularly administered progesterone of human pituitary gonadotrophin.' *Proc. Mayo Clin.* **33**, 197.

Stevens, V. C. and Vorys, M. (1967). 'The regulation of pituitary function by sex steroids.' *Obstet. Gynec. Survey* **22**, 781.

Stevenson, P. M. and Loraine, J. A. (1971). 'Pituitary gonadotropins—chemistry, extraction and immunoassay.' In *Advances in Clinical Chemistry,* Vol. 14, pp. 2–63, Ed. by O. Bodansky and A. L. Latner. New York; Academic Press.

Stewart, J. G., Skinner, L. G. and O'Connor, P. J. (1965). 'Hormone therapy in metastatic breast cancer: clinical response and urinary gonadotrophins.' *Acta endocr. (Kbh.)* **50**, 345.

Svendsen, E. K., Fotherby, K. and Fairweather, D. V. I. (1968). 'Gonadotrophin excretion in postmenopausal patients. The effects of Norgestrel.' *Clin. Trials J. (Lond.)* **5**, 1071.

Tsai, C. C. and Yen, S. S. C. (1971). 'Acute effects of intravenous infusion of 17β-estradiol on gonadotrophin release in pre- and postmenopausal women.' *J. clin. Endocr.* **32**, 766.

Yen, S. S. C., Llerena, O., Little, B. and Pearson, O. H. (1968). 'Disappearance rates of endogenous LH and chorionic gonadotrophin in man.' *J. clin. Endocr.* **28**, 1763.

— and Tsai, C. C. (1971a). 'The biphasic pattern in the feedback action of ethynyloestradiol on the release of pituitary FSH and LH.' *J. clin. Endocr.* **33**, 882.

— — (1971b). 'The effect of ovariectomy on gonadotrophin release.' *J. clin. Invest.* **50**, 1149.

# PART II

# Mechanisms in Neuroendocrine Regulation

# 7

# Regulation of Pituitary Function by Catecholamines

## Robert M. MacLeod

Secretion of most pituitary gland hormones is stimulated by regulating factors present in the hypothalamus. Prolactin secretion, however, is specifically inhibited through neurohumoral mechanisms. The existence of the inhibitory action of the hypothalamus on prolactin secretion is well documented by the frequent observations of lactation in experimental animals following the placement of hypothalamic lesions, and in humans following pituitary stalk section. When pituitary glands are incubated in organ or tissue culture, the synthesis and release of prolactin is maintained at a high level but production of other pituitary hormones is diminished, indicating that the presence of the hypothalamus is not required and, in fact, is inhibitory for prolactin secretion.

## INVOLVEMENT OF CATECHOLAMINES IN PROLACTIN SECRETION

The implication of catecholamines in the neural control of prolactin production was fostered by the findings of Kanematsu, Hilliard and Sawyer (1963), who showed that lactation was induced in oestrogen-primed ovariectomized rabbits following the injection of reserpine. Since lactation could not be produced by this treatment in rabbits with electrolytic lesions in the basal tuberal hypothalamus, it was concluded that prolactin release was mediated by a system in the hypothalamus. There is now abundant evidence that the catecholamines in the hypothalamus have an inhibitory effect on prolactin release.

The important function of the hypothalamic catecholamines was suggested by the finding that placement of electrolytic lesions in the ventro-medial nucleus significantly increased the *in vitro* synthesis and release of prolactin by the pituitary gland (MacLeod and Lehmayer, 1972). Partial destruction of this area or of the arcuate nucleus was without effect on prolactin production. Hence it is evident that discrete anatomical areas of the hypothalamus have an important function in regulating the secretion of prolactin. There is, however, considerable disagreement regarding the mechanism involved in inhibition of prolactin release. All workers agree that the catecholamines in the hypothalamus inhibit prolactin release, but whether they act directly on the pituitary gland or through an intermediary such as prolactin-inhibiting factor (PIF) which, in turn, inhibits prolactin release, is a subject for debate.

Hökfelt (1967) demonstrated that the termination of the tubero-infundibular dopamine neurons in the median eminence are adjacent to the portal vessels leading to the anterior pituitary. The dopamine released from these neurons may exert its effects on pituitary function either indirectly by causing the secretion of hypophysiotropic factors or by direct transport to the pituitary via the portal system.

## Direct inhibition of prolactin secretion

Van Maanen and Smelik (1968) demonstrated that dopamine was the predominant catecholamine in the ventro-hypothalamus and that, following reserpine administration, dopamine disappeared from the hypothalamus. They hypothesized that dopamine was released into the portal vessels leading to the pituitary gland where it exerted a direct inhibitory effect on prolactin release.

Support for this mechanism was provided by the findings of MacLeod (1969) and Birge et al. (1970), who conclusively demonstrated that catecholamines had a direct inhibitory effect on prolactin synthesis and release *in vitro*. These workers showed that small amounts of epinephrine, norepinephrine and dopamine caused an 80–90 per cent decrease in prolactin release. Since the incorporation of radioactive amino acids into the prolactin retained by the pituitary gland was increased in the presence of the catecholamines, while the amount of labelled prolactin in the incubation medium was greatly decreased, these agents apparently exert their primary effect on prolactin release rather than on synthesis *(Figure 7.1)*. The metabolites of the catecholamines were inactive.

Although addition of norepinephrine to pituitary glands incubated *in vitro* causes a prompt cessation of radioactive prolactin release, a constant exposure of the tissue to catecholamine for 60 minutes is necessary to effectively inhibit hormone release. A brief exposure of 15 minutes to norepinephrine followed by incubation in fresh medium without norepinephrine was ineffective in decreasing prolactin release (MacLeod and Lehmeyer, 1972). A longer exposure of three hours to catecholamine completely abolished prolactin release but subsequent incubation in fresh medium resulted in a normal rate of prolactin release within two hours. These findings suggest that the catecholamine is either poorly bound to the pituitary receptor or is rapidly metabolized. The latter possibility may be particularly important because the pituitary gland contains a monoamine oxidase capable of degrading two

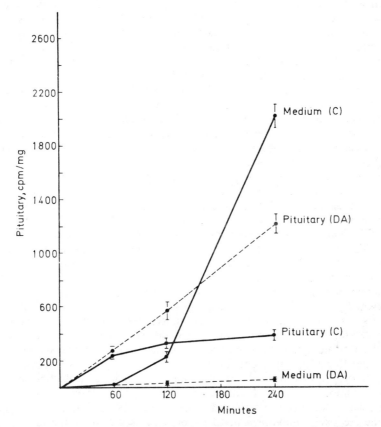

*Figure 7.1. In vitro effect of* $10^{-6}$M *dopamine on the incorporation of leucine* 4·5-$^3$H *into rat prolactin*

nanomoles of catecholamine per minute (MacLeod, Fontham and Lehmeyer, 1970). When the pituitary is incubated continuously in $10^{-6}$ M norepinephrine for several hours, the complete inhibition of prolactin release is abolished within two hours after transferring the glands into incubation medium devoid of catecholamine. Thus once again the transient inhibition caused by catecholamine on prolactin release is demonstrated and may be of some physiological importance.

Both α- and β-adrenergic blocking agents are partially effective in blocking the catecholamine-induced inhibition of prolactin release (Birge et al., 1970). A combination of both propranolol and phentolamine completely blocked in *in vitro* effects of norepinephrine. Unpublished data from our laboratory are in agreement with this data and, additionally, the inhibitory effect of dopamine on prolactin release was completely blocked by the *in vitro* or *in vivo* administration of haloperidol, an agent which specifically blocks the effect of dopamine in other tissues. These findings clearly demonstrate that the pituitary gland is highly sensitive to the direct inhibitory action of catecholamine and is responsive to the classic adrenergic and dopaminergic blocking agents.

The direct inhibitory action of catecholamines on prolactin release correlates well with the well-established changes in serum prolactin following drug-induced changes in brain catecholamines. We have previously demonstrated that prior injection of reserpine or α-methyl tyrosine resulted in an increase in *in vitro* prolactin release and synthesis by the pituitary gland (MacLeod and Abad, 1968). Lu et al. (1970) showed that reserpine, chlorpromazine and α-methyl tyrosine, agents that effectively decrease brain catecholamine function, caused an increase in serum prolactin levels while administration of L-DOPA, a precursor of brain catecholamines, caused a decrease in serum prolactin concentration (Lu and Meites, 1971; Donoso et al., 1971). Very recently these findings were extended to humans where the tranquillizing drugs caused a prompt increase in serum prolactin (Frantz, Kleinberg and Noel, 1972). In another study, patients with Forbes-Albright syndrome were administered L-DOPA and a dramatic decrease in the elevated circulating prolactin concentration was observed (Turkington, 1972).

Elevated plasma levels of prolactin caused by the implantation of pituitary tumours cause a suppression of prolactin synthesis by the host's pituitary gland. Although the tumour hormones do not cause any increase in hypothalamic norepinephrine or dopamine concentration, brain catecholamine levels may have an important function in regulating prolactin release since injection of perphenazine or reserpine into rats bearing prolactin-secreting pituitary tumours restored the decreased synthesis and release of prolactin to normal rates (MacLeod, Fontham and Lehmeyer, 1970). These data suggest that the feedback inhibition caused by prolactin secreted by the tumour on pituitary gland prolactin production is mediated by a catecholamine-dependent mechanism.

Translation of these *in vitro* findings into plausible physiological terms is possible, and they are consonant with the hypothesis that the hypothalamic catecholamines are transported via the portal vessels to the pituitary gland where they cause an inhibition of prolactin release. Interruption of the flow of catecholamine by stalk section, electrolytic lesion or by pharmacological manipulation releases the pituitary gland from its chronic inhibition and results in an increased production of prolactin.

## Indirect inhibition of prolactin secretion

The pioneering work of Pasteels (1962) and of Talwalker, Ratner and Meites (1963) provided evidence that PIF was present in hypothalamic extracts and, when added to cultures of pituitary glands, produced an inhibition in the amount of prolactin released into the incubation medium. It is presumed that hypothalamic PIF is released into the portal vessels leading to the pituitary gland. Extracts of hypothalami from rats treated with reserpine are less effective in causing inhibition of prolactin release (Ratner, Talwalker and Meites, 1965). From this and other data, it was concluded that reserpine depletes the hypothalamus of PIF. Subsequently, Coppola et al. (1965) suggested that, in reserpine-treated rats, the absence of brain norepinephrine impaired the synthesis and release of PIF, but this was not documented. Arimura, Dunn and Schally (1972) have recently demonstrated that in rats anaesthetized with pentobarbital, infusion of rat stalk median eminence or cerebral cortex extracts produced a pronounced decrease in serum prolactin concentration. If, however, the rats were treated with perphenazine or reserpine prior to pentobarbital injection, neither brain extract decreased serum prolactin. Since the brain extracts did not decrease serum prolactin levels in rats bearing hypothalamic lesions the authors concluded that the extracts decreased serum prolactin by causing the release of hypothalamic PIF and not by acting directly on the pituitary gland. Their conclusion partially assumes that perphenazine and reserpine block PIF release and have no effect at the pituitary level. These conclusions must be viewed with caution since pre-treatment of rats with perphenazine has been shown to render the pituitary gland completely refractory to the *in vitro* inhibitory effects of dopamine (MacLeod and Lehmeyer, 1972). Although reserpine does not block the *in vitro* effects of dopamine, it exerts its effect by eliminating the stores of brain catecholamine.

The findings of Kamberi, Mical and Porter (1971a) contributed significantly to the establishment of the importance of brain catecholamines in regulating prolactin release. When dopamine was infused into the third ventricle of male rats, anaesthetized with pentobarbital, a prompt decrease in plasma prolactin followed. Epinephrine and norepinephrine were also active but only in large doses. Catecholamine perfusion of the pituitary gland via the portal vessels, peduncular artery or infundibular artery was not successful in decreasing plasma prolactin levels. In an interesting pharmacological study, Donoso et al. (1971) also concluded that dopamine was the inhibitory transmitter which suppresses prolactin release.

Recent evidence presented by Kamberi, Mical and Porter (1971b) shows that neutralized acid extracts of hypothalamic fragments significantly reduce the plasma prolactin concentration when perfused directly into these portal vessels. A progressive fall in plasma prolactin was observed for the duration of hypothalamic infusion, but a prompt rise to control values was observed one hour after stopping the infusion, thus suggesting the transient nature of the inhibiting factor. The biological half-life of plasma prolactin was calculated to be $14 \cdot 4 \pm 0 \cdot 2$ minutes.

The authors proposed that brain catecholamines, especially dopamine, stimulate the neurosecretory granules to release PIF which, in turn, inhibits prolactin release. Evidence for increased PIF activity in stalk median eminence plasma following dopamine injection into the third ventricle was subsequently presented (Kamberi, Mical and Porter, 1971c). When this stalk plasma was infused into the hypophysial portal vessel of other rats a prompt and significant decrease in circulating prolactin was observed. Similar results have also been observed when stalk plasma was incubated *in vitro* with pituitary glands (Kamberi, Mical and Porter, 1970a).

It is difficult to reconcile these results with the dramatic and direct *in vitro* inhibitory effects that catecholamines exert on prolactin release (MacLeod, 1969; Birge et al., 1970). There is the possibility, however, that the pentobarbital used by Kamberi, Mical and Porter (1971b) to anaesthetize his animals altered their response to catecholamine. Unpublished work from our laboratory confirms that of Wuttke and Meites (1970) and Arimura, Dunn

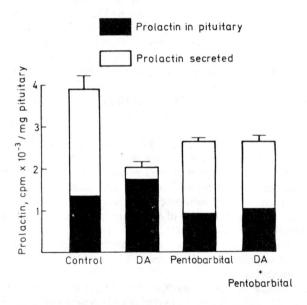

*Figure 7.2. Effect of pentobarbital injection on the in vitro secretion of newly-synthesized prolactin in the presence of* $5 \times 10^{-7}$M *dopamine. Pentobarbital (40 mg/kg) injected 30 minutes before sacrifice*

and Schally (1972) who demonstrated that pentobarbital significantly increases plasma prolactin. No such increase was reported by Kamberi, Mical and Porter (1971b). Additionally, the data in *Figure 7.2* show that the pituitary glands of rats injected with pentobarbital are refractory to the inhibitory effects of dopamine on prolactin release.

We believe, therefore, that since the direct *in vitro* effects of dopamine and norepinephrine on inhibition of prolactin release are well established, the hypothesis that catecholamines exert their inhibitory action exclusively through mechanisms involving the release of PIF deserves further investigation.

## Mechanism of stimulatory action of perphenazine on prolactin secretion

Among the numerous tranquillizers developed, several cause abnormal lactation after administration to women and animals. Although their mammotropic and sedative effects are associated biological activities they are independent of each other and the mammotropic effects are resistant to energizers which block the tranquillizing properties of the drugs (Khazan et al., 1966). Perphenazine is among the group of chlorpromazine derivatives which has received special attention because of its potent lactogenic activity. Mammogenesis was not observed when hypophysectomized rats were injected with perphenazine, thus indicating the involvement of pituitary hormones. Recently Ben-David, Danon and Sulman (1970) have demonstrated that perphenazine increases the secretion of prolactin within one hour of injection. Their conclusion that perphenazine stimulates the synthesis of prolactin agrees with the findings of MacLeod, Fontham and Lehmeyer (1970), who demonstrated that the drug increased the incorporation of radioactive amino acids into prolactin. The drug-induced increased synthesis and release of prolactin were observed in male and female rats which minimizes the direct role of gonadal hormones in the synthesis of prolactin. More recently, increase in serum prolactin in adrenalectomized rats following perphenazine injection was observed. Since the mammotropic effects of the drug were not observed in endocrine-ablated animals, an ability of perphenazine to specifically stimulate prolactin secretion is indicated.

A mechanism whereby the tranquillizer increases prolactin production was suggested by Danon, Dikstein and Sulman (1963) who found that hypothalamic fragments from rats treated with perphenazine failed to block prolactin release *in vitro*, or following the injection of hypothalamic extracts (Danon and Sulman, 1970). The interpretation of their results was that perphenazine caused an acute inhibition of PIF release initially, but after long-term treatment, the drug caused a subsequent decrease in PIF synthesis.

We propose an alternative explanation of the increase in prolactin synthesis and release following perphenazine injection. The results presented in *Figure*

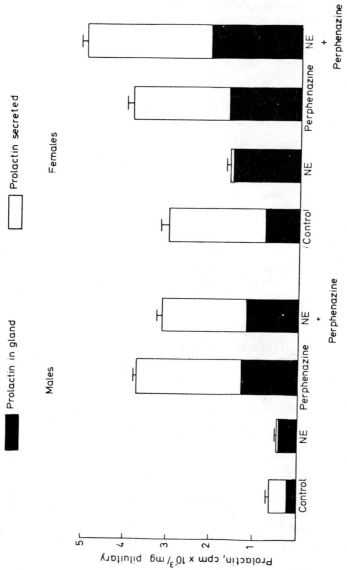

Figure 7.3. *Effect of perphenazine injection on the in vitro secretion of newly-synthesized prolactin in the presence of $2 \times 10^{-6}$M norepinephrine. Perphenazine (5 mg/kg) injected daily for five days*

*7.3* indicate that *in vitro* prolactin synthesis and release were increased in acids into prolactin. The drug-induced increased synthesis and release of prolactin were observed in male and female rats which minimizes the direct pituitary glands of rats following injection with perphenazine. Although catecholamine greatly decreased prolactin production in the control group, the drug had no significant effect on prolactin synthesis or release in glands from

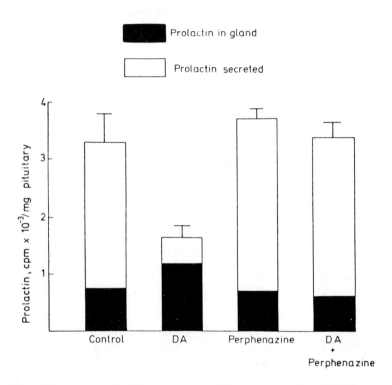

*Figure 7.4. In vitro blockade by perphenazine of the dopamine-induced inhibition of prolactin secretion; $5 \times 10^{-7}M$ dopamine and $2.5 \times 10^{6}M$ perphenzaine per 1 ml incubation medium*

rats receiving perphenazine. These results are consistent with the hypothesis that perphenazine decreases the responsiveness of the pituitary gland to the inhibiting effects of catecholamines and thereby increases prolactin production. Direct evidence for this hypothesis is presented in *Figure 7.4,* where it is observed that the inhibitory effect of dopamine on prolactin release was completely blocked by the simultaneous addition of perphenazine to the incubation medium.

### Inter-relationships of neurohormones, reproductive cycle and ovarian steroids

It has long been known that natural and synthetic oestrogens cause hypertrophy of the pituitary gland and increase prolactin production (Ratner, Talwalker and Meites, 1963; Baker and Zanotti, 1966). More recently it was demonstrated that spayed rats synthesize less prolactin than intact females, and injection with oestrogen restores in *in vitro* synthesis of the hormone by the pituitary gland (Catt and Moffat, 1967; MacLeod, Abad and Eidson, 1969). Although the fundamental mechanism whereby oestrogens stimulate prolactin production is unclear, Ratner and Meites (1964) presented evidence that the PIF activity in the hypothalamus of rats receiving the steroid was reduced and therefore permitted an increased synthesis of the protein hormone.

With the advent of the radioimmunoassay for prolactin a much clearer understanding of prolactin dynamics is emerging. There is complete agreement that low or moderate amounts of oestrogen stimulate prolactin production, but it is believed that large amounts of oestrogen are inhibitory to prolactin

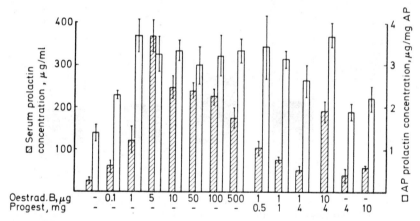

*Figure 7.5. Effects of different doses of oestradiol benzoate and/or progesterone on serum and anterior pituitary prolactin concentration in ovariectomized rats*
[Reproduced from Chen and Meites (1970) by courtesy of the Editor of *Endocrinology, Philadelphia*]

release. Until recently the latter supposition was not well investigated. Chen and Meites (1970) administered 17-β-oestradiol benzoate in increasing daily doses of 0·1 to 500 μg to ovariectomized rats, and observed that 5 μg oestradiol caused the maximum stimulation of plasma prolactin concentration. Higher amounts of oestradiol caused lesser stimulation of serum prolactin levels, but even 500 μg of steroid caused a very large increase in serum prolactin. *(Figure 7.5)*. Thus, the authors' results do not support the concept that large doses of oestrogen are inhibitory to prolactin synthesis and release. The injection of 4 or 10 mg of progesterone caused a modest increase in serum prolactin, but it was less than that caused by 0·1 μg of oestradiol, suggesting that the former steroid has a minor function in regulating prolactin production. When a combination of oestradiol and progesterone was injected, a slight but insignificant decrease in plasma prolactin levels was observed.

Sar and Meites (1967), Neill (1970), Niswender et al. (1969), Kwa and Verhofstad (1967), and Amenomori, Chen and Meites (1970) made the important observation that on the afternoon of pro-oestrus there is a large increase in serum prolactin concentration. Rats in other stages of the oestrus cycle had basal levels that were similar to levels observed in male rats. The work of Ieiri, Akikusa and Yamamoto (1971) demonstrated that the *in vitro* incorporation of radioactive amino acid into prolactin was three fold greater in pituitary glands of rats in oestrus than in rats in other phases. Since prolactin synthesis and release are controlled by inter-related but independent mechanisms, the neuroendocrine stimulus for prolactin release probably provokes a subsequent initiation of prolactin synthesis to replenish that previously released.

The pro-oestrus surge of prolactin release is a rhythmic, internally-mediated response governed by ovarian hormones and neurohormones. The essential nature of oestradiol in the release of prolactin during pro-oestrus was demonstrated by the finding that the administration of antiserum to oestradiol on the second day of di-oestrus abolished the expected subsequent increase in plasma prolactin (Neill, Freeman and Tillson, 1971). The simultaneous injection of the antiserum and diethylstilboesterol reversed the inhibitory effects of the antiserum. The authors were careful to avoid defining the site(s) of oestrogen action but reintroduced the findings of Kanematsu and Sawyer (1963), who demonstrated that implantation of the median eminence with oestradiol caused an increase in pituitary prolactin. Hökfelt and Fuxe (1972) and Ahren et al. (1971) point out that the increased turnover of dopamine neurons during di-oestrus is correlated with the low serum prolactin levels and the decreased dopamine turnover correlated with the elevated serum prolactin levels of pro-oestrus. They suggest that the tubero-infundibular dopamine neurons are part of a feedback system involved in the regulation of prolactin secretion. In the experimental rat, brain catecholamine synthesis was prevented by the injection of α-methyl-p-tyrosine methyl ester and subsequent prolactin injection was then found to increase the rate of disappearance from dopamine nerve terminals. These effects seem rather specific since they were observed in castrated female rats, thereby eliminating the possible interaction of the ovarian steroids. Although no evidence was obtained for the afferent hypothalamic norepinephrine or the nigro-neostriatal dopamine neurons, the tubero-infundibular dopamine neurons may stimulate the release of PIF from the hypothalamus which, in turn, inhibits prolactin secretion. Thus, these neurons would be a link in the feedback system whereby serum prolactin influences PIF secretion. Weiner et al. (1972) failed to observe any change in norepinephrine content of the basal hypothalamus, anterior hypothalamus or amygdala during different stages of the reproductive cycle. This agrees with the work of Sandler (1968) but not with that of Stefano and Donoso (1967), who found minimum catecholamine levels at oestrus and maximum levels at pro-oestrus. Complete deafferentation of the medial basal hypothalamus resulted in total depletion of norepinephrine within the deafferented island but no change in catecholamine concentration in the residual hypothalamic fragment (Hökfelt and Fuxe, 1972). Blake, Weiner and Sawyer (1972) have recently studied pituitary prolactin secretion in rats made persistently oestrus or di-oestrus by hypothalamic deafferentation. Persistent-oestrus rats, produced by extended anterior cuts in the brain, showed elevated serum and pituitary concentrations of prolactin that were approximately the same as observed on the afternoon of pro-oestrus. It is likely that the increased prolactin production is due to the action of oestrogen. Complete deafferentation, which caused a complete disappearance of norepinephrine but not of dopamine, decreased serum prolactin levels and pituitary prolactin concentration.

It may be, however, that the measurement of brain catecholamine concentration or content is not the appropriate parameter for study. The rates of catecholamine turnover may be the physiological determinate in regulating prolactin secretion.

The influence of progesterone on the production of prolactin has not been established. Sar and Meites (1968) reported that the daily injection of 10 mg of progesterone for 21 days caused 51 per cent increase in pituitary prolactin and a decrease in hypothalamic PIF. Other groups did not find that progesterone influenced prolactin synthesis (MacLeod, Abad and Eidson, 1969; Jones et al., 1965).

The administration of testosterone to rats caused a significant increase in pituitary gland prolactin and its *in vitro* synthesis (MacLeod, Abad and Eidson, 1969; Sar and Meites, 1968). Since testosterone is readily converted into oestrogens, it is possible that this is a partial explanation for these observations and accounts for the measurable plasma prolactin levels in males (Amenomori, Chen and Meites, 1970; Neill, 1970).

## ROLE OF NEUROHORMONES IN GONADOTROPHIN SECRETION

The concept that the hypothalamus regulates pituitary gonadotrophin secretion has received widespread support. Regulation of LH and FSH secretion is directly controlled by a gonadotrophin-releasing polypeptide

(Schally et al., 1972) which is synthesized in the hypothalamus. After being transported to the pituitary gland via the portal system, this polypeptide causes the release of LH and FSH. Over the past several years it has become increasingly evident that the hypothalamic releasing factors are themselves regulated by other neurohormones. Markee, Everett and Sawyer (1952) were among the first to demonstrate that brain catecholamines have an important function in the ultimate secretion of pituitary gonadotrophins when they showed an increase in LH secretion following elevation of brain catecholamine levels. Subsequently Sawyer (1963) and Barraclough and Sawyer (1957) found that neural activity changes accompanied the administration of drugs which decreased brain catecholamine content or blocked their action at the receptor site and inhibited ovulation and LH secretion.

Weiner et al. (1972, 1973) and Blake et al. (1972) recently observed that catecholamine injection increased the multiple unit activity of the rat hypothalamus. Norepinephrine and epinephrine had similar potency but dopamine was inactive. Surgical deafferentation of the median basal hypothalamus resulted in disappearance of norepinephrine but not of dopamine from the hypothalamic island and a decreased plasma LH concentration. They concluded that the concomitant changes in electrical activity of the hypothalamus and plasma LH concentration indicate that catecholamine may have an important function in the neuroendocrine control of tonic and phasic aspects of pituitary gonadotrophin secretion.

These concepts correlate well with the pharmacological studies conducted by Lippmann et al. (1967) and Coppola (1968). Reduction of hypothalamic catecholamines following the administration of reserpine or α-methyl tyrosine induced pseudo-pregnancy and blocked ovulation. Pre-treatment of the rats with central monoamine oxidase inhibitors, thus maintaining catecholamine levels, blocked the biological effect of the drugs. Although these studies substantiate and extend the concept that depletion of hypothalamic catecholamine levels results in decreased gonadotrophin and increased prolactin secretion, these studies provide support for the hypothesis that pituitary function is regulated by a sympathetic tone or rate of catecholamine turnover in the hypothalamus. In these studies reserpine produced a prompt fall of 50 per cent in the catecholamine content of the hypothalamus; no further decrease was observed. Despite the low catecholamine concentration, ovulation could be induced in all rats by the injection of pregnant mare's serum after a short interval of time. The findings suggested to the authors that the newly-synthesized catecholamines were of primary importance in stimulating gonadotrophic release. These studies were extended (Coppola, 1969) by the finding that ovariectomy caused a large increase in hypothalamic catecholamine content and turnover. The injection of oestrone or progesterone into ovariectomized female rats restored hypothalamic catecholamine pool size and turnover to normal.

## Inter-relationship of neurohormones and releasing factors

*In vitro* studies by Schneider and McCann (1969) have presented convincing evidence that elevation of LH secretion is mediated by dopamine. This catecholamine presumably exerts its action by increasing the release of LRH from the hypothalamus. Alone, dopamine was inactive but in the presence of hypothalamic fragments it promoted LH release. It is important to note that, in these studies, norepinephrine and epinephrine were not effective. These investigators concluded that dopamine is the synaptic transmitter for LRH release because its effects were completely abolished by the α-blocking agent phentolamine. Alpha-receptors are apparently not involved in the response of pituitary tissue to LRH since phentolamine did not inhibit the direct effect of LRH.

The importance of the median eminence in mediating the *in vivo* effects of dopamine on gonadotrophin release was clearly demonstrated by the studies of Kamberi, Mical and Porter (1970b, 1971d). Using anaesthetized male rats they found that injection of 1·25 µg dopamine into the third ventricle caused a marked increase in serum LH and FSH. Norepinephrine, epinephrine, serotonin and melatonin were inactive. Direct perfusion of the portal blood vessels leading to the pituitary gland with dopamine did not produce an increase in gonadotrophin release. These studies and those of Schneider and McCann (1969) suggest that dopamine has the function of a synaptic transmitter to stimulate or facilitate the release of LRH and, secondarily, the release of LH and FSH.

Direct evidence that dopamine produces an increase in LRH was demonstrated by Schneider and McCann (1970a) and Kamberi, Mical and Porter (1969) who introduced catecholamine into the third ventricle of hypophysectomized rats. Alpha-adrenergic receptors appeared to mediate the dopamine effects because phentolamine or phenoxybenzamine completely blocked the dopamine response. Haloperidol, a neuroleptic agent, also completely blocked the effects of dopamine (Schneider and McCann, 1970b). The finding that dopamine simultaneously increases both LH and FSH suggests that these hormones may share a similar releasing or regulatory mechanism. This is consonant with the suggestion by Schally et al. (1972) that LRH is responsible for the release of both gonadotrophins.

Interesting data on the antagonistic actions of dopamine and oestradiol on LH secretion are accumulating. The negative feedback effect that oestradiol exerts on pituitary gonadotrophin secretion has long been recognized but its function in neuroendocrine regulation was substantiated by the findings of Schneider and McCann (1970a) who found that injection of the steroid into the third ventricle completely inhibited the dopamine-mediated discharge of LRH. Using *in vitro* techniques, these workers (Schneider and McCann, 1970c) obtained similar results. Puromycin and cyclohexamide, inhibitors of protein synthesis, blocked the inhibitory action of oestradiol and permitted the stimulatory effect of added dopamine on LRH release, thus increasing LH secretion.

## Effect of synthetic and ovarian steroids on neurohormones

The mechanisms through which the anti-fertility steroids block ovulation have been studied extensively. Early work by Schally et al. (1968) presented evidence that various oestrogens and progestins block the release of LH by an action on the hypothalamus. Administration of large doses of chlormadinone acetate (5–10,000 µg) and mestranol (50–200 µg) separately and in combination lowered plasma LH concentration. Intravenous injection of LRF into rats pre-treated with these drugs resulted in a prompt increase in plasma LH values. Other progestins, norethynodrel, ethynodial diacetate, nore-thindrone, dimethisterone and medroxyprogesterone acetate given alone in high doses and in combination with mestranol or ethynyl oestradiol suppressed plasma LH in ovariectomized rats but did not block the response to LRF. Much smaller amounts of these substances have similar effects on plasma gonadotrophin levels. These studies complement the similar findings of Harris and Sherratt (1969) who studied ovulation in the rabbit. Although these results clearly implicate the hypothalamus as the site of ovarian steroid feedback inhibition of LH release, more recent data by Arimura and Schally (1970) substantiate the claim by Hilliard et al. (1966) that sites in the pituitary gland are implicated in the progesterone suppression of LH in the intact rat and rabbits.

Although elevated progesterone levels are generally regarded as exerting an inhibitory action on LH secretion, Everett (1964) demonstrated that administration of progesterone to constant-oestrus rats can produce ovulation. Nallar, Antunes-Rodrigues and McCann (1966) and, more recently, Caligaris, Astrada and Taleisnik (1971) have presented evidence that the injection of progesterone into rats at an appropriate time of the cycle, specifically pro-oestrus, or into ovariectomized rats primed previously with oestrogen produced the greatest increase in gonadotrophin release.

The mechanisms whereby the ovarian steroids influence pituitary function are being elucidated. Several experimental approaches have implicated the hypothalamic catecholamines, dopamine and norepinephrine. The turnover rates of norepinephrine were found to be increased at pro-oestrus by some workers (Stefano and Donoso, 1967; Donoso and DeGuiterres Moyano, 1970) but not by others (Weiner et al., 1972; Sandler, 1968). Castration of male or female rats caused an increase in norepinephrine turnover as measured by isotopic methods (Wurtman, Anton-Tay and Anton, 1969; Anton-Tay and Wurtman, 1968) which resulted in an increase in the amount of catecholamine present in the hypothalamus (Coppola, 1968). One interpretation of these studies is that the absence of the ovarian hormones caused an increase in the hypothalamic catecholamine synthesis. Anton-Tay, Pelham and Wurtman (1969) concluded, however, that the increased catecholamine synthesis was not caused by the absence of ovarian steroids in the castrated rat but by the increased FSH secreted by the pituitary. Their conclusion is based on the finding of increased catecholamine synthesis in rats injected with purified FSH.

Bapna, Neff and Costa (1971) have studied the rates of catecholamine and serotonin synthesis and the steady-state levels in ovariectomized rats injected with oestradiol-3 benzoate (0·2 mg/kg) and progesterone (2·0 mg/kg). Neither the amine nor serotonin concentrations were altered by the ovarian steroids. Steroid treatment, however, caused a considerable decrease in the rate of norepinephrine synthesis and a very slight increase in serotonin synthesis in the anterior hypothalamus.

The essential involvement of the adrenergic system in the secretion of gonadotrophins and their regulation by ovarian steroids was clearly demonstrated by Kalra et al. (1972). The elevated plasma levels of LH were decreased by the injection of 5 μg oestradiol benzoate. Injection of 1·5 mg progesterone, 48 hours later, resulted in a five to ten fold increase in plasma LH concentration and a lesser increase in plasma FSH. If, prior to progesterone injection, phenoxybenzamine, an α-adrenergic receptor blocker, was administered, the action of the progesterone was blocked. Haloperidol, an agent which blocks both dopamine and norepinephrine receptors, has a similar inhibiting action. Propranolol, a β-blocker, had no inhibitory action. The progesterone-induced increase in plasma gonadotrophins was blocked if the brain catecholamine levels were decreased by inhibitors of tyrosine hydroxylase. While restoration of dopamine synthesis alone was ineffective in promoting the effect of progesterone, selective restoration of norepinephrine synthesis caused the expected increase in plasma gonadotrophins following progesterone treatment. It would appear then that norepinephrine mediates the progesterone-induced release of gonadotrophins. These steroid-sensitive neurons located in the pre-optic area (Taleisnik, Velasco and Astrada, 1970) lead directly or indirectly to the neuron regulating gonadotrophin-releasing factor and their stimulation results in elevated plasma gonadotrophins and ovulation.

## SUMMARY

Abundant evidence has accumulated implicating adrenergic mechanisms in the control of prolactin and gonadotrophin release. It is quite clear that any pharmacological or steroidal manipulation which results in alterations in the turnover or concentration of specific central catecholamine stores will produce subsequent changes in prolactin and gonadotrophin production. The administration of DOPA, which increases brain dopamine concentration, causes a decrease in prolactin release while administration of reserpine, perphenazine, or adrenergic blocking agents—drugs which lower brain catecholamine concentration or block their action in the pituitary gland—is stimulatory to prolactin release. Anatomical and pharmacological considerations suggest that a dopaminergic mechanism is involved in the inhibition of prolactin release. When stimulated, these axons, terminating in the median eminence, may release *(a)* hypothalamic catecholamines or *(b)* prolactin-inhibiting factor into the portal blood perfusing the pituitary gland and thereby inhibit prolactin release. Strong evidence for both mechanisms has been offered, thus presenting the possibility of a dual inhibitory control of prolactin release.

The stimulation of gonadotrophin release apparently also occurs via a neuronal mechanism. These nerve terminals presumably stimulate the discharge of gonadotrophin-releasing hormone from neurosecretory storage granules. There is no evidence for a direct stimulatory effect of catecholamines on gonadotrophin release.

## REFERENCES

Ahren, K., Fuxe, K., Hamberger, L. and Hökfelt, T. (1971). 'Turnover changes in the tubero-infundibular dopamine neurons during the ovarian cycle of the rat.' *Endocrinology* **88**, 1415.

Amenormori, Y., Chen, C. L. and Meites, J. (1970). 'Serum prolactin levels in rats during different reproductive states.' *Endocrinology* **86**, 506.

Anton-Tay, F., Pelham, R. W. and Wurtman, R. J. (1969). 'Increased turnover of $^3$H-norepinephrine in rat brain following castration or treatment with ovine follicle-stimulating hormone.' *Endocrinology* **84**, 1489.

— and Wurtman, R. J. (1968). 'Norepinephrine: turnover in rat brains after gonadectomy.' *Science* **159**, 1245.

Arimura, A., Dunn, J. D. and Schally, A. V. (1972). 'Effect of infusion of hypothalamic extracts on serum prolactin levels in rats treated with nembutal, CNS depressants or bearing hypothalamic lesions.' *Endocrinology* **90**, 378.

— and Schally, A. V. (1970). 'Progesterone suppression of LH-releasing hormone-induced stimulation of LH release in rats.' *Endocrinology* **87**, 653.

Baker, B. L. and Zanotti, D. B. (1966). 'Electrophoresis of pituitary proteins after treatment of rats with norethynodrel.' *Endocrinology* **78**, 1037.

Bapna, J., Neff, N. H. and Costa, E. (1971). 'A method for studying norepinephrine and serotin metabolism in small regions of rat brain: effect of ovariectomy on amine metabolism in anterior and posterior hypothalamus.' *Endocrinology* **89**, 1345.

Barraclough, C. A. and Sawyer, C. H. (1957). 'Blockage of the release of pituitary ovulating hormone in the rat by chlorpromazine and reserpine: possible mechanism of action.' *Endocrinology* **61**, 341.

Ben-David, M., Danon, A. and Sulman, F. G. (1970). 'Acute changes in blood and pituitary prolactin after a single injection of perphenazine.' *Neuroendocrinology* **6**, 336.

155

Birge, C. A., Jacobs, L. S., Hammer, C. T. and Daughaday, W. H. (1970). 'Catecholamine inhibition of prolactin secretion.' *Endocrinology* **86**, 120.

Blake, C. A., Weiner, R. I., Gorski, R. A. and Sawyer, C. H. (1972). 'Secretion of pituitary luteinizing hormone and follicle stimulating hormone in female rats made persistently estrous or diestrous by hypothalamic deafferentation.' *Endocrinology* **90**, 855.

— Weiner, R. I. and Sawyer, C. H. (1972). 'Pituitary prolactin secretion in female rats made persistently estrous or diestrous by hypothalamic deafferentation.' *Endocrinology* **90**, 862.

Caligaris, L., Astrada, J. J. and Taleisnik, S. (1971). 'Biphasic effect of progesterone on the release of gonadotropin in rats.' *Endocrinology* **89**, 331.

Catt, K. and Moffat, B. (1967). 'Isolation of internally labeled rat prolactin by preparative disc electrophoresis.' *Endocrinology* **80**, 324.

Chen, C. L. and Meites, J. (1970). 'Effects of estrogen and progesterone on serum and pituitary prolactin levels in ovariectomized rats.' *Endocrinology* **86**, 503.

Coppola, J. A. (1968). 'The apparent involvement of the sympathetic nervous system in the gonadotrophin secretion of female rats.' *J. Reprod. Fertil.,* Suppl. **4**, 35.

— (1969). 'Turnover of hypothalamic catecholamines during various states of gonadotrophin secretion.' *Neuroendocrinology* **5**, 75.

— Leonardi, R. G., Lippmann, W., Perrine, J. W. and Ringler, I. (1965). 'Induction of pseudopregnancy in rats by depletors of endogenous catecholamines.' *Endocrinology* **77**, 485.

Danon, A., Dikstein, S. and Sulman, F. G. (1963). 'Stimulation of prolactin secretion by perphenazine in pituitary hypothalamus organ culture.' *Proc. Soc. expl Biol. Med.* **114**, 366.

— and Sulman, F. G. (1970). 'Storage of prolactin-inhibiting factor in the hypothalamus of perphenazine-treated rats.' *Neuroendocrinology* **6**, 295.

Donoso, A. O., Bishop, W., Fawcett, C. P., Krulich, L. and McCann, S. M. (1971). 'Effects of drugs that modify brain monoamine concentrations on plasma gonadotrophin and prolactin levels in the rat.' *Endocrinology* **89**, 774.

— and DeGuiterrez Moyano, M. B. (1970). 'Adrenergic activity in hypothalamus and ovulation.' *Proc. Soc. expl Biol. Med.* **135**, 633.

Everett, J. W. (1964). 'Central neural control of reproductive functions of the adenohypophysis.' *Physiol. Rev.* **44**, 373.

Frantz, A. G., Kleinberg, D. L. and Noel, G. L. (1972). 'Physiological and pathological secretion of human prolactin studied by *in vitro* bioassay.' In *CIBA Foundation Symposium on Lactogenic Hormones,* p. 137, Ed. by G. E. W. Wolstenholme and J. J. Knight. Edinburgh; Churchill Livingstone.

Harris, G. W. and Sherratt, R. M. (1969). 'The action of chlormadinone acetate (6-chloro $\Delta^6$ dehydro-17 and acetoprogesterone) upon experimentally induced ovulation in the rabbit.' *J. Physiol. (Lond.)* **203**, 59.

Hilliard, J., Croxatto, H. B., Hayward, J. N. and Sawyer, C. H. (1966). 'Norethindrone blockade of LH release to intrapituitary infusion of hypothalamic extract.' *Endocrinology* **79**, 411.

Hökfelt, T. (1967). 'The possible ultrastructural identification of tubero-infundibular dopamine-containing nerve endings in the median eminence of the rat.' *Brain Res.* **5**, 121.

— and Fuxe, K. (1972). 'Effects of prolactin and ergot alkaloids on the tubero-infundibular dopamine (DA) neurons.' *Neuroendocrinology* **9**, 100.

Ieiri, T., Akikusa, Y. and Yamamoto, K. (1971). 'Synthesis and release of prolactin and growth hormone *in vitro* during the estrous cycle of the rat.' *Endocrinology* **89**, 1533.

Jones, A. R., Fisher, J. N., Lewis, U. J. and VanderLaan, W. P. (1965). 'Electrophoretic comparison of pituitary glands from male and female rats.' *Endocrinology* **76**, 578.

Kalra, P. S., Kalra, S. P., Krulich, L., Fawcett, C. P. and McCann, S. M. (1972). 'Involvement of norepinephrine in transmission of the stimulatory influence of progesterone on gonadotropin release.' *Endocrinology* **90**, 1168.

Kamberi, I. A., Mical, R. S. and Porter, J. C. (1969). 'LHRF activity in hypophysial stalk blood and elevation by dopamine.' *Science* **166**, 388.

— — — (1970a). 'PIF activity in hypophysial stalk blood and elevation by dopamine.' *Experientia* **26**, 1150.

— — — (1970b). 'Effect of anterior perfusion and intraventicular injection of catecholamines and indoleamines on LH release.' *Endocrinology* **87**, 1.

— — — (1971a). 'Effect of anterior pituitary perfusion and intraventricular injection of catecholamine on prolactin release.' *Endocrinology* **88**, 1012.

— — — (1971b). 'Pituitary portal vessel infusion of hypothalamic extract and release of LH, FSH, and prolactin.' *Endocrinology* **88**, 1294.

— — — (1971c). 'Hypophysial portal vessel infusion: *in vivo* demonstration of LRF, FRF, and PIF in pituitary stalk plasma.' *Endocrinology* **89**, 1042.

— — — (1971d). 'Effect of anterior pituitary perfusion and intraventricular injection of catecholamines on FSH release.' *Endocrinology* **88**, 1003.

Kanematsu, S., Hilliard, J. and Sawyer, C. H. (1963). 'Effect of reserpine on pituitary prolactin content and its hypothalamic site of action in the rabbit.' *Acta endocr.* **44**, 467.

— and Sawyer, C. H. (1963). 'Effects of intrahypothalamic and intrapituitary estrogen implants on pituitary prolactin and lactation in the rabbit.' *Endocrinology* **72**, 243.

Khazan, N., Ben-David, M., Mishkinsky, J., Khazan, K. and Sulman, F. G. (1966). 'Dissociation between mammotropic and sedative effects of non-hormonal hypothalamic tranquilizers.' *Archs int. Pharmacodyn.* **164**, 258.

Kwa, H. G. and Verhofstad, F. (1967). 'Radioimmunoassay of rat prolactin.' *Biochem. biophys. acta* **133**, 186.

Lippmann, R. L., Ball, J. and Coppola, J. A. (1967). 'Relationship between hypothalamic catecholamines and gonadotrophin secretion in rats.' *J. Pharmac. expl Ther.* **156**, 258.

Lu, K. H., Amenormori, Y., Cheng, C. L. and Meites, J. (1970). 'Effects of central acting drugs on serum and pituitary prolactin levels in rats.' *Endocrinology* **87**, 667.

— and Meites, J. (1971). 'Inhibition of L-Dopa and monamine oxidase inhibitors of pituitary prolactin release; stimulation by methyldopa and d-amphetamine.' *Proc. Soc. expl Biol. Med.* **137**, 480.

MacLeod, R. M. (1969). 'Influence of norepinephrine and catecholamine-depleting agents on the synthesis and release of prolactin and growth hormone.' *Endocrinology* **85**, 916.

MacLeod, R. M. and Abad, A. (1968). 'On the control of prolactin and growth hormone synthesis in rat pituitary glands.' *Endocrinology* **83**, 799.

— — and Eidson, L. L. (1969). '*In vivo* effect of sex hormones on the *in vitro* synthesis of prolactin and growth hormone in normal and pituitary tumor-bearing rats.' *Endocrinology* **84**, 1475.

— Fontham, E. H. and Lehmeyer, J. E. (1970). 'Prolactin and growth hormone production as influenced by catecholamines and agents that affect brain catecholamines.' *Neuroendocrinology* **6**, 283.

— and Lehmeyer, J. E. (1972). 'Regulation of the synthesis and release of prolactin.' In *CIBA Foundation Symposium on Lactogenic Hormones*, p. 53, Ed. by G. E. W. Wolstenholme and J. J. Knight. Edinburgh; Churchill Livingstone.

Markee, J. E., Everett, J. W. and Sawyer, C. H. (1952). 'The relationship of the nervous system to the release of gonadotropin and the regulation of the sex cycle.' *Recent Progr. Hormone Res.* **7**, 139.

Nallar, R., Antunes-Rodrigues, J. and McCann, S. M. (1966). 'Effect of progesterone on the level of plasma luteinizing hormone (LH) in normal female rats.' *Endocrinology* **79**, 907.

Neill, J. D. (1970). 'Effect of "stress" on serum prolactin and luteinizing hormone levels during the estrous cycle of the rat.' *Endocrinology* **87**, 1192.

— Freeman, M. E. and Tillson, S. A. (1971). 'Control of the proestrous surge of prolactin and LH secretion by estrogens in the rat.' *Endocrinology* **89**, 1448.

Niswender, G. D., Chen, C. L., Midgley, A. R. Jnr, Meites, J. and Ellis, S. (1969). 'Radioimmunoassay for rat prolactin.' *Proc. Soc. expl. Biol. Med.* **130**, 793.

Pasteels, J. L. (1962). 'Administration of hypothalamic extracts to the rat pituitary *in vitro*, with a view to controlling the secretion of prolactin.' *C. R. Acad. Sci (Paris)* **254**, 2664.

Ratner, A. and Meites, J. (1964). 'Depletion of prolactin-inhibiting activity of rat hypothalamus by estradiol or suckling stimulus.' *Endocrinology* **75**, 377.

— Talwalker, P. K. and Meites, J. (1963). 'Effect of estrogen administration *in vivo* on prolactin release by rat pituitary *in vitro*.' *Proc. Soc. expl Biol. Med.* **112**, 12.

— — — (1965). 'Effect of reserpine on PIF activity of rat hypothalamus.' *Endocrinology* **77**, 315.

Sandler, R. (1968). 'Concentration of norepinephrine in the hypothalamus of the rat in relation to the estrous cycle.' *Endocrinology* **83**, 1383.

Sar, M. and Meites, J. (1967). 'Changes in pituitary prolactin release and hypothalamic PIF content during the estrous cycle of rats.' *Proc. Soc. expl Biol. Med.* **125**, 1018.

— — (1968). 'Effects of progesterone, testosterone, and cortisol on hypothalamic PIF and pituitary prolactin content.' *Proc. Soc. expl Biol. Med.* **127**, 426.

Sawyer, C. H. (1963). 'Mechanisms by which drugs and hormones activate and block release of pituitary gonadotropins.' In *Proceedings of the First International Pharmacological Meeting*, Vol. 1, p. 27. Oxford; Pergamon Press.

Schally, A. V., Carter, W. H., Saito, M., Arimura, A. and Bowers, C. Y. (1968). 'Studies of the site of action of oral contraceptive Steroids. I. Effect of antifertility steroids on plasma LH levels and on the response to luteinizing hormone-releasing factor in rats.' *J. clin. Endocr.* **28**, 1747.

— Redding, T. W., Matsuo, H. and Arimura, A. (1972). 'Stimulation of FSH and LH release *in vitro* by natural and synthetic LH and FSH releasing hormone.' *Endocrinology* **90**, 1561.

Schneider, H. P. G. and McCann, S. M. (1969). 'Possible role of dopamine as transmitter to promote discharge of LH-releasing factor.' *Endocrinology* **85**, 121.

— — (1970a). 'Release of LHRF into the peripheral circulation hypophysectomized rats by dopamine and its blockage by estradiol.' *Endocrinology* **87**, 249.

— — (1970b). 'Dopami:.ergic pathways and gonadotropin releasing factors.' In *Aspects of Neuroendocrinology*, p. 177, Ed. by W. Bargmann and B. Scharrer. Berlin; Springer-Verlag.

— — (1970c). 'Estradiol and the neuroendocrine control of LH release *in vitro*. *Endocrinology* **87**, 330.

Stefano, F. J. E. and Donoso, A. O. (1967). 'Norepinephrine levels in the rat hypothalamus during the estrous cycle.' *Endocrinology* **81**, 1405.

Taleisnik, S., Velasco, M. E. and Astrada, J. J. (1970). 'Effect of hypothalamic deafferentation on the control of luteinizing hormone secretion.' *J. Endocr.* **46**, 1.

Talwalker, P. K., Ratner, A. and Meites, J. (1963). '*In vitro* inhibition of pituitary prolactin synthesis and release by hypothalamic extract.' *Am. J. Physiol.* **205**, 213.

Turkington, R. W. (1972). 'Inhibition of prolactin secretion and successful therapy of the Forbes-Albright syndrome with L-DOPA.' *J. clin. Endocr.* **34**, 306.

Van Maanen, J. H. and Smelik, P. G. (1968). 'Induction of pseudopregnancy in rats following local depletion of monoamines in the median eminence of the hypothalamus.' *Neuroendocrinology* **3**, 177.

Weiner, R. I., Gorski, R. A. and Sawyer, C. H. (1973). 'Hypothalamic catecholamines and pituitary gonadotropic function.' In Press.

— Shryne, J. E., Gorski, R. A. and Sawyer, C. H. (1972). 'Changes in the catecholamine content of the rat hypothalamus following deafferentation.' *Endocrinology* **90**, 867.

Wurtman, R. J., Anton-Tay, F. and Anton, S. (1969). 'On the use of synthesis inhibitors to estimate brain norepinephrine synthesis in gonadectomized rats.' *Life Sci.* **8**, 1015.

Wuttke, W. and Meites, J. (1970). 'Effects of ether and pentobarbital on serum prolactin and LH levels in proestrous rats.' *Proc. Soc. expl. Biol. Med.* **135**, 648.

# 8

# Hypothalamic Control of Prolactin Secretion

## James A. Clemens and Joseph Meites

### INTRODUCTION

A number of reviews on the control of prolactin secretion have appeared in recent years (Meites and Nicoll, 1966; Meites, 1966, 1970; Nicoll, 1971; Meites et al., 1972; Meites and Clemens, 1972). The considerable current interest in prolactin is due in part to the recognition that it has an important role in development and growth of mammary and pituitary tumours in addition to its role in normal mammary growth and lactation, that it has multitudinous functions in submammalian species, that it exists as a distinct and separate hormone in human and other primate species, that it can now be measured quantitatively in the blood of humans and other species by specific radioimmunoassays, and that it has a unique control system.

Prolactin synthesis and release are regulated mainly by the hypothalamus, although some hormones and drugs can act directly on the pituitary to influence prolactin secretion. Unlike other anterior pituitary hormones, prolactin (and GH) secretion is not inhibited by hormones from any target tissue. Interestingly, however, high circulating levels of prolactin can depress pituitary prolactin secretion via hypothalamic mechanisms. The hypothalamus appears to exert predominantly an inhibitory influence over prolactin secretion under most conditions by releasing a prolactin-inhibiting factor (PIF) into the hypothalamo-pituitary portal system. However, there is some evidence that the hypothalamus also contains a prolactin-releasing factor (PRF), suggesting that prolactin secretion may be under dual control by the hypothalamus. Biogenic amines present in the hypothalamus also have been shown to be important in regulation of PIF release from the hypothalamus, thereby indirectly influencing prolactin secretion by the pituitary.

With the increased knowledge gained in the past 15 years of the control of prolactin secretion, it is now possible to inhibit or increase prolactin secretion at will, most simply by use of appropriate drugs but also by direct manipulation of the hypothalamus (induced lesions, implants of hormones or drugs, or by electrical stimulation) and by use of appropriate environmental agents. It is possible by these means to inhibit or accelerate growth of mammary and pituitary tumours in murine species, to depress or increase normal mammary growth and lactation, to inhibit or stimulate functions of the corpora lutea in rats and mice, and to regulate other actions of prolactin in the body. This presents interesting possibilities to study the involvement of this hormone in health and disease.

## NEURAL INFLUENCES ON PROLACTIN SECRETION

### Effects of removal of hypothalamic connections to the pituitary

Removal of the pituitary from the sella turcica and autografting it beneath the kidney capsule results in continuous prolactin secretion, as indicated by prolonged maintenance of luteal function in rats (Desclin, 1950; Everett, 1954). Secretion of the other anterior pituitary hormones is profoundly reduced, as judged by appearance of the target organs and decreased body growth. Many investigations have confirmed these observations and also have shown that the pituitary is capable of autonomous secretion of prolactin after pituitary stalk section, after placement of lesions in the hypothalamus and upon culture or incubation of the pituitary (Meites, Nicoll and Talwalker, 1963; Meites and Nicoll, 1966). These, as well as studies with recently developed radioimmunoassays, indicate that the predominant action of the mammalian hypothalamus on prolactin secretion is inhibitory in nature.

Transplantation of one to four heterologous anterior pituitaries underneath the kidney capsule of hypophysectomized–ovariectomized rats, resulted in continuous prolactin secretion for 10 weeks (Chen et al., 1970). Rats with no grafts had barely detectable levels of serum prolactin, whereas rats with one graft had levels as high as on the day of oestrus. Rats with four grafts had about four times as much serum prolactin during most of the ten-week period of observation as rats with one graft.

Destruction of the median eminence, or parts of the anterior or posterior hypothalamus of ovariectomized rats, resulted in significant elevations of serum prolactin levels above control values (Chen et al., 1970) *(Figure 8.1)*. This suggests that a rather diffuse area participates in regulation of prolactin secretion. Interestingly, all these lesioned areas lie in the 'hypophysiotropic area' of the hypothalamus as defined by Halasz et al. (1962). The 'hypophysiotropic area' is believed to control the basal secretion of anterior pituitary hormones, while cyclic secretory changes are mediated by other brain areas. Welsch et al. (1971) demonstrated that placement of bilateral lesions in the median eminence in intact female rats resulted in a ten-fold

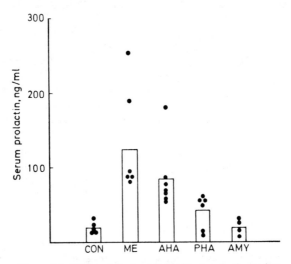

*Figure 8.1. Effects of placing bilateral lesions in the median eminence (ME), anterior hypothalamus (AHA), posterior hypothalamus (PHA) or amygdala (AMY) on serum prolactin (after Chen et al., 1970)*

increase in serum prolactin by the end of 30 minutes and a subsequent fall to levels still above those of controls. This elevation persisted during six months of observation. Earlier studies demonstrated that lesions placed in the medial basal hypothalamus were found to result in initiation of lactation in the rabbit (Haun and Sawyer, 1960), cat (Grosz and Rothballer, 1961) and rat (DeVoe, Ramirez and McCann, 1966).

It is clear from the above observations that removal of the link between the anterior pituitary gland and the hypothalamus by lesions or transplantation results in unattenuated prolactin secretion by the anterior pituitary, and that the predominant influence of the hypothalamus on prolactin secretion is inhibitory.

## Presence of a prolactin-inhibiting factor (PIF) in the hypothalamus

After the many indications of the inhibitory nature of the hypothalamus on prolactin release, it became of interest to determine whether a factor was present in the hypothalamus that could inhibit prolactin secretion. Addition of crude hypothalamic extracts to incubations (Meites, Nicoll and Talwalker,

1961; Talwalker, Ratner and Meites, 1963) or cultures (Pasteels, 1961) of rat pituitary, decreased prolactin release. Hypothalamic extracts from the sheep, bovine, pig and human also were demonstrated to inhibit release of prolactin (Schally et al., 1967). Kragt and Meites (1965) were able to demonstrate a negative dose–response relationship between the amount of rat hypothalamic extract added to an incubation medium containing pituitary halves from male rats, and the amount of prolactin released into the medium. Several workers have reported that hypothalamic extracts can inhibit prolactin release *in vivo* (Schally et al., 1967; Amenomori and Meites, 1970; Watson, Krulich and McCann, 1971).

The prolactin-inhibiting factor (PIF) (Talwalker, Ratner and Meites, 1963) from the hypothalamus has not been characterized chemically although it may be a small polypeptide like the other hypothalamic hypophysiotropic hormones. Recent work by Nicoll (1971) demonstrated that $3',5'$-cyclic AMP could overcome the inhibitory action of hypothalamic extract on pituitary prolactin release *in vitro*, and that hypothalamic extract is as effective in inhibiting prolactin release in the absence as in the presence of theophylline. These results suggest that an action of PIF on the adenyl cyclase–phosphodiesterase system is unlikely. Nicoll (1971) indicated that PIF acts on the prolactin-secreting cell membrane to inhibit calcium (Ca) influx. The cell is believed to depolarize spontaneously when it is freed from hypothalamic influence, with a resultant increase in Ca entry into the cell and consequent release of secretory granules. Therefore, PIF may act by preventing spontaneous depolarization of prolactin cells.

## Possibility of existence of a prolactin-releasing factor (PRF) in the hypothalamus

It had been hypothesized that oxytocin might be the hypothalamic factor responsible for prolactin release, based on the observation that injections of oxytocin, like prolactin, could inhibit involution of the mammary glands in post-partum rats after litter removal (Benson and Folley, 1956). They suggested that oxytocin induced prolactin release, although prolactin was not actually measured. Subsequent studies demonstrated that oxytocin prevented mammary involution by a different action than prolactin, and that it did not alter pituitary prolactin levels (Meites, Nicoll and Talwalker, 1963). Recently, Greenwood (1971) reported that oxytocin had little effect on blood prolactin levels in sheep. Thus oxytocin does not appear to be a significant factor in prolactin release.

Injections of crude hypothalamic extracts have been shown to induce lactation in oestrogen-primed female rats (Meites, Talwalker and Nicoll, 1960; Mishkinsky, Khazan and Sulman, 1968). However, it could not be concluded from these studies that the extracts contained a prolactin-releasing factor (PRF), since many other agents initiated lactation in the oestrogen-primed rat.

More recently Nicoll (1971) reported that when they incubated rat pituitary tissue with hypothalamic extract, inhibition of prolactin release was observed for the first four hours and increased prolactin release during the subsequent four hours. They concluded that their hypothalamic extracts contained both PIF and PRF activities. Using a somewhat different system of incubation, Meites (1970) observed only inhibition of prolactin release throughout an eight-hour period of incubation. Krulich, Quijada and Illner (1971) sectioned freshly frozen rat hypothalami, and reported that PIF activity was predominant in the dorsolateral part of the pre-optic area, and that PRF activity was predominant in the median eminence area. The latter observation is difficult to reconcile with the many observations indicating that placement of lesions in the median eminence area results in increased release of prolactin (Meites, 1970). If PRF activity resides in the median eminence it might be expected that lesions in this area would result in decreased prolactin release. It is noteworthy that the pre-optic area, which Krulich, Quijada and Illner (1971) reported contains PIF activity, has been observed to be concerned with the release of LH but not of prolactin by Everett and Quinn (1966) and Kordon (1966). The latter workers showed that stimulation of the pre-optic area produced ovulation but not pseudo-pregnancy in the rat.

Recent reports have suggested that synthetic TRH can induce release of prolactin in rats and humans. Tashjian, Barowsky and Jensen (1971) observed that addition of TRH to an incubation medium containing two clonal strains of cells from rat pituitary tumours, stimulated release of prolactin and inhibited release of GH. They also reported that extracts of hypothalamus, cerebral cortex, liver and kidney similarly increased prolactin release but inhibited release of GH. This casts some doubt on the specificity of the TRH action on rat pituitary cells. Lu et al. (1970) added several doses of synthetic TRH to an incubation medium containing pituitary halves, and observed no effect on prolactin release. Single injections of TRH also failed to alter serum prolactin levels, but when TRH was injected daily for six days there was a small increase in pituitary and serum prolactin levels. These increases of prolactin were not observed when TRH was injected into thyroidectomized rats, suggesting that its effects were mediated through the TSH–thyroid system. It has been reported that thyroid hormones can be stimulatory to prolactin secretion in the rat (Chen and Meites, 1969) and can act directly on the rat anterior pituitary to increase prolactin release (Nicoll and Meites, 1963). In women and men, injection of synthetic TRH was reported to induce a rapid elevation of serum prolactin values (Hwang, Guyda and Friesen, 1971; Jacobs et al., 1971; Bowers et al., 1972). Although these studies show that TRH can increase prolactin levels in human subjects, its mechanism of action remains to be elucidated. It is possible that TRH is similar to the postulated prolactin-releasing factor (PRF) or that it acts by inhibiting the action of PIF on the pituitary.

## Extrahypothalamic influences on prolactin secretion

Areas that lie outside of the hypothalamus appear to be able to influence prolactin secretion. The amygdaloid nuclei were considered to have a role in the control of prolactin secretion by Tindal, Knaggs and Turvey (1967). They found that oestrogen implants in the amygdaloid nuclei induced lactation in pseudo-pregnant rabbits. Later Mena and Beyer (1968) induced lactation in rabbits by temporal lobe lesions in the amygdaloid complex. They concluded that the amygdaloid complex exerted an inhibitory influence on prolactin secretion.

Rubenstein and Sawyer (1969) proposed a stimulatory role for the hippocampus in the control of prolactin secretion in the rat. They found that electrochemical stimulation of the dentate gyrus induced pseudo-pregnancy. The possibility exists that the primary effect of the lesions, implants or stimulation changed the secretion of some other hormone that secondarily influenced prolactin.

Tindal and Knaggs (1969) attempted to trace the ascending pathways in the brain responsible for prolactin release. The lactogenic responses of the mammary glands were rated and used as an index of prolactin release. The pathway ascended through the mid-brain and was located medially at the level of the posterior hypothalamus. They reported in a subsequent study that the pathway ascended through the lateral hypothalamus and also appeared to be associated with the orbitofrontal cortex (Tindal and Knaggs, 1970). This latter finding is very interesting in that it provides the anatomical substrate through which emotional and stressful stimuli may influence prolactin release.

## Biological rhythms and prolactin secretion

A number of different rhythms have been reported for prolactin secretion in the rat. The pattern of the rhythm appears to change according to the animal's physiological state. In both male and female rats, and in ovariectomized rats, a diurnal rhythm in serum prolactin has been observed, with values about twice as high in the late afternoon as in the morning (Koch, Chou and Meites, 1971) (Table 8.1). A similar diurnal rhythm in blood prolactin levels has been observed in lactating cows, with values between 4 and 7 p.m. about twice as high as values between 4 and 10 a.m. (Koprowski et al., unpublished). Dunn, Arimura and Scheving (1972) reported a periodicity in serum prolactin levels in both 'stressed' and 'unstressed' male rats. In the 'stressed' rats the peak of prolactin secretion appeared at about 5 p.m., while in the 'unstressed' rats the peak was at 11 p.m. Both groups demonstrated the nadir at about 8 a.m. The lights were on from 4 a.m. to 6 p.m. A similar rhythm was reported by Butcher, Fugo and Collins (1972) with the additional observation of a nocturnal surge of prolactin during early gestation.

TABLE 8.1

Morning and Afternoon Serum Prolactin Concentrations and Secretion Rates

| Experimental group | No. of rats | Serum prolactin (ng/ml) | | Secretion rate (ng/min) | |
|---|---|---|---|---|---|
| | | 9.45–10.15 a.m. | 5.45–6.15 p.m. | a.m. | p.m. |
| Di-oestrus | 23 | 24·6 ± 2·4* | 55·4 ± 4·9 | 32·4 | 73·1 |
| Pro-oestrus | 23 | 26·0 ± 3·0 | 178·6 ± 14·3 | 34·3 | 235·8 |
| Oestrus | 19 | 48·8 ± 7·6 | 105·1 ± 11·1 | 64·4 | 138·7 |
| Met-oestrus | 24 | 26·8 ± 2·5 | 53·5 ± 3·7 | 35·4 | 70·6 |
| Ovariectomized | 10 | 20·0 ± 1·8 | 42·5 ± 5·9 | 26·4 | 56·2 |
| Males | 15 | 25·7 ± 2·5 | 46·2 ± 4·5 | 33·9 | 60·0 |

After Koch et al., 1971.
* Mean ± SE.

Freeman and Neill (1972), using cannulated female rats, observed no diurnal rhythm in prolactin secretion. The only significant peak was during pro-oestrus. In contrast, daily nocturnal surges of prolactin were noted in pseudo-pregnant rats. The lights were on from 5 a.m. to 5 p.m. Thus it appears that there are definite periodicities in prolactin secretion, and that the pattern for any particular animal may depend on its physiological state as well as on the light schedule.

## ROLE OF BIOGENIC AMINES

### Catecholamines

A large number of early studies suggested that biogenic amines were involved in the control of anterior pituitary function. Some workers suggested that the biogenic amines might be releasing factors for anterior pituitary hormones. Mizuno, Talwalker and Meites (1964) observed that iproniazid, a recognized monoamine oxidase inhibitor and therefore a depressor of catecholamine metabolism, inhibited post-partum lactation in rats. It was concluded that iproniazid inhibited prolactin secretion. Subsequently, iproniazid was shown to increase hypothalamic PIF and reduce serum prolactin levels in rats (Lu and Meites, 1971).

Norepinephrine and serotonin are highly concentrated in the hypothalamus (Vogt, 1954; Brodie, Spector and Shore, 1959) and the median eminence is rich in dopaminergic nerve terminals (Fuxe, 1964; Carlsson et al., 1965). It subsequently was shown that various drugs and different physiological states altered catecholamine concentration in the hypothalamus and median eminence area, and secretion of prolactin, LH and FSH (Mizuno, Talwalker and Meites, 1964; Schneider and McCann, 1970; Lu et al., 1970). Changes were observed in hypothalamic PIF (Ratner et al., 1965), LRF and FRF (Schneider and McCann, 1970; Kamberi, Mical and Porter, 1970) subsequent to alteration of catecholamine levels. From these and other related observations the concept evolved that hypothalamic catecholamines act as

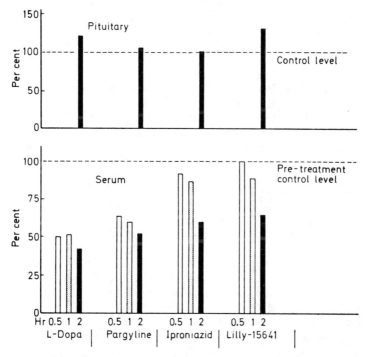

Figure 8.2. Effects of L-Dopa and three monoamine oxidase inhibitors on serum and pituitary prolactin values. All drugs decreased serum prolactin but only L-Dopa and Lilly 15641 increased pituitary prolactin content (after Lu and Meites, 1971)

neurotransmitters to control the release of the hypothalamic hypophysiotropic hormones and their entry into the hypothalamo-pituitary portal vessels, which in turn regulate the release of anterior pituitary hormones (Coppola, 1968; Fuxe and Hökfelt, 1969; Wurtman, 1970).

Administration of catecholamine precursors and monoamine oxidase inhibitors results in elevation in hypothalamic PIF content and reduction in serum prolactin concentration (Figure 8.2). Single injections of drugs that inhibit hypothalamic catecholamine activity, including reserpine, chlorpromazine, alpha-methyl-para-tyrosine, alpha-methyl-meta-tyrosine, methyl-dopa and d-amphetamine, all markedly increased serum prolactin levels (Lu et al.,

1970; Lu and Meites, 1971). These observations support the hypothesis that the hypothalamic catecholamines act as neurotransmitters to increase PIF release and this results in reduced release of prolactin. Evidence supporting this hypothesis has also been derived from human studies. Administration of levodopa was shown to suppress prolactin secretion in patients with galactorrhoea (Malarkey, Jacobs and Daughaday, 1971; Turkington, 1971).

Horn and Snyder (1971) suggested that the neuroleptic activity of chlorpromazine might be due to its ability to fit the dopamine receptor. This is presumably due to the conformational similarities between the two compounds. The ability to block the effects of dopamine at the receptor site appears to be greater than the ability to block at the norepinephrine receptor (Carlsson and Lindquist, 1963; Nyback and Sedvall, 1968; Anden et al., 1970). Pimozide, a very potent neuroleptic drug, can block the action of dopamine at its receptor without exerting an appreciable effect on the interaction between norepinephrine and its receptor (Janssen et al., 1968). As a norepinephrine antagonist, it is about 63 to 364 times less potent than chlorpromazine. The following study was performed to test the effects of these drugs on prolactin secretion (Clemens et al., unpublished): adult female rats were ovariectomized and on the tenth day after ovariectomy they were treated with chlorpromazine, 9·2 mg/kg; pimozide, 2·5 mg/kg; disulfiram (an inhibitor of norepinephrine synthesis), 200 mg/kg; and d1-2,3-dichloro-α-methyl benzylamine HCl (an inhibitor of epinephrine synthesis), 30 mg/kg.

Table 8.2 shows the results of this study. The epinephrine inhibitor did not influence prolactin levels. This is suggestive of little or no participation by epinephrine in the inhibition of prolactin secretion. Both agents that theoretically block the dopamine-receptor interaction (chlorpromazine and pimozide) significantly stimulated prolactin secretion. The potency of these compounds as norepinephrine antagonists had no relationship to their ability

TABLE 8.2

Effects of Several Drugs on Prolactin Release in Ovariectomized Rats

| Treatment | No. of rats | Prolactin* levels (ng/ml) |
|---|---|---|
| Controls, saline treated | 10 | 13·1 ± 1·1 |
| Chlorpromazine, 9·2 mg/kg | 10 | 75·2 ± 2·2 |
| Pimozide, 2·5 mg/kg | 10 | 62·2 ± 3·9† |
| Disulfiram, 200 mg/kg | 10 | 7·0 ± 0·9‡ |
| d1-2,3-dichloro-α-methylbenzylamine HCl, 30 mg/kg | 8 | 10·5 ± 1·2 |

After Clemens et al., unpublished.
* Expressed as ng NIAMD-prolactin-RP-1 per ml.
† $p < 0.0001$, treated vs. control using Student's t test.
‡ $p < 0.001$.

to stimulate prolactin. These results provide strong support for the view that dopaminergic neurons tonically stimulate PIF secretion, and that this tonic stimulation of PIF is not a non-specific alpha-adrenergic phenomenon. In addition, it is possible that norepinephrine is stimulatory to prolactin secretion under normal conditions, since disulfiram caused a significant inhibition of prolactin release. This is in agreement with the results recently reported by Donoso et al. (1971).

### Other biogenic amines

Apparently there are indolamines that are capable of exerting a stimulatory influence on prolactin secretion. Kamberi, Mical and Porter (1971) showed that a single injection of serotonin or melatonin into the third ventricle of rats elevated serum prolactin concentration. Systemic administration of serotonin had no definite effect on serum prolactin levels (Lu et al., 1970), but injection of tryptophan and 5-hydroxytryptophane (precursors of serotonin) produced significant elevations of serum prolactin (Lu and Meites, unpublished). Hypothalamic serotonin and catecholamines appear to act in opposition on prolactin release. The diurnal changes mentioned previously with regard to prolactin levels may be the result of the net change in activity of serotonergic and catecholaminergic nervous transmission. It is noteworthy that the effects of indolamines and catecholamines on LH and FSH are opposite to their effects on prolactin (Kamberi, Mical and Porter, 1970, 1971). The involvement of cholinergic fibres in the hypothalamic inhibition of prolactin secretion was suggested by Gala, Markariah and O'Neill (1970). They found that implantation of atropine into the hypothalamus induced deciduomata formation in rats. The influence of other biogenic amines in the hypothalamus on PIF and prolactin release remain to be investigated.

## NEGATIVE FEEDBACK OF PROLACTIN ON PROLACTIN SECRETION

### Effects of prolactin implantation into the median eminence

Perhaps the principal endocrine inhibitory mechanism for controlling prolactin secretion is the feedback of prolactin upon its own secretion. The negative feedback of prolactin was demonstrated by showing that implantation of small amounts of prolactin into the median eminence of mature intact and ovariectomized rats resulted in increased hypothalamic PIF content and reduced pituitary weight and prolactin concentration (Clemens and Meites, 1968) (Table 8.3). In addition, the prolactin implants produced marked mammary gland regression. A similar reduction in pituitary prolactin levels after median eminence prolactin implants was observed by Mishkinsky, Nir

TABLE 8.3

Effects of a Prolactin Implant into the Median Eminence on Pituitary Prolactin Concentration and Hypothalamic PIF Content

| Treatment | AP*<br>Weight (mg) | AP prolactin<br>concentration<br>(i.u./100 mg) | PIF content<br>(AP prolactin<br>released in vitro) |
|---|---|---|---|
| Intact controls (13) | 8·1 ± 0·2 | 2·36 ± 0·50 | 1·77 ± 0·30 |
| Intact prolactin-implanted (10) | 6·2 ± 0·4 | 1·32 ± 0·20 | 0·81 ± 0·14 |
| OVX† controls (6) | 11·3 ± 0·6 | 3·31 ± 0·23 | 1·09 ± 0·40 |
| OVX, prolactin-implanted (6) | 9·05 ± 0·5 | 2·35 ± 0·56 | 0·32 ± 0·15 |

After Clemens and Meites (1968).
* AP = anterior pituitary.
† OVX = ovariectomy, ( ) = number of rats.

and Sulman (1969). Human growth hormone, which has some intrinsic prolactin activity, also was shown to decrease serum prolactin levels when implanted into the median eminence of female rats (Voogt et al., 1971).

The importance of the so-called 'short loop' feedback is emphasized by observations that prolactin implants in the median eminence can block every physiological process known to be dependent on prolactin. It has been demonstrated that prolactin implants can inhibit pseudo-pregnancy (Chen et al., 1970), pregnancy (Clemens, Sar and Meites, 1969a) and lactation (Clemens, Sar and Meites, 1969b). Spies and Clegg (1971) suggested that prolactin may be capable of inhibiting its own secretion by acting directly on the pituitary. However, Nicoll (1971) concluded on the basis of *in vitro* experiments that prolactin does not act directly on the pituitary to inhibit its own secretion, and additional results of Sud and Meites (unpublished) are in agreement with those of Nicoll (1971).

An interesting relationship exists between the 'short loop' feedback of prolactin and the secretion of LH and FSH. An example of this is the advancement of puberty in rats by prolactin implants in the median eminence or by injections of prolactin (Clemens et al. 1969). Voogt, Clemens and Meites (1969) reported that implants of prolactin in the median eminence evoked a highly significant release of FSH. More recently, Voogt and Meites (1971) demonstrated that an implant of prolactin in the median eminence of pseudo-pregnant rats approximately doubled the serum levels of LH and FSH (Table 8.3). It therefore appears probable that the main inhibitory controlling mechanism on pituitary prolactin secretion is the internal feedback by prolactin.

Apparently prolactin inhibits its own secretion by acting on hypothalamic catecholamines (Fuxe and Hökfelt, 1970). They demonstrated that prolactin injections into rats markedly activated the tubero-infundibular dopaminergic neuron system. Apparently prolactin acts *via* the hypothalamus to increase dopaminergic neuron activity, resulting in increased release of PIF into the portal vessels and inhibition of prolactin release.

## Effects of pituitary grafts, prolactin secreting pituitary tumours and injections of prolactin on prolactin secretion by the *in situ* pituitary

Other evidence for a 'short loop' feedback for the control of prolactin secretion is that prolactin and growth hormone secreting pituitary tumours are able to reduce the prolactin content in the *in situ* pituitary (MacLeod, Smith and DeWitt, 1966; Chen, Minaguchi and Meites, 1967). Chen, Minaguchi and Meites (1967) also found more PIF in the hypothalamus of rats bearing pituitary tumour transplants.

Daily injection of 1 or 10 mg of NIH-P-S7 prolactin markedly reduced pituitary weight and prolactin concentration in adult female rats (Sinha and Tucker, 1968). Multiple pituitary grafts under the kidney capsule for two weeks lowered pituitary weight and prolactin concentration of the *in situ* pituitary in intact and overiectomized rats (Sinha and Tucker, 1968). In contrast, long-term pituitary grafts (two months) decreased pituitary prolactin content and concentration but did not change hypothalamic PIF content in ovariectomized rats (Welsch, Negro-Villar and Meites, 1968).

Prolactin secretion is also inhibited by pituitary grafts placed in the hypothalamus (Averill, 1969). Many of the grafts were distant from the median eminence and portal vessels, and the grafts themselves did not produce luteotropic effects similar to grafts placed underneath the kidney capsule. This is strongly indicative of a local feedback between the graft and neural tissue that produces PIF.

## DIRECT EFFECTS OF DRUGS AND HORMONES ON PROLACTIN SECRETION

Many ergot drugs are capable of exerting strong inhibitory influences on prolactin secretion. Incubation of rat anterior pituitary with ergocornine for a period of 12 hours resulted in marked inhibition of prolactin release and accumulation of prolactin in the pituitary (Lu and Meites, 1971). Ergocornine also prevented an increase in prolactin release when oestradiol was placed into the incubation medium. Injections of ergocornine into rats also partially or completely inhibited stimulation of prolactin release by oestrogen and prevented enlargement of the pituitary. In addition to its direct action on the pituitary, ergocornine was shown to increase hypothalamic PIF activity in rats (Wuttke et al., 1971), indicating that it acts both *via* the hypothalamus and directly on the pituitary to depress prolactin secretion.

A number of different ergot alkaloids were shown to inhibit prolactin secretion, as evidenced by inhibition of lactation and lowered serum prolactin levels (Shaar and Clemens, 1972) (Table 8.4). Lactational performance of the female rats was assessed by litter weight gains. Most of the ergot alkaloids markedly suppressed lactation as indicated by loss of litter weight when compared with the litters of the control group. All treated rats exhibited lowered serum prolactin levels. Lutterbeck et al. (1971) and Wenner and Varga (1972) reported that 2-Br-alpha-ergocryptine treatment terminated galactorrhoea in women. Their study provides evidence that ergots can inhibit prolactin secretion in humans.

TABLE 8.4

Effects of Various Ergot Alkaloids on Mother Body Weight, Litter Weight and Serum Prolactin Levels of Post-partum Lactating Female Rats

| Group and treatment | No. of animals | Mean net body weight gain (g) | Mean net litter weight gain (g) | Mean serum prolactin levels (ng/ml) |
|---|---|---|---|---|
| I. Control—corn oil 0·1 mg/day | 16 | $+12.7 \pm 1.8$ | $+50.3 \pm 2.5$* | $56.3 \pm 6.9$ |
| II. 0·5 mg ergocornine hydrogenmalienate | 8 | $-3.8 \pm 2.7$† | $-2.3 \pm 8.0$† | $11.6 \pm 2.6$† |
| III. 1·0 mg ergocornine hydrogenmalienate | 8 | $-13.4 \pm 4.2$† | $-9.2 \pm 3.3$† | $12.4 \pm 2.6$† |
| IV. 4·0 mg ergonovine maleate | 8 | $-4.8 \pm 4.1$† | $+20.8 \pm 4.3$† | $15.3 \pm 1.7$† |
| V. 1·0 mg dihydro-ergocornine | 8 | $-6.0 \pm 2.5$† | $-4.0 \pm 7.3$† | $12.9 \pm 3.1$† |
| VI. 4·0 mg ergotamine tartrate | 9 | $-9.1 \pm 4.7$† | $-4.7 \pm 6.9$† | $28.4 \pm 8.3$‡ |
| VII. 0·5 mg ergocryptine | 6 | $-22.8 \pm 4.5$† | $-10.7 \pm 4.9$† | $13.2 \pm 7.3$† |

* Mean ± SE.
† Significantly different from control value (P < 0·001).
‡ Significantly different from control value (P < 0·02),

A few hormones have direct stimulatory effects on prolactin release. Of these, oestradiol appears to be the most effective. Oestrogen stimulates prolactin secretion by anterior pituitary grafts placed beneath the kidney capsule in hypophysectomized rats (Desclin, 1954; Chen et al., 1970). Thyroxine and triiodothyronine also can increase prolactin release from the rat anterior pituitary *in vitro* (Nicoll and Meites, 1963).

## SUMMARY

The primary influence of the hypothalamus on prolactin secretion appears to be inhibitory. Interference with hypothalamic pathways to the anterior pituitary results in augmented prolactin release. The biogenic amines appear to exert an important regulatory influence on hypothalamic PIF secretion. Catecholamines appear to stimulate PIF release, and indolamines to inhibit PIF release into the portal vessels that feed the anterior pituitary. The presence of a PRF in mammals has not yet been definitely established, although there is much circumstantial evidence for its existence. The ability of synthetic TRH to stimulate prolactin release in humans is well established, but its mode of action remains unclear. It remains to be demonstrated that it acts directly on the pituitary or via other mechanisms. The inhibitory action of prolactin on its own secretion appears to be mediated *via* the hypothalamus by increasing dopaminergic and PIF activity. Ergot drugs, catecholamine precursors (particularly 1-dopa), and monoamine oxidase inhibitors are able to inhibit prolactin secretion in a number of species including humans. This work may provide a basis for treatment of endocrine responsive mammary and pituitary tumours, and for inhibiting or increasing breast growth and lactation.

## ACKNOWLEDGMENTS

Work from the laboratory of J. Meites was supported in part by a grant from Eli Lilly and Co., Indianapolis, Indiana, and by NIH research grants AM–4784 and CA–10771.

## REFERENCES

Amenomori, Y. and Meites, J. (1970). 'Effect of a hypothalamic extract on serum prolactin levels during the estrous cycle and lactation.' *Proc. Soc. expl Biol. Med.* **134**, 492.

Anden, N. E., Butcher, S. G., Carrodi, H., Fuxe, K. and Ungerstadt, U. (1970). 'Receptor activity and turnover of dopamine and noradrenaline after neuroleptics.' *Europ. J. Pharmac.* **11**, 303.

Averill, R. L. W. (1969). 'Failure of luteotrophic function due to pituitary grafts in the rat hypothalamus.' *Neuroendocrinology* **5**, 121.

Benson, G. K., and Folley, S. J. (1956). 'Oxytocin as stimulator for the release of prolactin from the anterior pituitary.' *Nature, Lond.* **177**, 700.

Bowers, C. Y., Friesen, H. G. and Folkers, K. (1972). 'On the mechanism of the TRH-induced prolactin release.' *Clin. Res.* **20**, 71.

Brodie, B. B., Spector, S. and Shore, P. A. (1959). 'Interaction of drugs with norepinephrine in the brain.' *Pharmac. Rev.* **11**, 548.

Butcher, R. L., Fugo, N. W. and Collins, W. E. (1972). 'Semi-circadian rhythm in plasma levels of prolactin during early gestation in the rat.' *Endocrinology* **90**, 1125.

Carlsson, A and Lindquist, M. (1963). 'Effect of chlorpromazine or haloperidol on formation of 3-methoxytyramine and normetanephrine in mouse brain.' *Acta pharmac. toxicol.* **20**, 140.

— Dahlström, A., Fuxe, K. and Hillarp, N. (1965). 'Failure of reserpine to deplete noradrenaline neurons of α-methylnoradrenaline formed from α-methyl dopa.' *Acta pharmac. toxicol.* **22**, 270.

Chen, C. L., Amenomori, Y., Lu, K. H., Voogt, J. L. and Meites, J. (1970). 'Serum prolactin levels in rats with pituitary transplants or hypothalamic lesions.' *Neuroendocrinology* **6**, 220.

— and Meites, J. (1969). 'Effects of thyroxine and thiouracil on hypothalamic PIF and pituitary prolactin levels.' *Proc. Soc. Exp. Biol. Med.* **131**, 576.

— Minaguchi, H. and Meites, J. (1967). 'Effects of transplanted pituitary tumors on host pituitary prolactin secretion.' *Proc. Soc. expl Biol. Med.* **126**, 317.

Clemens, J. A. and Meites, J. (1968). 'Inhibition by hypothalamic prolactin implants of prolactin secretion, mammary growth and luteal function.' *Endocrinology* **82**, 876.

— — (1971). 'Neuroendocrine status of old constant-estrous rats.' *Neuroendocrinology* **7**, 249.

— Sar, M. and Meites, J. (1969a). 'Inhibition of lactation and luteal function in postpartum rats by hypothalamic implantation of prolactin.' *Endocrinology* **84**, 868.

— — — (1969b). 'Termination of pregnancy in rats by a prolactin implant in the median eminence.' *Proc. Soc. expl Biol. Med.* **130**, 628.

— Minaguchi, H., Storey, R. and Meites, J. (1969). 'Advancement of puberty in rats by prolactin injections and hypothalamic prolactin implants.' *Neuroendocrinology* **4**, 150.

Coppola, J. A. (1968). 'The apparent involvement of the sympathetic nervous system in the gonadotrophin secretion of female rats.' *J. Reprod. Fertil.* Suppl. **4**, 35.

DeVoe, W. F., Ramirez, V. D. and McCann, S. M. (1966). 'Induction of mammary secretion by hypothalamic lesions in male rats.' *Endocrinology* **78**, 158.

Desclin, L. (1954). 'Apropos du mécanisme d'action des oestrogènes sur le lobe antérieur de l'hypophyse chez le rat.' *Annls Endocr.* **11**, 656.

Donoso, A. O., Bishop, W., Fawcett, C. P., Krulich, L., and McCann, S. M. (1971). 'Effects of drugs that modify brain monoamine concentrations on plasma gonadotropin and prolactin levels in the rat.' *Endocrinology* **89**, 774.

Dunn, J. D., Arimura, A. and Scheving, L. E. (1972). 'Effect of stress on circadian periodicity in serum LH and prolactin concentration.' *Endocrinology* **90**, 29.

Everett, J. W. (1954). 'Luteotrophic function of autografts of the rat hypophysis.' *Endocrinology* **54**, 685.

— and Quinn, D. L. (1966). 'Differential hypothalamic mechanisms inciting ovulation and pseudopregnancy in the rat.' *Endocrinology* **78**, 141.

Freeman, M. E. and Neill, J. D. (1972). 'The pattern of prolactin secretion during pseudopregnancy in the rat: A daily nocturnal surge.' *Endocrinology* **90**, 1292.

Fuxe, K. (1964). 'Cellular localization of monoamines in the median eminence and the infundibular stem of some mammals.' *A. Zellforsch.* **61**, 710.

— and Hökfelt, T. (1969). 'Catecholamines in the hypothalamus and the pituitary gland.' In *Frontiers in Neuroendocrinology*, pp. 47–96, Ed. by W. F. Ganong and L. Martini. New York and London; Oxford University Press.

— — (1970). 'Central monoaminergic systems and hypothalamic function.' In *The Hypothalamus*, p. 123, Ed. by L. Martini, M. Mota and F. Fraschini. New York; Academic Press.

Gala, R. R., Markarian, P. B. and O'Neill (1970). 'The influence of neural blocking agents implanted into the hypothalamus of the rat on induced deciduomata formation.' *Life Sci.* **9**, 1055.

# REFERENCES

Greenwood, F. (1971). *Lactogenic Hormones,* pp. 197–206. Ciba Foundation Symposium.

Grosz, H. J. and Rothballer, A. B. (1961). 'Hypothalamic control of lactogenic function in the cat.' *Nature, Lond.* **190,** 349.

Halasz, B. (1962). 'Hypophysiotropic area in the hypothalamus.' *J. Endocr.,* **25,** 147.

Haun, C. K. and Sawyer, C. H. (1960). 'Initiation of lactation in rabbits following placement of hypothalamic lesions.' *Endocrinology* **67,** 270.

Horn, A. S. and Snyder, S. (1971). 'Chlorpromazine and dopamine: Conformational similarities that correlate with antischizophrenic activity of phenothiazine drugs.' *Proc. natn Acad. Sci. U.S.A.* **68,** 2325.

Hwang, P., Guyda, H. and Friesen, H. (1971). 'Human prolactin (HPr): Purification and clinical studies.' *Clin. Res.* **19,** 772.

Jacobs, L. S., Snyder, P., Wilber, J., Utiger, R. and Daughaday, W. (1971). 'Increased serum prolactin after administration of synthetic thyrotrophin releasing hormone.' *J. clin. Endocrin.* **33,** 996.

Janssen, P. A. J., Niemegeers, C. J. E., Schellekens, K. H. L., Dresse, A., Lenaerts, F. M., Pinchard, A., Schaper, W. K. A., Van Nueten, J. M. and Verbruggen, F. J. (1968). 'Pimozide, a chemically novel, highly potent and orally long-acting neuroleptic drug.' *Arzneimittel Forschung* **3,** 261.

Kambari, I. A., Mical, R. S. and Porter, J. C. (1970). 'Effect of anterior pituitary perfusion and intraventricular injection of catecholamines and indoleamines on LH release.' *Endocrinology* **87,** 1.

— — — (1971). 'Effects of melatonin and serotonin on the release of FSH and prolactin.' *Endocrinology* **88,** 1288.

Koch, Y., Chou, Y. F. and Meites, J. (1971). 'Metabolic clearance and secretion rates of prolactin in the rat.' *Endocrinology* **89,** 1303.

Kordon, C. (1966). Thesis, University of Paris.

Kragt, C. L. and Meites, J. (1965). 'Stimulation of pigeon pituitary prolactin release by pigeon hypothalamic extract *in vitro.*' *Endocrinology* **76,** 1169.

Krulich, L., Quijada, M. and Illner, P. (1971). 'Localization of prolactin-inhibiting factor (PIF), p-releasing factor (PRF), growth hormone-RF (GRF) and GIF activities in the hypothalamus of the rat.' Proceedings of the 53rd Meeting, Endocrine Society, P. A-83, San Francisco.

Lu, K. H. and Meites, J. (1971). 'Inhibition by L-dopa and monoamine oxidase inhibitors of pituitary prolactin release; stimulation by methyldopa and d-amphetamine.' *Proc. Soc. expl Biol. Med.* **137,** 480.

— Amenomori, Y., Chen, C. L. and Meites, J. (1970). 'Effects of central acting drugs on serum and pituitary prolactin levels in rats.' *Endocrinology* **87,** 667.

— Koch, Y. and Meites, J. (1971). 'Direct inhibition by ergocornine of pituitary prolactin release.' *Endocrinology* **89,** 229.

Lutterbeck, P. M., Pryor, J. S., Varga, L. and Wenner, R. (1971). 'Treatment of non-puerperal galactorrhea with an ergot.' *Br. Med. J.* **3,** 228.

MacLeod, R. M. (1969). 'Influence of norepinephrine and catecholamine-depelting agents on the synthesis and release of prolactin and growth hormone.' *Endocrinology* **85,** 916.

— Smith, M. C. and DeWitt, G. W. (1966). 'Hormonal properties of transplanted pituitary tumors and their relation to the pituitary gland.' *Endocrinology* **79,** 1149.

Malarkey, W. B., Jacobs, L. S. and Daughaday, W. H. (1971). 'Levodopa suppression of prolactin secretion in non-puerperal galactorrhea.' *New Engl. J. Med.* **285**, 1160.

Meites, J. (1963). 'Pharmacological control of prolactin secretion and lactation.' In *Pharmacological Control of Release of Hormones Including Antidiabetic Drugs* (Proceedings of First International Pharmacological Meeting), Vol. 1, pp. 151–181, Ed. by R. Guillemin and P. Lindgren. New York; Pergamon Press.

— (1966). 'Control of mammary growth and lactation.' In *Neuroendocrinology*, Vol. 1, pp. 664–708, Ed. by L. Martini and W. F. Ganong. New York; Academic Press.

— (1967). 'Control of prolactin secretion.' *Archs Anat. Microscop. Morphol. Exp.* **56**, Suppl. 3–4, 516.

— (Ed.) (1970). 'Direct studies of the secretion of the hypothalamic hypophysiotropic hormones.' In *Hypophysiotropic Hormones of the Hypothalamus*, pp. 261–281. Baltimore; Williams and Wilkins.

— and Clemens, J. A. (1972). 'Hypothalamic control of prolactin secretion.' *Vitamins and Hormones* **30**, 165.

— and Nicoll, C. S. (1966). 'Adenohypophysis: prolactin.' *Ann. Rev. Physiol.* **28**, 57.

— — and Talwalker, P. K. (1961). Symposium on Neuroendocrinology, Miami, Florida.

— Lu, K. H., Wuttke, W., Welsch, C. W., Nagasawa, H. and Quadri, S. K. (1972). 'Hypothalamic control of prolactin secretion.' *Recent Progr. Hormone Res.* **28**, 471.

— — — (1963). 'The central nervous system and secretion and release of prolactin.' In *Advances in Neuroendocrinology*, pp. 238-277, Ed. by A. V. Nalbandov. Urbana, Ill.; University of Illinois Press.

— Talwalker, P. K. and Nicoll, C. S. (1960). 'Initiation of lactation in rats with hypothalamic or cerebral tissue.' *Proc. Soc. expl Biol. Med.* **103**, 298.

Mena, F. and Beyer, C. (1968). 'Induction of milk secretion in the rabbit by lesions in the temporal lobe.' *Endocrinology* **83**, 618.

Mishkinsky, J., Khazan, K. and Sulman, F. G. (1968). 'Prolactin releasing activity of the hypothalamus of postpartum rats.' *Endocrinology* **82**, 611.

— Nir, I. and Sulman, F. G. (1969). 'Internal feedback of prolactin in the rat.' *Neuroendocrinology* **5**, 48.

Mizuno, H., Talwalker, P. K. and Meites, J. (1964). 'Inhibition of mammary secretion in rats by iproniazid.' *Proc. Soc. expl Biol. Med.* **115**, 604.

Nicoll, C. S. (1971). 'Aspects of the neural control of prolactin secretion.' In *Frontiers in Neuroendocrinology*, pp. 291-330, Ed. by L. Martini and W. F. Ganong. Oxford University Press.

— and Meites, J. (1963). 'Prolactin secretion *in vitro: effects of thyroid hormones and insulin.' J. Endocr.* **72**, 544.

— Fiorindo, R. P., McKenee, C. T. and Parsons, J. A. (1970). 'Assay of hypothalamic factors which regulate prolactin secretion.' In *Hypophysiotropic Hormones of the Hypothalamus: Assay and Chemistry*, pp. 115–144, Ed. by J. Meites. Baltimore; Williams and Wilkins.

Nyback, H. and Sedvall, G. (1968). 'Effect of chlorpromazine on accumulation and disappearance of catecholamines formed from tyrosine-$C^{14}$ in brain.' *J. Pharmac. exp. Ther.* **162**, 294.

Pasteels, J. L. (1961). 'Sécrétion de prolactine par l'hypophyse en culture de tissus.' *Compt. Rend. Soc. Biol.* **253**, 2140.

Ratner, A., Talwalker, P., and Meites, J. (1965). 'Effect of reserpine on prolactin-inhibiting, activity of the rat hypothalamus.' *Endocrinology,* **77**, 315.

Rubenstein, L. and Sawyer, C. H. (1969). 'Changes in electrical activity of the rat hippocampus correlated with the initiation of pseudopregnancy.' Program of Fifty-First Meeting of Endocrine Society, p. 86.

Schally, A. V., Kastin, A. J., Lock, W. and Bowers, C. Y. (1967). In *Hormones in the Blood,* p. 492, Ed. by C. H. Gray and H. L. Bacharach. New York; Academic Press.

Schneider, H. P. G. and McCann, S. M. (1970). 'Mono- and indolamines and control of LH secretion.' *Endocrinology* **86**, 1127.

Shaar, C. J. and Clemens, J. (1972). 'Inhibition of lactation and prolactin secretion in rats by ergot alkaloids.' *Endocrinology* **90**, 285.

Sinha, Y. N. and Tucker, H. A. (1968). 'Pituitary prolactin content and mammary development after chronic administration of prolactin.' *Proc. Soc. expl Biol. Med.* **128**, 84.

Spies, H. G. and Clegg, M. T. (1971). 'Pituitary as a possible site of prolactin feedback in autoregulation.' *Neuroendocrinology* **8**, 205.

Talwalker, P. K., Ratner, A. and Meites, J. (1963). '*In vitro* inhibition of pituitary prolactin synthesis and release by hypothalamic extract.' *Am. J. Physiol.* **205**, 213.

Tashjian, A. H., Barowsky, N. J. and Jensen, D. K. (1971). 'Thyrotropin releasing hormone: Direct evidence for stimulation of prolactin production by pituitary cells in culture.' *Biochem. Biophys. Res. Commun.* **43**, 516.

Tindal, J. S., Knaggs, G. S. and Turvey, A. (1967). 'Central nervous control of prolactin secretion in the rabbit: Effect of local estrogen implants in the amygdaloid complex.' *J. Endocr.* **37**, 279.

— — (1969). 'An ascending pathway for release of prolactin in the brain of the rabbit.' *J. Endocr.* **45**, 111.

— — (1970). 'Release of prolactin in the rabbit after electrical stimulation of the forebrain.' *J. Endocr.* **48**, xxxii.

Turkington, R. W. (1971). 'Inhibition of prolactin secretion and successful therapy of the Forbes-Albright syndrome with L-Dopa.' *J. Lab. Clin. Med.* **78**, 824.

Vogt, M. (1954). 'The concentration of sympathin in different parts of the central nervous system under normal conditions and after the administration of drugs.' *J. Physiol.* **123**, 451.

Voogt, J. L., Chen, C. L. and Meites, J. (1970). 'Serum and pituitary prolactin levels before, during, and after puberty in female rats.' *Am. J. Physiol.* **218**, 396.

— and Meites, J. (1971). 'Effects of an implant of prolactin in median eminence of pseudopregnant rats on serum and pituitary LH, FSH and prolactin.' *Endocrinology* **88**, 286.

— Clemens, J. A. and Meites, J. (1969). 'Stimulation of pituitary FSH release in immature female rats by prolactin implant in the median eminence.' *Neuroendocrinology* **4**, 157.

— — Negro-Vilar, A., Welsch, C. and Meites, J. (1971). 'Pituitary GH and hypothalamic GHRF after median eminence implantation of ovine or human GH.' *Endocrinology* **88**, 1363.

Watson, J. T., Krulich, L. and McCann, S. M. (1971). 'Effect of crude rat hypothalamic extract on serum gonadotropin and prolactin levels in normal and orchidectomized male rats.' *Endocrinology* **89**, 1412.

Welsch, C. W., Jenkins, T., Amenomori, Y. and Meites, J. (1971). 'Tumorous development of in situ and grafted anterior pituitaries in female rats treated with diethylstil-besterol'. *Experientia* **27**, 1350.

— Negro-Vilar, A. and Meites, J. (1968). 'Effects of pituitary homografts on host pituitary prolactin and hypothalamic PIF levels'. *Neuroendocrinology* **3**, 238.

Wenner, R. and Varga, L. (1972). 'Prolactinhemmung mittels ergocryptin.' *Acta endocr.* **69**, Suppl. 159, 40.

Wurtman R. J. (1970). 'Brian catecholamines and the control of secretion from the anterior pituitary gland.' In *Hypophysiotropic Hormones of the Hypothalamus*, p. 184, Ed. by J. Meites. Baltimore; Williams and Wilkins.

Wuttke, W. and Meites, J. (1970). 'Effects of ether and pento-barbital on serum prolactin and LH levels in proestrous rats'. *Proc. Soc. expl Biol. Med.* **135**, 648.

— Cassell, E. and Meites, J. (1971). 'Effects of ergocornine on serum prolactin and LH, and on hypothalamic content of PIF and LRF.' *Endocrinology*, **88**, 737.

# 9

# Assay of Human Prolactin and Factors Affecting its Serum Concentrations

## P. Hwang, H. G. Friesen and H. J. Guyda

## INTRODUCTION

Prolactin, a pituitary hormone which is necessary for normal lactation, was first identified in 1928 (Striker and Grueter). Since then, extensive studies have been carried out on the chemistry and physiology of the hormone in several subprimate species (Apostolakis, 1968). Knowledge on human prolactin lagged behind, mainly because attempts to isolate it from human pituitary glands have been unsuccessful (Lyons et al., 1968). Indeed it was only very recently that the existence of this hormone in man has been firmly established by a number of immunological and histochemical studies, confirming conclusions drawn from clinical observations made earlier. The evidence has been recently summarized by Sherwood (1971).

This development has opened up questions on the physiological function of prolactin in man and studies in this direction have progressed fairly rapidly following the development of specific and sensitive bio- and radio-immunoassay for human prolactin by several groups of investigators (Kleinberg and Frantz, 1971; Forsyth and Myers, 1971; Loewenstein et al., 1971; Turkington, 1971; Bryant et al., 1971; Jacobs, Mariz and Daughaday, 1972; Hwang, Guyda and Friesen, 1971a). Most of the recently accumulated data concerns the measurement of variations in serum prolactin concentrations under different physiological or pathological conditions or after the administration of various drugs.

The physiological function of prolactin in man is still far from clear, and the relationship between prolactin and human breast cancer, if any, remains to be elucidated. Numerous studies have suggested that prolactin may be involved in the development of breast tumours in animals (Furth, 1969; Meites, 1972; Pearson et al., 1969), and that suppression of prolactin secretion could reduce the incidence as well as cause the regression of these tumours (Cassell, Meites and Welsch, 1971; Yanai and Nagasawa, 1971; Quadri and Meites, 1971). With the availability of sensitive and specific assays for human prolactin, parallel studies in relation to human breast carcinoma are being carried out.

## METHODS FOR MEASURING HUMAN SERUM PROLACTIN

In animal studies, prolactin has been quantitated by both biological and immunological procedures and the assays generally employed until recently have been adequately summarized in a recent review (Apostolakis, 1968). At that time, no biological assay was sufficiently sensitive for measuring prolactin concentrations in human biological fluids and no immunoassay could be developed since human prolactin was not available. In the past few years, however, several apparently specific assays with sufficient sensitivity for measuring serum prolactin concentrations in man have been reported.

### Biological assays

The currently available bioassays which appear suitable for measuring human serum prolactin concentrations are all based on the *in vitro* incubation of mammary tissue explants obtained from pregnant or pseudo-pregnant mice or rabbits. When such breast tissue slices are incubated in the presence of prolactin, certain morphological and biochemical changes occur; the magnitude of these changes appears to be quantitatively related to the concentrations of prolactin in the incubation media.

Kleinberg and Frantz (1971) and Forsyth and Myers (1971) showed that the secretory changes observed in histological sections of the explants after incubation, when graded on a $1+$ to $4+$ scale, give a fairly reliable semi-quantitative estimate of the prolactin concentration. Loewenstein et al. (1971) and Turkington (1971), instead of histological criteria, employed as end points the increases in synthesis of N-acetyl-lactosamine and casein respectively.

In these four bioassays, it was found that, with sheep prolactin as standard, a satisfactory dose–response curve could be obtained, with the lower limit of detectability between 2 and 50 ng/ml. Precision of these assays is low, but with multiple assays variation is usually within a two fold range and may be as low as $\pm 10$ per cent. In all these bioassay systems, human growth hormone (HGH) and human chorionic somatomammotrophin (HCS) give positive responses and would interfere with the assay if present in significant amounts unless neutralized by their specific antisera. The major drawback of these procedures would appear to be the enormous labour involved in assaying multiple samples.

## Radioimmunoassays

Radioimmunoassays have been widely employed in the measurement of peptide hormones in the past decade. The great sensitivity, specificity and simplicity represent major advantages over bioassays. The principles and methods of radioimmunoassays are well discussed by Berson and Yalow (1964). The failure to purify human prolactin has been the major stumbling block in the development of a satisfactory immunoassay for this hormone. Attempts have therefore been made to measure human prolactin by immune systems in which the radioactive tracer used is thought to be immunologically related to human prolactin.

Jacobs, Mariz and Daughaday (1972) and Midgley (1971), employing pork or sheep prolactin tracer and antisera to sheep prolactin, detected increased concentrations of immunoreactive material in human sera which appeared to be prolactin. Bryant et al. (1971) described a preliminary and crude assay using human foetal pituitary tissue culture media as a source of prolactin. It had cross-reactivity with both HGH and HCS but appeared capable of detecting prolactin immunoreactivity in the small number of cases studied.

In our laboratory, monkey prolactin, purified from incubates of pregnant monkey pituitary glands (Guyda and Friesen, 1971) was originally employed as the antigen in the assay (Hwang, Guyda and Friesen, 1971a). Subsequently with the purification of human prolactin (Hwang, Guyda and Friesen, 1972) a completely homologous system was developed. HGH and HCS showed no significant cross-reaction in the assay. The sensitivity is satisfactory for measuring prolactin concentrations in serum without pre-treatment.

## Radioreceptor assays

A radioreceptor assay utilizing membrane receptors derived from mid-pregnant mouse mammary tissue has been reported (Frantz and Turkington, 1972). In our laboratory we have used mammary glands obtained from mid-pregnant rabbits treated with cortisone acetate and HCS for four days (Shiu and Friesen, unpublished observation). With this assay we have been able to detect a concentration of 5 ng/ml of prolactin in a 90-minute assay. Several other lactogenic hormones which inhibit binding of labelled human prolactin to the tissue receptors are HGH and HCS as well as some animal prolactins. The great advantage of this method is that assay results could be obtained very rapidly. The receptor preparation is stable for at least several weeks in the frozen state and large amounts of tissue can be obtained from a single animal. It is probable that this form of assay will replace the more tedious bioassays to a large extent.

When comparing bioassays, receptor assays and radioimmunoassays, several important factors require consideration: specificity, sensitivity, reproducibility, and cost and ease with which assays can be performed. It is clear that bioassays are not specific for human prolactin, but measure several lactogenic substances including HGH. The sensitivity of the radio-immunoassays and radioreceptors are very similar and significantly greater than that of most bioassays. The precision and reproducibility of radio-immunoassays are generally considerably better than bioassays.

The chief advantage of radioimmunoassays is the facility with which large numbers of samples can be assayed, and the major drawback of the method is that immunoreactivity of a hormone may not correlate with its biological activity. For example, prolactin may be inactivated in serum and any biologically inert breakdown products which are formed could still cross-react in an immunoassay if they contained the antigenic determinants. Fortunately, in the case of prolactin, Frantz and Kleinberg (1972) found extremely good correlation between the results obtained by bioassay and immunoassay in numerous samples.

It is not certain at present whether all the assays that have been developed for measuring human prolactin are measuring the same entity; some discrepancies have appeared when identical samples were assayed by the different groups (unpublished observations). Undoubtedly some of the discrepancies probably result from methodological differences, but real differences may still exist. There is, however, general agreement in many areas and the following is a summary of data which are fairly well established.

## SERUM PROLACTIN CONCENTRATIONS IN THE HUMAN

Since human prolactin is not yet generally available, arbitrary standards have been employed in the assays so far reported, and the concentrations of prolactin in human serum as reported in the literature may require revision now that a human prolactin standard has become available. An interim standard is being distributed by the Medical Research Council of Great Britain.

### Physiological factors affecting serum prolactin

*Age and sex*

Table 9.1 summarizes some of the results obtained in our laboratory. The average concentration in random serum samples of normal men is 5 ng/ml, while that in non-pregnant non-lactating women is 10 ng/ml. It is unusual to observe values above 30 ng/ml in normal adults at rest. In virtually all serum samples, including those from patients with hypopituitarism, prolactin is clearly detectable in our radioimmunoassay. Reports by other investigators that prolactin was undetectable in sera of normal subjects as well as of patients with breast cancer must be viewed with caution as in their assay systems

TABLE 9.1

Serum Prolactin Concentrations in Normal Subjects

| Group | Age | No. | Serum prolactin (ng/ml) Mean ± SEM |
|---|---|---|---|
| Adult ♂ | 16–84 | 26 | 4·9 ± 0·6 |
| Adult ♀ * | 16–84 | 47 | 10·8 ± 0·7 |
| Children† | 1–15 | 48 | 6·5 ± 0·7 |
| Newborn† | at birth | 19 | 257 ± 23·0 |
| | 24 hours | 7 | 192 ± 51·0 |
| | 1–2 weeks | 7 | 84 ± 25·0 |
| | 5–6 weeks | 5 | 20 ± 2·9 |

* Pre- and post-menopausal subjects have similar levels.
† No significant difference was observed between male and female.

serum from normal male subjects was added routinely to the incubation media containing the prolactin standard.

In nine adult females with normal menstruation, serum prolactin was assayed daily throughout the cycles. As can be seen in *Figure 9.1*, no consistent elevation was seen around the time of ovulation (as indicated by the LH peak) or during the luteal phase. In the rat, a sharp rise in serum prolactin was observed in the afternoon on the day of pro-oestrus and this surge has

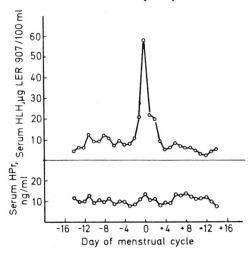

*Figure 9.1. Mean serum prolactin and luteinizing hormone concentrations in nine normal cyclic women*

been shown to be responsible for the regression of the corpora lutea formed during the previous cycle (Wuttke and Meites, 1971). In women, it is unknown what causes the regression of the corpus luteum, but our study would indicate that prolactin is probably not involved. This suggestion is supported by Midgley's (1972) observation that radioautographs failed to show any binding of labelled human prolactin to ovarian tissue, whereas binding by human chorionic gonadotrophin was readily demonstrable.

Insufficient data is available to know whether serum prolactin values in post-menopausal women decrease to male levels. We found no significant difference between pre- and post-menopausal hospital patients but interpretation is difficult as many of these patients were given medication, which might possibly affect prolactin secretion. L'Hermite, Stavric and Robyn (1971) reported lower values for post-menopausal women. This needs to be confirmed.

Serum prolactin concentrations show a diurnal variation, there being an elevation 2–3 hours after the onset of sleep to the early hours of the morning.

In the newborn at birth, serum prolactin concentrations are of the order of about 200 ng/ml. The concentration gradually falls to adult levels at the end of six weeks and thereafter remains fairly constant throughout childhood. Preliminary experiments in monkeys (Tyson, personal communication) indicate that prolactin does not cross the placental barrier readily. The high prolactin concentrations observed in the early neonatal period would therefore suggest that the pituitary gland of the neonate is very active in the synthesis and secretion of this hormone. The significance of this is not clear at present but the intriguing observation of Sinha, Lewis and VanderLaan (1971) that prolactin deficiency in newborn mice was associated with a high mortality and failure to grow suggests that prolactin may serve a critical role in the neonatal period.

It may also be speculated that since animal prolactins have been shown to be important in the regulation of electrolyte balance (Maetz et al., 1968) and to have HGH-like effects (McGarry, Rubinstein and Beck, 1968), human prolactin may conceivably play similar roles during the intra-uterine and early neonatal life in man. In this respect, it is particularly interesting that human amniotic fluid contains extremely high concentrations of prolactin (Hwang, Guyda and Friesen, 1971b) varying between 10 and 100 times those in maternal serum. Obviously the importance of prolactin in human reproduction still requires to be defined, and the various hypotheses could only be tested when human prolactin becomes available for metabolic studies.

### Pregnancy and lactation

*Figure 9.2* shows the results of a study on serum prolactin in over 300 normal females during various periods of pregnancy and the immediate post-partum period. Elevations of serum prolactin were evident as early as eight weeks' gestation, the average concentration in the first trimester being about 30 ng/ml. With advancing pregnancy, serum prolactin concentration progressively increased to a maximum of about 200 ng/ml at term. Post-partum,

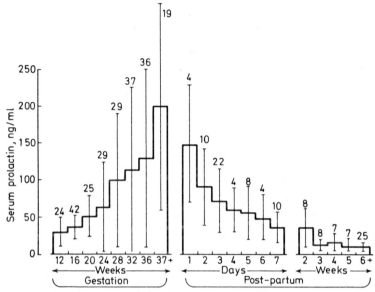

*Figure 9.2. Serum prolactin concentrations during pregnancy and post-partum period. The prolactin concentration is given as mean ± SD. The number of subjects in each group is indicated*

[Reproduced from Hwang, Guyda and Friesen (1971a) by courtesy of the Editor of *Proceedings of the National Academy of Sciences*]

in the absence of breast-feeding, the serum prolactin fell fairly rapidly and by the end of the first week had returned to 30 ng/ml.

There were large variations in prolactin concentration at each stage in pregnancy, particularly in the third trimester where values ranged from 40 to 600 ng/ml. The physiological significance of the progressive rise of serum prolactin during pregnancy remains unknown. In rodents, prolactin is necessary for the maintenance of corpus luteum function in early pregnancy, but thus far there is no evidence that human prolactin is in any way related to corpus luteum function either in early pregnancy or during the menstrual cycle.

It would appear that, whatever function prolactin might serve during pregnancy, it is clearly required for the initiation of post-partum lactation. In a recent study, Del Pozo et al. (1972) demonstrated that a single oral dose of 2-Br-α-ergocryptine, an ergot derivative which has been shown to suppress prolactin secretion specifically (see below), completely inhibited puerperal lactation in four post-partum women.

Suckling is a potent stimulus to prolactin secretion in women: *Figure 9.3* shows the changes in serum prolactin concentrations occurring in nursing

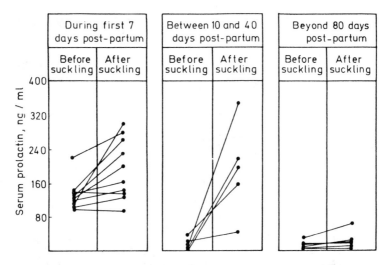

*Figure 9.3. Effect of suckling on serum prolactin concentration during different periods post-partum. Blood was sampled immediately before and 30 minutes after the initiation of breast-feeding*

[Reproduced from Tyson *et al.* (1972) by courtesy of the Editor of *American Journal of Obstetrics and Gynecology*]

mothers 30 minutes after feeding their infants. During the first post-partum week, serum prolactin increased from an average concentration of about 100 ng/ml before nursing to about 200 ng/ml after nursing. Between 10 and 40 days post-partum, the increases were far more dramatic, commonly ranging from 10 to 20 fold above the basal level. However, beyond 80 days, suckling had little or no effect on serum prolactin. These observations would suggest that, while prolactin may be important in the initiation of lactation, it may be less critical for maintenance of lactation especially at later periods, as experiments in cows would indicate (Schams, Reinhardt and Karg, 1972).

## Stress

Vigorous exercise and surgical stress appear to cause modest elevations of serum prolactin in man (Frantz and Kleinberg, 1973). The mechanism is unknown.

## Hypoglycaemia

In normal volunteers, insulin infusion causes significant elevations of serum prolactin, provided the blood glucose falls below 30–40 mg per cent (Frantz and Kleinberg, 1973).

## Pathological conditions associated with abnormal prolactin secretion

To date no distinct clinical entity has been clearly identified with deficient prolactin secretion since the currently available assays are not sufficiently sensitive to define the lower limit of normal serum prolactin concentration. Observations made by Turkington (1972a) and by Tolis et al. (1973) indicate that some patients with hypopituitarism and some mothers with difficulties in nursing may fail to respond to pharmacological agents which normally stimulate prolactin secretion, suggesting diminished pituitary prolactin reserve. Preliminary data in our laboratory would suggest that most patients judged to have hypopituitarism by other criteria have prolactin concentration within the normal range. Much more information is available relating to conditions associated with high serum prolactin levels.

## Hypothalamic–pituitary disorders

Tumours in the hypothalamic–pituitary area constitute one of the commonest causes for hyperprolactinaemia. Indeed, recent observations (D'Amour et al., 1973) indicate that about 20–30 per cent of all functional tumours arising from the pituitary (most commonly chromophobe adenomas) are associated with elevated serum prolactin concentration. It is not yet clear what proportion of these tumours produce excessive amounts of prolactin autonomously and what proportion secrete excess prolactin as a result of interference with the secretion of prolactin-inhibitory factor (PIF) from the hypothalamus.

In our experience, a serum prolactin concentration above 1,000 ng/ml would indicate that a prolactin-producing tumour is probably present. Indeed, such a level should strongly suggest the existence of a pituitary tumour even in the absence of clinical and radiological signs, for, to date, we have observed such high levels only in patients with pituitary tumours. Some but not all such cases were associated with galactorrhoea. Cases of hyperprolactinaemia without galactorrhoea is being recognized as a new clinical syndrome and indicate that prolactin is not sufficient in itself to induce galactorrhoea.

In addition to pituitary tumours, craniopharyngiomas and metastatic carcinomas in the hypothalamic area have been reported to be associated with raised serum prolactin concentration (Turkington, 1972b) presumably by interfering with hypothalamic function. The same mechanism operates when serum prolactin concentrations rise after pituitary stalk section (Turkington, Underwood and Van Wyk, 1971).

Elevated serum prolactin concentrations are also seen in patients with galactorrhoea following contraceptive or sedative medication or from no obvious cause (Hwang, Guyda and Friesen, 1971a) as well as in patients with the Chiari–Frommel syndrome (Turkington, 1972b). In the absence of any demonstrable pathology, such elevations could only be ascribed to functional disturbances in the hypothalamic control of prolactin secretion.

## Hypothyroidism

The clinical observation that hypothyroidism is occasionally associated with galactorrhoea has suggested that prolactin secretion may be abnormally increased in hypothyroid patients. This has been confirmed by Edwards, Forsyth and Besser (1971) in one case. Information is still very scanty and it is impossible to say what percentage of hypothyroid subjects have high serum prolactin concentrations and how frequently is galactorrhoea an associated feature.

## Renal failure

It has been independently observed by Frantz and Kleinberg (1972) and us (Marcovitz and Friesen, 1971) that patients with renal failure often have elevated serum prolactin concentrations. In our series, 15 of 77 patients (i.e. 20 per cent) had abnormally high prolactin (30–600 ng/ml). There was no correlation between the prolactin level and the degree of renal failure as reflected by the blood urea nitrogen. Haemodialysis did not significantly alter the serum prolactin concentration, but successful renal transplantation rapidly brought the level to within the normal range.

The mechanism responsible for elevation of serum prolactin in such patients in unknown. Recalling that sheep prolactin alters sodium excretion in man (Horrobin et al., 1971), this observation suggests that prolactin may be of importance in the regulation of renal function and that the kidneys may be important in feedback regulation of prolactin secretion. Alternatively, the kidneys may be involved in the metabolic breakdown of prolactin.

## Pharmacological agents affecting prolactin secretion

A number of drugs capable of increasing or decreasing serum prolactin concentration in man have been identified. Some of these have already proved to be valuable in the assessment of hypothalamic–pituitary function (Friesen et al., 1972a). Undoubtedly their usefulness would increase if, in future, diseases due primarily to excessive or deficient prolactin secretion could be identified.

*Agents increasing prolactin secretion*

These may act directly on the pituitary or through the hypothalamus. The only agent in this group which clearly has a direct action on the pituitary is thyrotrophic releasing hormone (TRH). This is a tripeptide, pyroglutamyl-histidyl-prolinamide, which has been identified as a physiological hypothalamic factor which causes the release of thyrotrophin (TSH) from the pituitary gland. Tashjian, Barowsky and Jensen (1971) first observed that, in addition to causing TSH release, TRH also increases prolactin secretion when incubated *in vitro* with cultures of pituitary tissue.

Subsequently, extensive studies carried out by Bowers et al. (1971) clearly showed that TRH was also active *in vivo* in man; serum prolactin concentration increased three to six fold 15–30 minutes after the intravenous administration of doses as low as 10 µg. The response appeared to be greater in females than males *(Figure 9.4)*. This sex difference appears to be

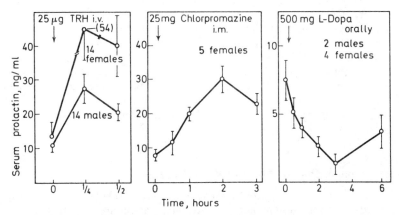

*Figure 9.4. Effect of administration of TRH, chlorpromazine and L-DOPA on serum prolactin in subjects with no endocrine disease. The mean and SE was shown in each case. In the L-DOPA suppression test, there was no significant difference in the responses of males and females*

oestrogen-related since the response of oestrogen-treated males was identical with that of the females. Hypothyroid patients showed the most dramatic response, increases of 10 to 20 fold being observed, whereas in thyrotoxicosis the response to TRH was only minimal. The apparent greater sensitivity of prolactin-producing cells to TRH in hypothyroidism may explain the galactorrhoea and hyperprolactinaemia seen in some cases of hypothyroidism.

Drugs which act via the hypothalamus interfere directly or indirectly with the secretion of prolactin-inhibitory factor (PIF). It is believed that an adrenergic tonus is required for PIF secretion (see Chapter 7) and depletion of catecholamines in the hypothalamus would lead to decreased PIF secretion and hence increased prolactin release. Thus, drugs such as reserpine, chlorpromazine, alpha-methyl-dopa and related drugs which either decrease the concentration or interfere with the action of monoamines in the hypothalamus have been found to raise serum prolactin in animals (Fuxe and Hökfelt, 1969); in man chlorpromazine is the only drug in this group which has been examined adequately and has been found to stimulate prolactin secretion fairly consistently (Kleinberg, Noel and Frantz, 1971). These same drugs have been implicated in the pathogenesis of some cases of galactorrhoea (Sulman, 1970).

Contraceptive medication has also been associated with some cases of galactorrhoea. In such cases, galactorrhoea often occurs soon after withdrawal of contraceptives; the explanation is unclear. The effect of gonadal steroids on prolactin secretion in man has not been adequately studied and reports are conflicting. In both animals (Friesen et al., 1972b) and man (Marcovitz and Friesen, 1971), some anaesthetics have been found to increase serum prolactin.

Up to the present time, only TRH and chlorpromazine have been used to any extent in tests of hypothalamic pituitary function with respect to prolactin secretion. Since TRH acts directly on the pituitary while chlorpromazine acts via the hypothalamus, it is possible to use these two agents to differentiate between hypopituitarism due to pituitary disease and that due to hypothalamic disease; failure to respond to chlorpromazine but not to TRH would localize the disease at the hypothalamic level while failure to respond to both probably means that the pituitary gland is involved.

## Agents that decrease serum prolactin

PIF is the physiologic agent that acts to decrease prolactin secretion. This is discussed in detail in Chapter 8. The chemical nature of PIF is not yet known. The use of PIF as a diagnostic or therapeutic agent must await its chemical synthesis.

At present, studies on the pharmacological suppression of prolactin secretion largely centre on derivatives of ergot and L-DOPA. Various studies have shown that these drugs consistently suppress prolactin secretion in animals (Wuttke and Meites, 1971; Liu and Meites, 1971), and man (Friesen et al., 1972a; Kleinberg, Noel and Frantz, 1971). Ergot alkaloids act on both the hypothalamus and pituitary to reduce serum prolactin (Wuttke, Cassell and Meites, 1971; Nicoll et al., 1970), while L-DOPA is thought to stimulate the release of PIF after being converted to catecholamines in the hypothalamus. Both drugs show promise as therapeutic agents in the symptomatic treatment of galactorrhoea (Friesen et al., 1972a; Malarkey, Jacobs and Daughaday, 1971; Turkington, 1972c; Lutterbeck et al., 1971), and are being tested as possible chemotherapeutic agents for human breast cancer (see below).

*Figure 9.4* shows changes in serum prolactin after administration of TRH, chlorpromazine and L-DOPA to a number of subjects free from endocrine disease in studies carried out in conjunction with Drs. Bowers and Tyson.

Table 9.2 summarizes conditions and pharmacological agents which cause changes in serum prolactin.

TABLE 9.2

Conditions or Agents which Change Serum Prolactin Levels

PHYSIOLOGICAL
    Neonatal period
    Pregnancy
    Suckling
    Stress
    Hypoglycaemia

PATHOLOGICAL
    Hypothalamic–pituitary disorders
      Tumours: primary and secondary
      Pituitary stalk section
      Functional disturbances:
      e.g.:  idiopathic galactorrhoea
            galactorrhoea on withdrawal of contraceptives
            Chiari–Frommel syndrome, etc.
    Hypothyroidism
    Renal failure
    Malignant tumours with ectopic prolactin production

PHARMACOLOGICAL
    Agents increasing serum prolactin
      Thyrotrophin releasing hormone (TRH)
      Catecholamine depleting agents
      Anaesthetics
    Agents decreasing serum prolactin
      Ergot derivatives, e.g. ergocryptine
      L–Dopa.

## Serum prolactin in breast diseases

Although much is known from animal experiments about the effects which prolactin has on breast development and function, there is only scanty information on serum prolactin concentration in human breast diseases. Galactorrhoea is the only condition which has been studied to some extent. More than 50 per cent of the reported cases have serum prolactin concentrations above normal (Frantz and Kleinberg, 1972; Hwang, Guyda and Friesen, 1971a; Turkington, 1971), but the range was extremely wide, varying from within the normal range to several thousand ng/ml.

There was no correlation between the severity of the symptoms and the serum prolactin concentration. The occurrence of galactorrhoea in some patients with prolactin levels in the normal range, and the absence of galactorrhoea in some patients with high serum prolactin concentrations (see above), clearly indicate that multiple factors are involved in galactorrhoea. Gynaecomastia does not appear to be associated with abnormally high serum prolactin (Turkington, 1972d).

Perhaps the most important aspect of prolactin in relation to breast disease is its possible role in the initiation or promotion of breast cancer. There is abundant evidence from experimental work done in rodents that prolactin is probably involved in mammary tumorigenesis (Furth, 1969; Pearson et al., 1969; Meites, 1972). The evidence may be summarized briefly. After the administration of the carcinogenic chemical dimethyl-benzanthracene, prolactin decreases the latent period of the appearance of tumours and increases the incidence and growth rate of the tumours. Increasing endogenous prolactin production with chlorpromazine increases the incidence and growth of the tumours, while lowering serum prolactin with ergot drugs decreases the incidence of both chemically induced and spontaneous mammary tumours.

The role which prolactin might play in human breast cancer is being actively investigated. The report (Turkington, Underwood and Van Wyk, 1971), that prolactin was undetectable in the sera of patients with advanced breast cancer, must be viewed with some scepticism since the assay system employed in that study was so designed that only values above the normal range could be detected. In a limited study in our laboratory, we found that breast cancer patients had essentially normal serum prolactin levels.

It would appear that an abnormally high serum prolactin concentration is not required for the development of breast cancer. Indeed, the available evidence indicates that there is probably no simple relationship between serum prolactin concentration and breast cancer. Hypophysectomy decrease serum prolactin while pituitary stalk section often increases it, yet both are capable of inducing regression of breast cancer. Undoubtedly other factors, such as the gonadal steroids, are involved.

In view of the beneficial effects which result from lowering serum prolactin levels in rodent tumours, studies using L-DOPA and ergocryptine have been started in human subjects with advanced breast cancer. While isolated reports are beginning to appear of objective remissions or subjective improvement induced by the administration of L-DOPA (Stoll, 1972; Minton and Dickey, 1972), the result of a trial on 19 patients with 2-br-α-ergocryptine was negative (European Breast Cancer Group, 1972) even though the doses of drug employed would be expected to lower markedly serum prolactin levels. In summary, the available evidence does not allow us to state unequivocally that prolactin is involved in the genesis or promotion of human breast cancer but it compels us to examine the possibility with the utmost attention.

## SUMMARY

The development of specific and sensitive assays for human prolactin has made it possible to measure serum concentrations of the hormone in man under physiological conditions and to define some of the factors controlling prolactin secretion. It is still premature to propose specific functions for human prolactin but it is now possible to test hypotheses formulated on the basis of animal studies. Particularly intriguing is the question of the function of prolactin during pregnancy and in the newborn. The assays have also provided the means for studying prolactin in relation to disease, especially of the hypothalamic–pituitary axis and of the breast. Already, several pharmacological agents have been found to be useful in the evaluation of hypothalamic pituitary function and in the treatment of abnormal lactation. The crucial question of what role prolactin plays in the development of breast cancer in women remains to be answered.

## ACKNOWLEDGMENTS

We wish to acknowledge the technical assistance of Mrs. J. Halmagyi, Mrs. J. Parodo and Miss Suzanne Peeters, and the secretarial help of Miss Francine Dupuis.

This work was supported by the MRC MA-1862 and USPHS HD-01727. P. Hwang is a recipient of a Fellowship from the Medical Research Council of Canada.

## REFERENCES

Apostolakis, M. (1968). 'Prolactin.' *Vitamins and Hormones* **26**, 197.

Berson, S. A. and Yalow, R. S. (1964). 'Immunossay of protein hormones.' In *The Hormones*, Vol. 4, p. 559, Ed. by G. Pincus, K. U. Thimann and E. B. Astwood. New York; Academic Press.

Bowers, C. Y., Friesen, H. G., Hwang, P., Guyda, H. and Folkers, K. (1971). 'Prolactin and thyrotropin release in man by synthetic pyroglutamyl-histidyl-prolinamide.' *Biochem. Biophys. Res. Commun.* **45**, 1033.

Bryant, G. D., Siler, T. M., Greenwood, F. C., Pasteels, J. L., Robyn, C. and Hubinont, P. O. (1971). 'Radioimmunoassay of a human pituitary prolactin in plasma.' *Hormones* **2**, 139.

Cassell, E. E., Meites, J. and Welsch, C. W. (1971). 'Effects of ergocornine and ergocryptine on growth of 7,12-dimethyl benzanthracine-induced mammary tumors in rats.' *Cancer Res.* **31**, 1051.

D'Amour, P. and Friesen, H. (1973). Unpublished observation.

Del Pozo, E., Brun del Re, R., Varga, L. and Friesen, H. (1972). 'The inhibition of prolactin secretion in man by CB-154 (2 Br-α-ergocryptine).' *J. clin. Endocr.* **35**, 768.

Edwards, C. R. W., Forsyth, I. A. and Besser, G. M. (1971). 'Amenorrhea, galactorrhea, and primary hypothyroidism with high circulating levels of prolactin.' *Br. med. J.* **3**, 462.

European Breast Cancer Group (1972). 'Clinical trial of 2-Br-α-ergocryptine (CB-154) in advanced breast cancer.' *Europ. J. Cancer* **8**, 155.

Forsyth, E. A. and Myers, R. P. (1971). 'Human prolactin: evidence obtained by the bioassay of human plasma.' *J. Endocr.* **51**, 157.

Frantz, A. G. and Kleinberg, D. (1972). *Recent Progr. Hormone Res.* **28**, 527.

Frantz, W. L. and Turkington, K. W. (1972). 'The prolactin receptor: studies on its hormonal binding, chemical and regulatory properties.' *Proceedings of the 54th Meeting of the Endocrinological Society*, p. 200. Washington D.C.

Friesen, H., Guyda, H., Hwang, P., Tyson, J. E. and Barbeau, A. (1972a). 'Functional evaluation of prolactin secretion: a guide to therapy.' *J. clin. Invest.* **51**, 706.

— — — — and Meyer, R. E. (1972b). In *Third Tenovus Symposium on Prolactin and Carcinogenesis*, Ed. by K. Griffiths. Tenovus Press.

Furth, J. (1969). 'Pituitary cybernetics and neoplasia.' *Harvey Lect.* **63**, 59.

Fuxe, K. and Hökfelt, T. (1969). 'Catecholamines in the hypothalamus and the pituitary gland.' In *Frontiers in Neuroendocrinology*, Ed. by W. F. Ganong and L. Martini. Oxford University Press.

Guyda, H. J. and Friesen, H. G. (1971). 'The separation of monkey prolactin from monkey growth hormone by affinity chromatography.' *Biochem. Biophys. Res. Commun.* **42**, 1068.

Horrobin, D. F., Burstyn, P. G., Lloyd, I. J., Durkin, N., Lipton, A. and Muiruri, K. L. (1971). 'Actions of prolactin on human renal function.' *Lancet* **2**, 352.

Hwang, P., Guyda, H. and Friesen, H. (1971a). 'A radioimmunoassay for human prolactin.' *Proc. nat Acad. Sci. U.S.A.* **68**, 1902.

— — — (1971b). 'Studies on human prolactin by radioimmunoassay.' *Proceedings of the 53rd Meeting of the Endocrine Society*, p. A-1. San Francisco.

— — — (1972). 'Purification of human prolactin.' *J. biol. Chem.* **247**, 1955.

Jacobs, L. S., Mariz, I. K. and Daughaday, W. H. (1972). 'A mixed heterologous radioimmunoassay for human prolactin.' *J. clin. Endocr.* **34**, 484.

Kleinberg, D. and Frantz, A. G. (1971). 'Human prolactin: measurement in plasma by in vitro bioassay.' *J. clin. Invest.* **50**, 1557.

— Noel, G. and Frantz, A. G. (1971). 'Chlorpromazine stimulation and L-DOPA suppression of plasma prolactin in man.' *J. clin. Endocr.* **33**, 873.

L'Hermite, M., Stavric, V. and Robyn, C. (1971). 'Human pituitary prolactin during pregnancy and post partum as measured in serum by a radioimmunoassay.' *Acta endocr.* Suppl. **159**, 37.

Liu, K. H. and Meites, J. (1971). 'Inhibition by L-DOPA and monoamine oxidase inhibitors of pituitary prolactin release; stimulation by methyl dopa and α-amphetamine.' *Proc. Soc. expl Biol. Med.* **137**, 480.

Loewenstein, J. E., Mariz, G. T., Peake, G. T. and Daughaday, W. H. (1971). 'Prolactin bioassay by induction of N-acetyl lactosamine synthetase in mouse mammary gland explants.' *J. clin. Endocr.* **33**, 217.

Lutterbeck, P. M., Pryor, J. S., Varga, L. and Wenner, R. (1971). 'Treatment of non-puerperal galactorrhea with an ergot alkaloid.' *Br. med. J.* **3**, 228.

Lyons, W. R., Li, C. H., Ahmad, N. and Rice-Wray, E. (1968). 'Mammotrophic effects of human hypophyseal growth hormone preparations in animals and man.' In *Growth Hormone*, p. 349, Ed. by A. Pecile and E. Muller. Excerpta Medica Foundation.

McGarry, E. E., Rubinstein, D. and Beck, J. C. (1968). 'Growth hormones and prolactins: biochemical, immunological and physiological similarities and differences.' *Ann. N.Y. Acad. Sci.* **148**, 559.

Maetz, J., Sawyer, W. H., Pickford, G. E. and Mayer, N. (1968). 'Evolution de la balance minerale du sodium chez fundulus heteroclitus au cour du transfert d'eau de mer en eau douce: effets de l'hypophysectomie et de la prolactine.' *Gen. Comp. Endocr.* **8**, 163.

Marcovitz, S. and Friesen, H. (1971). 'Regulation of prolactin secretion in man.' *Clin. Res.* **19**, 773.

Malarkey, W. B., Jacobs, L. S. and Daughaday, W. H. (1971). 'Levodopa suppression of prolactin in non-puerperal galactorrhoea.' *New Engl J. Med.* **285**, 1160.

Meites, J. (1972). In *Estrogen, Target Tissue, and Neoplasia* (Breast Cancer Workshop). Ed. by T. Dao. University of Chicago Press.

Midgley, R. (1971). Paper presented at N.I.H. Workshop Conference on Prolactin, Bethesda, Maryland.

— (1972). Paper presented at the Fourth International Congress of Endocrinology, Washington, D.C.

Minton, J. P. and Dickey, R. P. (1972). 'Prolactin FSH and LH in breast cancer: effect of L-DOPA and oophorectomy.' *Lancet* **1**, 1069.

Nicoll, C. S., Yaron, Z., Nutt, N. and Daniels, E. (1970). 'Effects of ergotamine tartrate on prolactin and growth hormone secretion by rat adenohypophysis in vitro.' *Biol. Reprod.* **5**, 59.

Pearson, O. H., Llerena, O., Llerena, L., Molina, A. and Butler, T. (1969). 'Prolactin-dependent rat mammary cancer: a model for man.' *Trans. Ass. Am. Phys.* **82**, 225.

Quadri, S. K and Meites, J. (1971). 'Regression of spontaneous mammary tumors in rats by ergot drugs.' *Proc. Soc. expl Biol. Med.* **138**, 999.

Schams, D., Reinhardt, V. and Karg, H. (1972). 'Effects of 2-Br-α-ergocryptine on plasma prolactin level during parturition and onset of lactation in cows.' *Experientia* **28**, 697.

Sherwood, L. (1971). 'Human prolactin.' *New Engl. J. Med.* **284**, 774.

Sinha, Y. N., Lewis, U. J. and VanderLaan, W. P. (1971). 'Effects of prolactin and growth hormone deficiency on the growth of neonatal mice.' *Proceedings of the 53rd Meeting of the Endocrine Society*, p. A-125. San Francisco.

Stoll, B. A. (1972). 'Brain catecholamines and breast cancer: a hypothesis.' *Lancet* **1**, 431.

Striker, P. and Grueter, F. (1928). 'Action du lobe anterieur de l'hypophyse sur la montee laiteuse.' *C.R. Soc. Biol. Paris* **99**, 1978.

Sulman, F. G. (1970). *Hypothalamic Control of Lactation* (Monographs on Endocrinology). Berlin; Springer-Verlag.

Tashjian, A. H., Barowsky, N. Y. and Jensen, D. K. (1971). 'Thyrotropin releasing hormone: direct evidence for stimulation of prolactin production by pituitary cells in culture.' *Biochem. Biophys. Res. Commun.* **43**, 516.

Tolis, G. and Friesen, H. Unpublished observation.

Turkington, R. W. (1971). 'Measurement of prolactin activity in human serum by the induction of specific milk proteins in the mammary gland in vitro.' *J. clin. Endocr.* **33**, 210.

— (1972a). 'Phenothiazine stimulation test for prolactin reserve: the syndrome of isolated prolactin deficiency.' *J. clin. Endocr.* **34**, 247.

— (1972b). 'Section of prolactin by patients with pituitary and hypothalamic tumors.' *J. clin. Endocr.* **34**, 159.

— (1972c). 'Inhibition of prolactin secretion and successful therapy of the Forbes-Albright syndrome with L-DOPA.' *J. clin. Endocr.* **34**, 306.

— (1972d). 'Serum prolactin levels in patients with gynecomastia.' *J. clin. Endocr.* **34**, 62.

— Underwood, L. E. and Van Wyk, J. J. (1971). 'Elevated serum prolactin levels after pituitary-stalk section in man.' *New Engl. J. Med.* **285**, 707.

Tyson, J. E., Hwang, P., Guyda, H. and Friesen, H. G. (1972). 'Studies of prolactin secretion in human pregnancy.' *Am. J. Obst. Gynec.,* **113**, 14.

Wuttke, W. and Meites, J. (1971). 'Luteolytic role of prolactin during the estrus cycle of the rat.' *Proc. Soc. expl Biol. Med.* **137**, 988.

— Cassell, E. and Meites, J. (1971). 'Effects of ergocornine on serum prolactin and LH, and on hypothalamic content of PIF and LRF.' *Endocrinology* **88**, 737.

Yanai, R. and Nagasawa, H. (1971). 'Inhibition by ergocornine and 2-Br-α-ergocryptine of spontaneous mammary tumor appearance in mice.' *Experienta* **27**, 934.

# 10

# Changes in Hypothalamic Sensitivity in Ageing and Cancer

## V. M. Dilman

## INTRODUCTION

Ageing appears to be an endogenous cause of cancer development, and age-associated hormonal changes may play a significant role in its pathological influence. The author suggests that the cause of the age-linked changes in the endocrine system is a failure of hormonal homeostasis. Homeostatic stability is normally maintained by rhythmic activity of the hypothalamus which is responsible for the control and integration of the main functions of the body. The most important method by which this integration is achieved is the negative feedback control.

Theoretically, there are three ways in which this mechanism of hormonal homeostasis may fail: (1) Elevation of the hypothalamic threshold to homeostatic suppression—a central type of homeostatic failure. A disturbance of this kind is observed in Cushing's disease where a lack of suppression by glucocorticoids is seen. (2) Decreased effect of peripheral hormones on the hypothalamus—a peripheral type of homeostatic failure. A disturbance of this kind is observed, for example, after subtotal castration (Lipschutz, 1957). (3) Impaired hormonal secretion or a qualitative shift in the spectrum of these hormones—a dysfunctional type of homeostatic failure. A disturbance of this kind is usually seen in congenital enzymatic defects—for example, the defect in hydroxylation of corticosteroids in congenital adrenal hyperplasia (Wilkins et al., 1955).

Experimental evidence suggests that failure of the homeostatic mechanism at any point may promote tumorigenesis, and the data summarized below suggest that all three types of homeostatic failure may develop in the course of normal ageing. Some years ago, the author put forward the hypothesis that the development of these changes is associated with age-related elevation of the hypothalamic threshold to feedback suppression (Dilman, 1958, 1968, 1971). As a result of this reduction in hypothalamic sensitivity, there is a compensatory increase in the activity of the peripheral endocrine glands which thus continue to maintain the feedback mechanism in spite of the elevation of the hypothalamic threshold. In time, however, it leads to loss of the rhythmic functioning of the major homeostatic systems and thus lays the foundations for specific age-related pathology and promotes tumorigenesis (Dilman, 1968, 1971).

Sensitivity of the hypothalamic feedback falls with age in the major homeostatic systems—in the energy, reproductive and adaptation systems. It may be possible in the future, by assays of the hypothalamic releasing hormones, to confirm this hypothesis. At present there is a large body of indirect evidence showing the presence of homeostatic failure in many breast and endometrial cancer patients, and this should be taken into account in attempts to improve the results of therapy in hormone-dependent cancer.

## HYPOTHALAMIC FEEDBACK AND THE EFFECT OF AGEING

### Energy homeostasis changes in ageing

An important process in energy homeostasis is the inhibition of growth hormone (GH) secretion after intake of glucose by an action on the hypothalamic receptors. On the other hand, during starvation GH secretion is increased and, by mobilizing fatty acids, provides the energy sources required by the organism (Glick et al., 1965). The functioning of this extremely important system becomes disturbed with ageing and, as can be seen from Table 10.1, a standard glucose load fails to inhibit the level of GH and FFA (free fatty acids) in middle-aged subjects (Dilman, 1970a).

These data suggest that in middle age the hypothalamic threshold to homeostatic suppression is increased in the case of the glucose–GH feedback system. The presence of this primary defect is sufficient to cause several age-related metabolic disturbances, such as gain of body-weight, relative insensitivity to insulin action, decreased tolerance to glucose, elevated FFA level, and hypercholesterolaemia. These are the metabolic abnormalities which are characteristic of both normal ageing and specific age-related pathology.

Table 10.2 demonstrates some metabolic differences in young and middle-aged subjects. Schematically, the relationship between these secondary metabolic disturbances and the primary disturbance of the hypothalamic regulatory mechanism may be represented as follows. The high GH level caused by the lack of a glucose suppression effect inhibits the utilization of glucose by the muscle tissue, mainly by the direct anti-insulin action of GH but

TABLE 10.1

Changes in GH and FFA Blood Level after Glucose Loading in Young and Middle-aged Subjects

| Group | Number of cases | Average age (years) | GH blood level (ng/ml) | | Change (%) | FFA blood level (µEq/l) | |
|---|---|---|---|---|---|---|---|
| | | | Before treatment | After treatment | | Before treatment | After treatment |
| Young | 15 | 26·6 | 14·4±2·4 | 9·1±1·6 | −37 | 356·0±19·0 | 191·0±19·5 |
| Young | 16 | 34·8 | 19·9±2·6 | 11·8±1·5 | −41 | — | — |
| Middle-aged | 17 | 52·7 | 29·8±5·0 | 44·6±9·1 | +50 | 460·0±17·2 | 427·0±18·0 |

Note: GH was determined radioimmunologically with the use of aminocellulose as immunosorbent (Bobrov and Patokin, 1971; Bobrov, Patokin and Dilman, 1971). Plasma FFA were titrated by Dole's method (1956).

199

TABLE 10.2

The Qualitative Difference in the Age-associated Metabolic Signs in Young and Middle-aged Subjects

| Signs | Young | Middle-aged | Significance |
|---|---|---|---|
| Average age | 34·8 (n = 35) | 52·7 (m = 115) | |
| GH level: | | | |
| basal (ng/ml) | 19·9 ± 2·6 | 29·8 ± 5·0 | |
| 1 hour after glucose load | 11·8 ± 1·5 | 44·6 ± 9·1 | |
| Insulin-glucose test (sugar level) | | | |
| 1 hour after glucose load | 112·6 ± 3·1 | 143·7 ± 3·5 | $p < 0.002$ |
| 2 hours | 89·3 ± 2·7 | 114·5 ± 3·1 | $p < 0.002$ |
| Average body weight (% variation from ideal weight) | + 4 | + 18·4 | |
| FFA level (μEq/1) | 393·0 ± 16·0 | 483·0 ± 16·1 | $p < 0.002$ |
| Sugar blood level | | | |
| 1 hour after glucose load | 114·9 ± 2·7 | 150·7 ± 2·5 | $p < 0.001$ |
| 2 hours after glucose load | 93·6 ± 6·0 | 131·0 ± 2·6 | $p < 0.001$ |
| after prednisolone glucose test | | | |
| 1 hour | 168·9 ± 4·6 | 215·3 ± 4·6 | $p < 0.002$ |
| 2 hours | 113·1 ± 4·4 | 158·3 ± 5·3 | $p < 0.002$ |
| Serum-cholesterol (mg/100 ml) | 181·8 ± 6·5 | 243·9 ± 5·0 | $p < 0.02$ |

Note: Blood cholesterol was tested by Sacket's method (1925), blood-sugar by the method of Hagedorn and Jensen.

also by an FFA-suppression effect on glucose transport and metabolism, the so-called Randle effect (Randle, 1965). This leads to the well-known phenomenon of age-associated decrease of glucose tolerance.

Under these conditions, compensatory over-production of insulin develops and, as a result, the excess of glucose is chiefly taken up in the fatty tissue where it is metabolized into fat. In this way, age-associated weight gain occurs with constant replenishment of fat stores, despite the intense lipolysis which is stimulated by the GH excess. Decreased glucose utilization in the muscle tissue causes in turn an excessive mobilization of FFA in addition, as is seen in starvation. Intensive oxidation of FFA leads to the accumulation of acetylcoenzyme A, which, owing to the disturbed glucose utilization, is metabolized to cholesterol to a greater degree than FFA because the synthesis of FFA requires considerably more NADP than that of cholesterol. Thus, hypercholesterolaemia develops concomitantly with normal ageing.

Similar changes may occur also in the regulation of appetite in the course of ageing. The activity of the hypothalamic appetite centre is known to be inhibited as the level of blood glucose rises, but clinical observations suggest that appetite often increases with age, and experimental data shows that food intake is elevated with advancing age in rats (Everitt, 1970). Since post-prandial blood glucose levels increase with age, it seems justifiable to conclude that advancing age is associated with a raised threshold in the hypothalamic appetite centre to the inhibitory effect of glucose (Dilman, 1958, 1968). This factor, coupled with the other age-related disorders of energy homeostasis, may predispose to serious metabolic disturbances.

The author suggests that all the above-mentioned metabolic disturbances increase the likelihood of tumorigenesis. It will be seen later that metabolic changes characteristic of ageing are more pronounced in breast and endometrial cancer patients than in age-matched controls, but it is not clear how such metabolic disturbances promote tumorigenesis. As far as the influence of cholesterol is concerned, it is possible that hypercholesterolaemia *per se* may play a significant role, since the rate of cell division seems to be connected with cholesterol level. Cholesterol synthesis is greatly increased in some malignant cells (Howard and Kritchevsky, 1969; Chevallier and Lutton, 1971), while on the other hand, many effective anti-tumour agents can inhibit cholesterol synthesis (Littman, Taguchi and Mosbach, 1966) and low cholesterol diets may suppress experimental tumour induction (Szepsenwol, 1966).

The pathogenic role of age-related-compensatory hyperinsulinaemia may also be important. The data derived from the study of Welborn, Stenhouse and Johnstone (1969) show increasing blood insulin response to glucose loading in the normal population with increasing age (Table 10.3). A high insulin level may be a key disturbance in the development of such types of age-related pathology as obesity, atherosclerosis and early adult onset of diabetes (for references see Dilman, 1971). The exaggerated blood insulin response to glucose loading seen with ageing must also be taken into account when considering the part metabolic disturbances may play in cancer predisposition, particularly in relation to breast cancer.

TABLE 10.3

Blood Insulin and Glucose Changes after Glucose Loading (50 g orally) (Wellborn, Stenhouse and Johnstone, 1969)

| Age group | $Log_{10}$ serum—insulin | | Blood glucose level (mg/100 ml) | |
|---|---|---|---|---|
| | Men | Women | Men | Women |
| 21–29 | $1 \cdot 506 \pm 0 \cdot 025$ | $1 \cdot 603 \pm 0 \cdot 019$ | $86 \pm 2$ | $95 \pm 2$ |
| 30–39 | $1 \cdot 534 \pm 0 \cdot 024$ | $1 \cdot 591 \pm 0 \cdot 021$ | $92 \pm 2$ | $91 \pm 2$ |
| 40–49 | $1 \cdot 573 \pm 0 \cdot 021$ | $1 \cdot 624 \pm 0 \cdot 017$ | $97 \pm 2$ | $102 \pm 2$ |
| 50–59 | $1 \cdot 618 \pm 0 \cdot 021$ | $1 \cdot 678 \pm 0 \cdot 018$ | $107 \pm 3$ | $106 \pm 2$ |
| 60–69 | $1 \cdot 729 \pm 0 \cdot 022$ | $1 \cdot 771 \pm 0 \cdot 019$ | $114 \pm 4$ | $121 \pm 4$ |
| 70 + | $1 \cdot 750 \pm 0 \cdot 029$ | $1 \cdot 816 \pm 0 \cdot 025$ | $131 \pm 6$ | $138 \pm 16$ |

## Reproductive homeostasis changes in ageing

Energy homeostasis is an 'open' system, and it could be claimed that the effects described above developed as a result of external factors. However, reproductive homeostasis is a closed-loop system and, as we shall see, analogous changes with ageing occur here too, ultimately leading to the menopause.

Table 10.4 shows that the level of excretion of total gonadotrophins and FSH increases with advancing age (Dilman and Pavlova, 1963a; Dilman et al. 1968). It is theoretically possible for such a change to be related either to a

TABLE 10.4

Age associated Changes in Total Gonadotrophin, FSH and Total Phenol-steroid Excretion

| Age (Years) | Number of cases | Total gonadotrophins (muu/24 hours) | FSH (mg/hour) | Total phenol-steroids (µg/24 hours) |
|---|---|---|---|---|
| 20–29 | 15 | 13·2 ± 0·4 | 1·05 ± 0·1 | 38·6 ± 4·12 |
| 30–39 | 15 | 41·0 ± 7·5 | — | 46·0 ± 4·84 |
| 40–49 | 15 | 84·1 ± 11·2 | 5·4 ± 0·4 | 55·6 ± 3·7 |
| 50–59 | 30 | 194·8 ± 13·0 | 12·7 ± 0·5 | 38·4 ± 2·7 |

Note: Total gonadotrophins were estimated by a modified method of Albert (1956) and results were expressed in mouse uterine units.

The method of Steelman and Pohley (1953) was used for FSH testing. The FSH value was estimated from the difference between the weights of the ovaries in experimental and control groups per 1 hour equivalent of 24 hours' urine output.

Total phenol-steroids which include both classical and non-classical oestrogens were measured by the method of Dikun-Pavlova (see Dilman et al., 1968).

decrease in the ovarian hormone level which acts as a physiological inhibitor of gonadotrophin release (peripheral type of homeostatic failure), or to an elevated resistance of the hypothalamic controlling centre to feedback suppression (central type of homeostatic failure). Since the rise in gonadotrophin excretion occurs concomitantly with elevation of total phenol-steroid excretion, it may be inferred that the cause of homeostatic failure is the elevation of the hypothalamic threshold to the suppressive effect of phenolsteroids, i.e. the central type of homeostatic failure.

It has been shown that the ovulatory surge of LH secretion depends on a rapid rise in oestrogen secretion during the late follicular phase of the ovulatory cycle (Tsai and Yen, 1971). Oestrogens can exert both positive and negative feedback effects. While the increased oestrogen level causes a fall in FSH concentration (usually between 12 and 24 hours before ovulation), it stimulates the release of LH at the same time, thus leading to ovulation.

These two effects, i.e. suppression of FSH and release of LH, are interconnected, and therefore if the hypothalamic threshold to the FSH inhibitory effect of oestrogen becomes extremely elevated, hypothalamic feedback effects begin to fall off and the menopause develops.

This suggested mechanism of age-associated switching-off of the menstrual cycle is consistent with existing concepts of the puberty mechanism. Donovan and van der Werff ten Bosch (1959) postulated that the fundamental change in advance towards sexual maturity is the reduction in the hypothalamic sensitivity to feedback effects of the gonadal hormones. These changes lead to an accelerated release of gonadotrophins and, eventually, to the attainment of puberty. Thus, both switching-on and switching-off of the reproductive cycle are attained by a common mechanism—the age-associated elevation of the hypothalamic threshold to homeostatic influence.

As far as breast cancer is concerned, two aspects of this mechanism should be emphasized. The first is the compensatory increase in the level of total phenol-steroid excretion which develops in response to over-stimulation by gonadotrophin. This permits, on the one hand, the reproductive cycle to continue functioning despite a constantly-rising hypothalamic threshold; but, on the other hand, it tends to exert a proliferative influence on the target epithelium in the reproductive system (see below).

Secondly, under the condition of gonadotrophic over-stimulation, the ovaries tend to secrete the so-called 'non-classical phenol-steroids' instead of the classical oestrogens, oestrone, oestriol and oestradiol (Dilman and Pavlova, 1963b; Dilman, 1968). This occurs after the menopause and has led to the false impression that oestrogenic activity, as judged by tests for classical oestrogens ceases in post-menopausal ovaries (MacBride, 1957; Brown, 1960). The output of non-classical phenol-steroids may be ascertained from the difference between the level of total phenol-steroids and that of the classical oestrogens. *Figure 10.1* shows the increasing difference in the ratio of total phenolsteroids to classical oestrogens in the course of ageing. (The adrenal cortex also secretes these oestrogen-like hormones and, in addition, classical oestrogens may metabolize to non-classical phenolsteroids in the liver.)

There is a large body of evidence that a shift in hormonal production from classical to non-classical phenol-steroids in the ovaries is connected with damage to follicular tissue. Thus, following radiation castration, lesions of follicular tissue develop in conjunction with hyperplasia of the thecal tissue and in such patients excretion of non-classical phenol-steroids is elevated despite a low excretion of classical oestrogen (Dilman and Pavlova, 1963b). Similar changes develop in the course of ageing, and it is assumed that the hyperplasia of thecal tissue and other observed changes in the follicular tissue are caused by gonadotrophin over-stimulation. The biological properties of non-classical phenol-steroids are still little understood but they may play a significant role in specific pathophysiological conditions in post-menopausal patients. In particular, these altered hormones have a less potent suppressive effect on hypothalamic levels, although they exert a proliferative influence on some target tissues in the reproductive system (Berstein et al., 1969).

It thus appears that in the course of normal ageing all three causes of

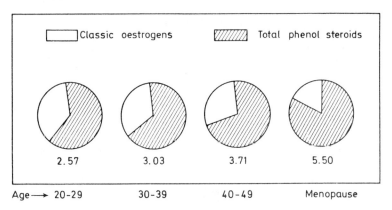

Age —→ 20-29      30-39      40-49      Menopause

*Figure 10.1. Changes in the ratio of excretion of total phenol steroids to classical oestrogens with normal ageing. Total phenol steroids include both classical and non-classical oestrogens. Determined by method of Dikun-Pavlova (Dilman et al., 1968). Classical oestrogens were determined by Brown method (1955)*

homeostatic failure may develop in the reproductive system: *(a)* elevation of the hypothalamic threshold to feedback action; *(b)* decreased production of classical oestrogens; *(c)* shifts in the spectrum of hormonal secretion, namely central, peripheral and dysfunctional types of homeostatic failure.

The above age-related changes in the reproductive system may exert a very important influence on energy homeostasis, and this is mainly related to the biological role of oestrogen. Oestrogens have the ability to improve the glucose tolerance, to reduce age-related hypercholesterolaemia and to increase the sensitivity to insulin (for references see Dilman, 1968). A transient decrease of reactive hyperinsulinaemia observed in women between the age of 30 and 39 is presumably due to this oestrogen effect (Table 10.3). On the other hand, the decreased oestrogen level produced by ovariectomy predisposes to the development of obesity and atherosclerosis.

Both in childhood, when reproductive homeostasis is not yet switched on, and at an advanced age, when it is switching off, the serum insulin level (Welborn, Stenhouse and Johnstone, 1969), blood cholesterol level (Adlersberg et al., 1956), serum FFA level (Pickens, Burkeholder and Womack, 1967), and blood sugar level (Danowski, 1957; Streeten et al., 1965) after food intake are much higher than in the intermediate stabilized age group.

Therefore, both in energy and reproductive homeostasis, analogous changes take place in the course of ageing; elevation of the hypothalamic threshold to homeostatic suppression accompanied by a secondary increase in the activity of peripheral endocrine glands. This results in excessive production of insulin and non-classical phenol-steroids. The operation of this common mechanism both in open and closed homeostatic systems is important evidence in favour of the endogenous origin of age-associated increase of the hypothalamic threshold.

## Adaptation system changes in ageing

Clinically, elderly people often manifest some Cushingoid signs. Patients with established Cushing's disease show resistance of the hypothalamus to feedback suppression and it is probable that similar but lesser changes occur with normal ageing. Experimental data obtained in our laboratory confirm that in rats the ability of prednisolone to suppress the blood corticosterone level progressively declines with age, and this suggests age-associated increase in the hypothalamic threshold to feedback mechanisms (Table 10.5).

TABLE 10.5

Age-associated Decrease of Hypothalamic Sensitivity to Prednisolone Suppression in Rats
(Dilman et al., 1972)

| Age (months) | Body weight (g) | Blood corticosterone level ($\mu g\%$) | | Inhibition (%) |
| --- | --- | --- | --- | --- |
| | | Before treatment | After treatment | |
| 3 | 100–149 | $15 \cdot 5 \pm 4 \cdot 9$ | $8 \cdot 5 \pm 2 \cdot 6$ | 48·9 |
| 4–7 | 150–199 | $21 \cdot 6 \pm 2 \cdot 6$ | $16 \cdot 1 \pm 2 \cdot 6$ | 20·4 |
| 8–6 | 200–300 | $23 \cdot 4 \pm 4 \cdot 1$ | $19 \cdot 7 \pm 3 \cdot 0$ | 15·8 |
| 16 | 250–300 | $30 \cdot 4 \pm 9 \cdot 3$ | $26 \cdot 3 \pm 3 \cdot 5$ | 13·5 |

Note: Prednisolone in a single dose of 0·05 mg/100 g body weight was administered intra-peritoneally at 10 a.m. and a sample of blood for corticosterone testing was taken at 12 noon.
Serum corticosterone was measured by routine fluorometric procedure.

This is corroborated by data suggesting the absence of diurnal rhythm in the plasma cortisol levels of middle-aged patients with ischaemic heart disease. In this group, the plasma cortisol level at 9 a.m. was found to be $16 \cdot 5 \pm 2 \cdot 2$ µg per cent and at 4 p.m. was $14 \cdot 6 \pm 1 \cdot 7$ µg per cent, whereas normally the fall would be approximately 50 per cent. Our data suggests that the effect of glucocorticoid hormones on the organism may rise with increasing age, although the absolute levels of blood cortisol may not increase. High levels of adrenal hormones may lead to myocardial, cerebral, renal and other damage (Wexler, 1971).

Apart from the immunosuppressive effect of excess glucocorticoid, age-associated disturbances in the reproductive homeostatic mechanisms may also exert an effect on the immune defence mechanism. Inhibition of the immunological response is seen in pregnancy, and it is interesting to note that the high excretion of oestriol-like non-classical oestrogens observed in pregnancy is also found in post-menopausal breast and endometrial cancer patients. Thus, age-linked changes in both glucocorticoid and oestrogen secretion might affect the immunological response.

## Other parts of the hypothalamo-pituitary system

It is well known that thyroid function declines with age. The cause of the change is unknown but recent data shows that the curve correlating thyrotrophin blood level with age is parabolic in shape, being higher in the early years and later decades of life (Mayberry et al., 1971). This distribution is similar to that defining age-dependent hypothalamo-pituitary function, although so far we have no direct data about age-linked changes in the hypothalamic threshold controlling thyrotrophic hormone secretion.

As is known, prolactin and MSH secretion are regulated chiefly by inhibitory hypothalamic hormones—so-called PIF and MIF. It would therefore be expected that in the course of ageing, elevation of the hypothalamic threshold will lead to *decrease* in the secretion of MSH and prolactin. Both decrease in the incidence of malignant melanoma, and greying of the hair with advancing age might then be a manifestation of age-associated decrease in the MSH level. These speculations are of course conjectural, because at present there is no direct evidence on the age dynamics of melanotrophin secretion. As far as prolactin secretion is concerned, recent measurements show that in the rat its level *increases* with age (Meites, 1972).

To evaluate the presence of hypothalamic changes in prolactin and MSH regulation, it is necessary to use an inhibitory test with levodopa or a stimulatory test with chlorpromazine (Kleinberg, Noel and Frantz, 1971), because the basal level of hormone secretion does not reflect the state of the regulatory system in all cases. This applies especially to prolactin regulation, which occurs not only at a hypothalamic level, but independently also on the pituitary level. The integrity of the system may be important if the prolactin regulation mechanism is to be manipulated in order to exert control on the growth of endocrine-dependent breast cancer (see later).

At present there are no data about the influence of ageing on oxytocin secretion although this might be interesting because oxytocin exerts an insulin-like effect on mammary gland tissue, and in particular stimulates the metabolism of glucose into fat (Braun and Hechter, 1969). Data on the hypothalamic regulation of lipotrophin are also lacking so far. Recent studies show that there is a negative feedback between secretion of GH and blood FFA level (Blackard et al., 1969; Taylor and Blackard, 1971), but it is unknown whether this mechanism plays any role in lipotrophin regulation.

There is now considerable evidence that in addition to the well known diabetogenic hormones, the pituitary gland also secretes a diabetogenic peptide which has no growth-prompting activity but which causes profound hyperinsulinaemia and hyperglycaemia co-existing with insulin resistance (Lawrence, Conn and Appelt, 1971). The biological role of this 'diabetogenic' factor is still unknown although its effect is similar to that of GH in many metabolic respects.

To complete the characterization of age-associated hypothalamic changes it must be noted that monoamine oxidase levels in brain increase with age and noradrenaline levels decrease with age (Robinson et al., 1972). The age-related changes in MAO activity undoubtedly exert a widespread effect on hypothalamic function and it is interesting to speculate on a possible relationship between age-associated change in MAO activity levels and age-associated changes both in the secretion of prolactin and in the ability of levodopa to suppress its secretion (see later).

In summary, it would seem that there is good evidence to support the hypothesis that the development of homeostatic failure with advancing years is a direct function of the elevated hypothalamic threshold associated with ageing (Dilman, 1971, 1972). For testing the major homeostatic systems the following tests are available. For the assessment of energy homeostasis, the measurement of blood GH level before and after glucose loading may be used; for reproductive homeostasis, the assay of total gonadotrophin and total phenol-steroid (or androgen) excretion levels; for the adaptation system, the determination of the diurnal rhythm of the cortisol level and the reaction to the dexamethasone suppressive test; for the prolactin releasing system, the use of levodopa suppression or chorpromazine stimulation tests. Not only inhibitory but also stimulatory tests may be used for assessing the degree of homeostatic failure. Insulin-induced hypoglycaemia, for instance, may be useful for the measurement of GH response, which usually increases under conditions of elevated hypothalamic activity.

It might be expected that individuals and human populations which are distinguished by a high risk of cancer might have a greater tendency to the development of metabolic disturbances associated with premature ageing. This will now be shown for patients with breast and endometrial cancer.

## HYPOTHALAMIC FEEDBACK IN BREAST AND ENDOMETRIAL CANCER PATIENTS

There is a large body of experimental evidence to suggest that changes in hormonal homeostasis create conditions promoting tumorigenesis. There is an increase in the incidence of mammary carcinoma in rats in the course of natural ageing, after transplantation of the ovary into the tail, or after treatment with DMBA. The hormonal imbalances which develop under these conditions have much in common (Table 10.6), and may be significant in carcinogenesis.

The data in Table 10.6 show that transplantation of the ovary into the tail of the rat or treatment with DMBA shifts the hormonal pattern towards that characteristic of ageing. It should be emphasized that hormonal imbalances developing after carcinogen administration inolve not only prolactin release, as has been demonstrated earlier (Furth, 1971), but also include a wide spectrum of changes in energy and reproductive homeostasis. The findings presented below support the suggestion that such changes normally associated with ageing may be even more pronounced in some types of human breast cancer.

### Reproductive homeostasis changes in cancer

The data in Table 10.7 show that the level of total phenol-steroid excretion in post-menopausal breast cancer patients is elevated, in contrast to the low level of excretion of classical oestrogens. It may be noted also that in breast cancer patients the excretion of total gonadotrophins is elevated as compared with healthy post-menopausal women. It suggests that both hypothalamo-pituitary activity and the compensatory ovarian response are increased. The late onset of menopause often observed in breast cancer patients may be explained on the basis of these data. As mentioned at the beginning of this chapter, compensatory over-secretion of ovarian oestrogens maintains the feedback ovulatory mechanism in the presence of a rising hypothalamic threshold to feedback suppression, but, at the same time, because of the hormonal excess, conditions conducive to tumour development are created.

The suggestion of an ovarian source for non-classical phenol-steroids is supported by the data presented in Table 10.8. This shows that ovariectomy performed in post-menopausal breast cancer patients leads to a decrease in non-classical phenol-steroid excretion, despite the constant excretion of classical oestrogens.

The data presented in Table 10.8 also suggest that the major proportion of total phenol-steroids in post-menopausal patients is contributed by non-classical oestrogens, and this is inconsistent with the generally-accepted assumption that non-classical oestrogens are chiefly products of the metabolism of the ovarian hormone oestradiol (Diczfalusy and Lauritzen, 1961). Our conclusion is supported by observations on x-ray castrated patients where the level of non-classical phenol-steroids is extremely high, in spite of low level of classical oestrogen excretion. These observations would suggest that the non-classical phenol-steroids are primary ovarian hormones which are produced independently of the synthesis of classical oestrogens.

The development of hyperplasia of ovarian thecal tissue, after x-ray castration, suggests that elevated production of non-classic phenol-steroids may be connected with its activity. Similar hyperplasia of the thecal tissue,

TABLE 10.6

The Incidence of Mammary Carcinoma and the Hormonal Pattern in Three Types of Carcinogenesis in Rats (Anisimov, 1971; Anisimov and Pavlova, 1972)

| Group | Age (months) | Mammary tumour incidence | Classical oestrogen excretion (μg/ 24 hours) | Pituitary FSH concentration (mg NIH standard) | Oestriol index* | Maximal increment of sugar level after glucose load (%) | Maximal decrease of FFA level after glucose loading (%) |
|---|---|---|---|---|---|---|---|
| Control group | 6 | — | 2.9 | 0.012 | 0.17 | 30 | 55 |
|  | 16 | 18 | 0.4 | 0.018 | 0.50 | 60 | 35 |
| Transplant group | 6 | — | 2.0 | 0.006 | 0.14 | 28 | 32 |
|  | 16 | 32 | 0.29 | 0.016 | 0.70 | 292 | 47 |
| Carcinogen-treated group | 6† | — | 0.04 | 0.003 | 0.40 | 161 | 44 |
|  | 14 | 50 | 0.04 | — | — | 82 | 39 |

* Oestriol index—the ratio of the sum of oestrone and oestradiol to oestriol measured by thin-layer chromatography method (see Dilman et al., 1968). This index indirectly reflects the production of non-classic phenol-steroids (see Dilman, 1968) or atypical oestrogens (Jellinck, 1966).
† Tests were made four days after carcinogen administration.

209

TABLE 10.7

The Level of Total Gonadotrophins, FSH, Total Phenol-steroids and Classical Oestrogen Excretion in Post-menopausal Breast Cancer Patients

| Group | Total gonadotrophins (muu/24 hours) | FSH (mg/hour) | Total phenol-steroids (μg/24 hours) | Classical oestrogens (μg/24 hours) |
|---|---|---|---|---|
| Menopausal controls | 194·8 ± 13·0 | 15·7 ± 1·3 | 38·4 ± 2·7 | 7·0 ± 0·7 |
| Breast cancer (menopausal) | 273 ± 9·8 | 14·2 ± 0·8 | 57·3 ± 3·0* 69·9 ± 5·6 | 12·2 ± 2·4* 8·9 ± 0·6 |

* Patients in menopause for less than two years.

TABLE 10.8

The Effect of Ovariectomy on the Level of Excretion of Total Gonadotrophins, Total Phenol-steroids and Classical Oestrogens in Post-menopausal Breast Cancer Patients

| Group | Total phenol-steroids (μg/24 hours) | Classical oestrogens (μg/24 hours) | Total gonadotrophins (mμ/24 hours) |
|---|---|---|---|
| Breast cancer patients | 69·9 ± 5·6 | 8·9 ± 0·6 | 281·0 ± 24·0 |
| Breast cancer patients + ovariectomy | 35·8 ± 3·5 | 6·0 ± 1·5 | 334·2 ± 29·0 |
| Breast cancer patients + x-ray castration | 72·5 ± 7·4 | 5·2 ± 2·2 | 235·4 ± 24·0 |

according to our data, is noted in 81·5 per cent of pre-menopausal breast cancer patients and in 88 per cent of post-menopausal patients as compared with 29·6 per cent and 49·0 per cent in age-matched control groups, respectively (Dilman, 1968). The high incidence of hyperplasia of thecal tissue is probably correlated with the elevated level of non-classical phenol-steroid excretion observed in breast cancer patients.

The high incidence of hyperplasia of ovarian thecal tissue in pre-menopausal breast cancer patients appears to be correlated also with elevation of total gonadotrophin excretion. Aveage levels were 66·0 ± 23·8 muu/24 hours for patients between 30 and 39 years and 130·0 ± 36·0 muu/24 hours for patients between 40 and 49 years, as compared with 41·0 ± 7·5 and 81·0 ± 10·2 in corresponding control groups.

Presumably, the excess of gonadotrophins in the pre-menopausal patients is the cause of the increased ovarian activity which manifests by an increased excretion of non-classical oestrogens. The synthesis of non-classical phenol-steroids instead of classical oestrogen is thus an example of qualitative alterations in the spectrum of secreted isohormones, when endocrine glands are subjected to intensive stimulation.

The signs of elevated hypothalamic threshold in the pre-menopausal homeostatic system are also evident in a large group of endometrial cancer patients, but the pattern of disturbance is more complicated. The association of endometrial hyperplasia with a low level of classical oestrogen excretion has been found difficult to explain in the past. The pathology may be explained on the basis of our findings of elevated levels of *non-classical* phenol-steroids in post-menopausal patients with endometrial carcinoma (Table 10.9).

However, total gonadotrophin excretion levels in endometrial cancer patients are significantly lower than those in breast cancer patients and even below those in normal control women. This observation is in contrast to such signs of increased activity in the target tissue as hyperplasia of ovarian thecal tissue, elevated excretion of non-classical phenol-steroids and endometrial hyperplasia all of which are frequently observed in patients with endometrial carcinoma (Hertig and Sommers, 1949; Dilman et al., 1968). The reason for the association of these signs of over-stimulation of the target tissue with a low level of total gonadotrophin excretion is unknown. It may be that the gonadotrophic effect is altered due to shift in the LH/FSH ratio, as high levels of immunoreactive LH excretion are observed in these patients (Table 10.9).

There is evidence that qualitative shifts in the pattern of hormones produced may occur as a result of over-stimulation of any endocrine gland (Dilman, 1968). The abnormal pattern of gonadotrophin excretion in women with endometrial cancer may be accounted for in the light of this suggestion as a result of pituitary over-stimulation following elevation of the hypothalamic threshold.

Some indirect evidence from our laboratory shows changes in gonadotrophin properties in endometrial cancer patients demonstrated by a lower level of carbohydrate content in gonadotrophin residue obtained from the urine (Table 10.10): Results of 'finger-print' assay of gonadotrophins in healthy post-menopausal women and patients with endometrial cancer also reveal substantial differences *(Figure 10.2)*.

It is interesting to note that both in breast and endometrial cancer patients, anti-gonadotrophic factors are much less frequently detected, despite different levels of gonadotrophin excretion (Table 10.11). A decrease in inhibitory anti-gonadotrophic effect seen in these groups of cancer patients may contribute to the gonadotrophic over-stimulation of the ovaries.

## TABLE 10.9

The Level of Classical Oestrogens, Total Phenol-steroids, Total Gonadotrophins, FSH and LH Excretion in Post-menopausal Endometrial Cancer Patients (Dilman, 1968; Dilman et al., 1968; Golubev, 1972)

| Group | Classical oestrogens (μg/24 hours) | Total phenol-steroids (μg/24 hours) | FSH (mg/hour) | Total gonadotrophins (muu/24 hours) | LH-immunologically reactive (i.u. HCG) | LH-hormonally active (i.u. HCG) |
|---|---|---|---|---|---|---|
| Menopausal control | 7·0±0·7 | 38·5±2·7 | 15·7±1·3 | 194·8±13·0 | 21·6±3·1 | 21·8± 3·4 |
| Endometrial cancer (menopausal) | 6·4±0·4 | 52·8±2·4 | 12·7±0·8 | 114·1± 9·5 | 25·6±2·8 | 107·0±12·1 |

Note: LH-immunologically reactive was tested by the method of Wide and Gemsell (1962); LH-hormonally active by Parlow's method (1958).

TABLE 10.10

Content of Carbohydrate Components in Kaolin-acetone Residues of Gonadotrophin in Healthy Women and in Patients with Endometrial Cancer (Ostroumova, 1970)

| Group | Content (% from protein concentration) | | |
| --- | --- | --- | --- |
| | Sialic acids | Hexosamines | Total hexoses |
| Healthy controls | 4·5 | 4·6 | 11·8 |
| Endometrial cancer | 1·6 | 2·8 | 6·3 |

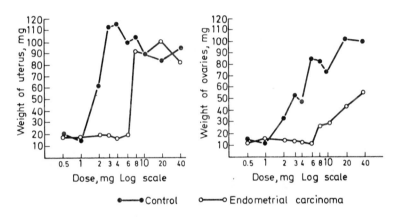

Figure 10.2. 'Finger-print' assay of gonadotrophins isolated from the urine of healthy women and endometrial carcinoma patients. Left: the influence of gonadotrophic extracts (isolated by Albert method) on the uterine weight of immature rats. Right: the same influence on the weight of the ovaries (minimal effective dose of control is 2 mg, but four times greater in gonadotrophin preparation from endometrial cancer group)

TABLE 10.11

Frequency of Anti-gonadotrophic Factor Detection in Controls and Patients with Breast and Endometrial Cancer (Ostroumova, 1972)

| Group | Detection (%) | Significance |
| --- | --- | --- |
| Menopausal controls | 80·0 | — |
| Menopausal breast cancer | 35·5 | $p < 0·02$ |
| Menopausal endometrial cancer | 11·8 | $p < 0·001$ |

## Energy homeostasis changes in cancer

The data recorded in Table 10.12 show that standard glucose loading fails to inhibit the STH level in patients with breast and endometrial cancer. It suggests that in these patients the hypothalamic threshold of sensitivity to homeostatic inhibition is increased.

This derangement of the homeostatic feedback is sufficient to facilitate or to cause a whole series of subsequent metabolic changes and the table shows these to be more pronounced in endometrial and breast cancer patients than in age-matched controls. The frequency of metabolic abnormalities in the endometrial cancer group was nearly 70–75 per cent, although the breast cancer group is not so homogenous (see below).

TABLE 10.12

Disturbances of Energy Homeostasis in Patients with Breast and Endometrial Carcinoma

| Tests | Control group | Breast carcinoma | Endometrial carcinoma |
|---|---|---|---|
| STH basal level* | $19.9 \pm 2.6$ | $22.6 \pm 2.9$ | $20.4 \pm 6.4$ |
| STH level 1 hour after glucose load | $11.8 \pm 1.5$ | $27.4 \pm 3.2$ | $22.0 \pm 6.8$ |
| Body weight (% ideal weight) | $+4.7$ | $+30.2$ | $+37.0$ |
| Insulin basal level ($\mu$U/ml) | $8.5 \pm 3.7$ | $36.9 \pm 11.6$ | $19.8 \pm 2.6$ |
| Insulin level 1 hour after glucose load | $38.0 \pm 3.3$ | $99.3 \pm 16.4$ | $38.0 \pm 5.3$ |
| Incidence of subclinical, latent and overt diabetes (%) | 20 | 36 | 63 |
| FFA level ($\mu Eq$/l) | $408 \pm 16$ | $604 \pm 75$ | $915 \pm 91$ |
| Cholesterol level (mg %) | $203 \pm 8.2$ | $270 \pm 19.5$ | $279 \pm 16.3$ |

Note: Recent estimation of STH by the double-antibody method has shown an absolute lower blood STH level, which is consistent with the values published in the literature. However, the lack of responsiveness to suppressive action of glucose had also been confirmed. The STH blood level determined by this standard technique was 2·4 ng/ml before and 2·4 ng/ml after glucose load in breast cancer patients, and 1·7 ng and 1·7 ng in endometrial cancer patients, respectively.

* STH was determined in the group of normal subjects under 35.

Consideration of the data shows a significant resemblance in the metabolic disturbances of both breast and endometrial carcinoma and leads to the suggestion that the primary cause of metabolic shift is common for both cancers. However, the insulin response is far more exaggerated in breast than in endometrial carcinoma. This difference may be related to an observed lower incidence of diabetes in breast cancer patients as compared with those with endometrial carcinoma. It may be suggested that the high insulin level in breast carcinoma patients plays a role in tumorigenesis because mammary gland tissue is very sensitive to the growth-promoting influence of insulin, and this might be taken into account in new attempts to improve the results of therapy in endocrine-dependent breast cancer.

It must also be pointed out that there is an early paradoxical increase in STH concentration within the first hour both in breast and endometrial cancer patients. A similar observation was made by Benjamin et al. (1969) in endometrial carcinoma. The cause of this 'paradoxical response' is unknown.

Some data obtained in our laboratory support the view that metabolic abnormalities which may pave the way to tumorigenesis, develop many years before cancer manifestations. It can be seen from Table 10.13 that among

TABLE 10.13

Frequency of Births of Large Babies in Two Age-distinct Cancer Groups (Berstein, 1973)

| Age at diagnosis of cancer | % with birth weight of children 4·0 kg or more | | | | |
|---|---|---|---|---|---|
| | Endometrial carcinoma | Breast cancer | Cancer of colon | Cancer of stomach | Mastopathia |
| 20–49 | 0 | 23·8 | 27·8 | 20·0 | 13·4 |
| Over 50 | 50 | 40·3 | 51·0 | 43·5 | 18·2 |

patients with cancer manifesting after 50 years of age, the proportion of women who gave birth to children weighing 4·0 kg or more was greater than in the younger patients. The frequent birth of large babies to diabetic mothers is well known (Mølsted-Pedersen, 1972) and these results may be interpreted to suggest that metabolic alterations related to pre-diabetes may possibly precede manifestations of cancer by many years.

## Adaptation system changes in cancer

It was suggested at the beginning of this chapter that normal ageing may be accompanied by a rise in the hypothalamic threshold to glucocorticoid feedback suppression. This change has been shown also in many patients with breast cancer (Bishop and Ross, 1970; Saez, 1971). In addition, these investigations reported that the average production rate of cortisol was higher than in normal subjects and the elevation seemed to correlate with the stage of the disease. Furthermore it was noted that the response to dexamethasone suppression was less marked in those patients who did not show good response to the treatment of cancer. It is noteworthy that, as the tumour progressed, the resistance of the hypothalamic feedback to suppression rose and was greater at stage 4 than that at stages 1 and 2 (Bishop and Ross, 1970).

The 'discriminant function' is claimed to be connected with such characteristics of breast cancer as individual predisposition, duration of recurrence-free interval and responsiveness to endocrine surgery (Bulbrook et al., 1962; Bulbrook, Hayward and Thomas, 1964; Bulbrook, Hayward and Spicer, 1971). It tends to become negative with ageing due to the discrepancy between age-associated decrease in androgen production, on the one hand (Bulbrook et al., 1962), and the relatively constant production of glucocorticoids, on the other. Therefore, after 65 years of age, women are most likely to enter the group at high cancer risk.

The significance of a similar discriminant function has been demonstrated also in relation to endometrial carcinoma (De Waard et al., 1969), and lung cancer (Rao, 1970). Furthermore, with regard to the former tumour, our laboratory data show signs of relative resistance to dexamethasone suppression in endometrial cancer patients compared to a control group of women with climacteric uterine bleeding (Table 10.14). However, differences

TABLE 10.14

The Effect of Dexamethasone Test on 17-oxysteroid and 17-ketosteroid Excretion Levels in Endometrial Cancer and Climacteric Bleeding Groups

| Group | Age (years) | 17-OHCS excretion | | | 17-KS excretion | | |
|---|---|---|---|---|---|---|---|
| | | Before | After | Change (%) | Before | After | Change (%) |
| | | Dexamethasone | | | Dexamethasone | | |
| Climacteric uterine bleeding | 44 | 7·0 | 4·8 | 30·0 | 11·1 | 6·8 | 39·9 |
| Endometrial carcinoma | 58 | 7·9 | 6·6 | 15·5 | 7·3 | 5·5 | 27·4 |

Note: Dexamethasone was given 0·5 mg/day for three successive days.

in average age in the study and control groups cannot be ruled out as the cause of the observed distinction, since it is impossible to distinguish between homeostatic failure occurring in the course of normal ageing and that in age-related pathology.

The absolute and relative excess of glucocorticoids in breast cancer patients probably exerts an unfavourable effect by its depressive action on the immunological defence mechanism (Mackay et al., 1971). In addition, the adrenal cortex also secretes a large fraction of oestrogenic phenol-steroids in breast cancer patients. The data in Table 10.15 show that dexamethasone

TABLE 10.15

Age-associated Variation in Inhibiting Effect of Dexamethasone in Breast Cancer Patients

| Test group | No. of patients | Total phenol-steroids (mg/24 hours) | 17-ketosteroids (mg/24 hours) | 17-oxysteroids (mg/24 hours) |
|---|---|---|---|---|
| Reproductive group | 9 | 93·0 | 7·87 | 6·66 |
| | | 42·6 | 5·05 | 3·42 |
| Variation (%) | | −54·0 | −36·4 | −48·7 |
| Menopausal group | 7 | 55·7 | 3·33 | 5·3 |
| | | 80·7 | 2·80 | 5·5 |
| Variation (%) | | +45·0 | −16·0 | +3·8 |

Note: Total phenol-steroids were determined in this study without chromatographic purification of $Al_2O_3$ column; absolute values are therefore higher than those for standard test methods (see above).

The first figure for each test represents the level prior to administration of dexamethasone (0·5 mg/day) for three days, and the second the level after treatment.

treatment significantly decreases the level of phenol-steroid excretion, thus indicating the adrenal origin of this fraction.

It should be pointed out, however, that the suppression of glucocorticoid excretion is higher in the reproductive age group than in post-menopausal patients, and with certain doses of dexamethasone, phenol-steroid excretion failed to decrease at all in the latter group. Thus, the high phenol-steroid production commonly seen in breast cancer patients is probably connected with an elevated hypothalamic threshold to suppression, since the rate of secretion of these hormones (like that of glucocorticoids) is influenced by the secretion of ACTH. It is interesting to note that data from our laboratory suggested that survival time of breast cancer patients is longer, when basal excretion of total phenol-steroids is low and when a ten-day course of prednisolone reduces this to a still lower level (Table 10.16).

In addition, it was noted that patients who had a recurrence-free interval of less than one year showed a level of phenol-steroid excretion significantly higher than that in patients with a more favourable clinical course. High levels of endogenous oestrogen may affect the immunological response in breast cancer.

To summarize this section, both breast and endometrial cancer patients frequently reveal changes in the -major homeostatic systems—in the reproductive, energy and adaptation systems. These changes appear to be associated with an elevation of the threshold of hypothalamic sensitivity to

TABLE 10.16

Correlation of Survival Time of Breast Cancer Patients and Level of Total Phenol-steroid Excretion

| Group | Number of cases | Age range | Total phenol-steroids (μg/24 hours) | |
|---|---|---|---|---|
| | | | Before prednisolone | After prednisolone |
| Survival time less than 3 years | 15 | 33–54 | $56 \cdot 5 \pm 7 \cdot 0$ | $35 \cdot 7 \pm 5 \cdot 3$ |
| Survival time more than 3 years | 26 | 29–50 | $40 \cdot 0 \pm 3 \cdot 2$ | $24 \cdot 0 \pm 2 \cdot 3$ |

homeostatic suppression. This in due course leads to a compensatory over-stimulation of the corresponding group of target endocrine glands (ovaries, beta-cells of pancreas and adrenal glands). Similar but less marked changes are seen also in the course of normal ageing.

The hormone sensitive section of breast cancer patients can be subdivided into two types. One type is characterized by the predominance of oestrogen-dependent tumours, and can be called the early-onset breast cancer type. The second type is characterized by an elevation of the hypothalamic threshold and can be called the late-onset breast cancer type. In patients with this latter type of tumour, we often observe signs of central homeostatic failure such as insufficient suppression of growth hormone secretion by glucose, hyper-insulinaemia, frequent births of large babies, excess of body weight, hypercholesterolaemia and a raised FFA level, resistance to the effect of insulin, a decrease in glucose tolerance, increased excretion of gonadotrophins and of non-classical phenol-steroids, elevated blood glucocorticoid level and resistance to inhibition by dexamethasone.

Although the latter type of tumour is more frequently observed in post-menopausal women and the former type in pre-menopausal women, many patients who are pre-menopausal also tend to show signs of age-associated change in hormonal homeostasis. These disturbances take the form of failure to inhibit blood GH levels after glucose loading, increased excretion of total gonadotrophins and increase in blood 17-oxysteroid levels.

Therefore, although carcinogenesis primarily depends on genetic trans-formations, metabolic disturbances arising in the course of ageing may substantially affect the clinical manifestations of tumorigenesis. Any influence which leads to increase in the hypothalamic threshold to feedback and its consequent compensatory responses, will tend to promote the development of breast cancer of the late-onset type. The following section considers the measures which might be utilized to correct the hormonal milieu found in patients with this type of cancer.

## ATTEMPTS TO INCREASE HYPOTHALAMIC SENSITIVITY AND TO RE-ESTABLISH HOMEOSTASIS

Elevation of the hypothalamic threshold to feedback in the major homeostatic systems is observed in some breast cancer patients, and it may be important to increase the hypothalamic sensitivity to regulating influences. It appears likely that the pineal gland secretes one or several hormones which can raise hypothalamic responsiveness. The data in Table 10.17 suggests that pineal extract can raise the sensitivity of the hypothalamo-adrenal system in rats to prednisolone-induced suppression. It is unlikely that the pineal gland secretes specific hormones for each individual controlling system in the hypothalamus, as shown by the following observation. Continuous lighting, which affects the hypothalamo-endocrine system mainly via the pineal gland, will lead to increased secretion of all pituitary trophic hormones controlled by a releasing mechanism but to decreased secretion of those controlled by an inhibitory mechanism.

TABLE 10.17

The Effect of Pineal Extract on Hypothalamo-adrenal Sensitivity to Prednisolone-induced Suppression in Rats (Ostroumova, 1972)

| | Blood corticosterone level ($\mu g$ %) | | |
|---|---|---|---|
| Treatment | Before treatment | After treatment | Significance |
| Prednisolone | $22.8 \pm 3.8$ | $22.2 \pm 2.6$ | NS |
| Prednisolone + pineal extract | $27.0 \pm 3.6$ | $11.1 \pm 2.8$ | $p < 0.05$ |

In this respect, it is very intriguing to compare the pharmacological effects of levodopa on the hypothalamus with those of pineal extracts. Levodopa, an agent which crosses the blood–brain barrier and is decarboxylated to dopamine has been shown to suppress the secretion of prolactin (Malarkey and Daughaday, 1971) and, possibly, MSH, but stimulates the secretion of STH, gonadotrophins and thyrotrophin (Eddy et al., 1971). Recently, Stoll (1972) has put forward a hypothesis leading to the use of levodopa treatment in breast cancer on the basis of the concept of age-associated elevation of hypothalamic controlling centres, and thus inhibit prolactin release from the pituitary.

Combined administration of levodopa and an inhibitor of its transformation to dopamine in peripheral tissue will probably enhance its effectiveness in the brain, as has been noted in the treatment of parkinsonism (Papavasiliou et al., 1972). Perhaps, in the future, combined administration of pineal hormones and levodopa should be investigated.

Hypothalamic changes are followed, as we have seen, by compensatory over-stimulation of some endocrine glands leading to a series of metabolic disorders. The possibility of affecting breast cancer by restoring intermediary metabolism to normal has not been investigated until quite recently. Compensatory increase in insulin secretion is a very important factor in age-associated metabolic disturbances, and it is a key factor in the development of obesity, late-onset diabetes mellitus, atherosclerosis and possibly even of the age-associated incidence of many tumours (Dilman, 1960, 1968, 1970a, b, 1971, 1972).

Some experimental observations may be relevant to this last suggestion, such as the selective uptake of insulin in some tumours (Davies, 1970), low cholesterol diet-induced suppression of a number of experimental tumours (Szepsenwol, 1966) and suppression of the growth of some experimental tumours in alloxan-induced diabetes. Relevant clinical observations include, on the one hand, a low cancer incidence in severe diabetes (Werner, 1955) and, on the other, a high incidence of decreased glucose tolerance in many types of cancer, particularly in endometrial and breast cancer.

At present, however, there are no means of reliably suppressing the rising insulin level. Nor are we in possession of insulin derivatives that could counter its hormonal effects, although our studies have shown that the hypoglycaemic and anti-lipolytic properties of insulin may be dissociated (Dilman et al., 1971b). Nevertheless, compensatory hyperinsulinaemia may be reduced by treatment with phenethylbiguanide (phenformin, dibotin) which increases glucose transport into the muscle tissue and, therefore, eliminates compensatory hyperinsulinism. It thereby reduces the cholesterol and triglyceride levels, and reduces excess body weight in aged patients (Schwartz, Mirsky and Schaefer, 1966).

On the basis of this effect, the author has suggested the use of dibotin for the treatment of metabolic lipid abnormalities characteristic of atherosclerosis (Dilman, 1968). Such an effect has been independently reported by Tzagourhis, Seidensticker and Hamwi (1968). Bearing this in mind the use of phenformin might be investigated for its ability to suppress the development not only of atherosclerosis, but also of tumour progression. In this respect it is interesting that phenformin treatment decreases blood cholesterol level and body weight in cancer patients who do not reveal clinical manifestations of diabetes.

It may be noted that two anti-epileptogenic preparations—diphenyl-hydantoin (phenytoin) and aminoglutetemide (eliptene)—have been shown in our laboratory (Dilman et al., 1969, 1971a) to decrease total gonadotrophin and LH excretion. They are also inhibitors of adrenal steroidogenesis, and therefore long-term administration of these agents may help to suppress the excessive production of glucocorticoids in breast cancer.

Protein hormone derivatives, or the so-called 'anahormones', should also be studied with a view to using them to reduce excessive secretion of protein hormones. Anahormones are chemically-modified derivatives of protein hormones which are deprived of specific hormonal effects but are either still capable of participating in hormonal homeostasis (anahormone-inhibitors), or retain specific antigenicity (anahormone-antigens), or binding affinity for the target tissue (competitive anahormones) (Dilman, 1966; Kovaleva, Rischka and Dilman, 1972).

TABLE 10.18

Suppression of Hormonal Activity of Human Pituitary Gonadotrophins by Immune Serum Against Sheep Anahormone of LH (Dilman et al., 1971b)

| Test | Weight of uterus (mg) | Significance |
|------|:---------------------:|:------------:|
| 3 μg of human LH + 0·5 ml of normal serum | $30·2 \pm 3·2$ | |
| 3 μg of human LH + 0·5 ml of serum against anahormone of sheep LH | $9·3 \pm 0·9$ | $p < 0·001$ |

An anahormone-antigen obtained by acetylation of sheep luteinizing hormone (LH) may be useful in combating over-stimulation of the sex glands (Dilman et al., 1971b). As shown in Table 10.18, an immunoserum against such a derivative of LH deprived of gonadotrophic effect is capable of neutralizing the hormonal effect of human LH. As was shown some years ago, treatment of humans with sheep gonadotrophins results in immunological neutralization of endogenous LH and suppression of the hormonal function of the sex glands (Leatham, 1949). For this reason, one might expect LH anahormone to produce the same effect, without any risk of stimulating the sex glands in the course of immunization.

Blockage of GH effects by administration of an immune serum against its anahormone (Table 10.19) suggests the advisability of studying the effect of the active immunization of humans by somatotrophin anahormone (Golubev et al., 1969; Sofronov et al., 1972). Suppression of ACTH secretion may be achieved experimentally by means of acetylated ACTH which acquires the properties of an anahormone-inhibitor (Table 10.20). Acetylated ACTH might therefore be studied with a view to using it for suppression of the adrenal function.

Acetylated ovine prolactin is capable of counteracting the lipolytic action of human growth hormone (Kovaleva, Rischka and Dilman, 1972), i.e. it possesses the properties of a competitive anahormone. However, since

TABLE 10.19

Decrease in Blood Sugar Level as a Result of Administration of Immune Serum to Anahormone of Somatotrophin (Dilman et al., 1971b)

| Tests | Days of treatment | | | | | | |
|---|---|---|---|---|---|---|---|
| | 1 | 4 | 5 | 6 | 8 | 11 | 13 |
| Blood sugar level at 8.30 a.m. | 252 | 249 | 214 | 254 | 203 | 204 | 153 |
| Blood sugar level at 12.30 a.m. | 190 | 158 | 204 | 170 | 155 | 122 | 132 |
| Insulin dose | 140 | 140 | 120 | 112 | 112 | 112 | 112 |

TABLE 10.20

Decrease in Blood Corticosterone Levels Achieved by Treatment with Acetylated ACTH and Blockage of Stressor Release of ACTH (Bulovskaya et al., 1969)

| Group | Pituitary level of corticotrophins (mU/mg) | Blood corticosterone (µg %) | Significance |
|---|---|---|---|
| Controls | $5 \cdot 4 \pm 0 \cdot 63$ | $8 \cdot 0 \pm 1 \cdot 0$ | |
| Operation | $3 \cdot 3 \pm 0 \cdot 69$ | $18 \cdot 6 \pm 0 \cdot 8$ | $p < 0 \cdot 001$ |
| Operation + acetylated ACTH | $6 \cdot 0 \pm 0 \cdot 85$ | $11 \cdot 3 \pm 1 \cdot 4$ | $p < 0 \cdot 002$ |

preparations of human prolactin are not available, it is not established whether the competitive effect is retained with respect to the latter, in addition.

More opportunities are offered by the use of newly-developed variants of anahormones, e.g. anahormone-chimaeras (Berstein et al., 1972). We have chosen this term to designate anahormones produced by conjugation of heterogeneous hormones as, for example, a conjugate of human somatotrophin and porcine ACTH. Another variant of anahormone-chimaeras was produced by conjugation of a protein hormone with a steroid hormone. Immunization against both ovarian and adrenal oestrogens by means of such anahormones deserves further study. Yet, it is still to be established whether an immune serum to a conjugate of a protein and steroid hormone, e.g. oestrone, is capable of neutralizing the biological effect of other phenol-steroids.

There is evidence that acetylated oxytocin can compete with natural oxytocin (Smyth, 1967). Studies of anahormones developed on the basis of such polypeptides as hypothalamic hormones are of great interest, considering the effectiveness by oral administration of such hypothalamic hormones as thyrotrophin-releasing factor.

## CONCLUSION

The incidence of specific hormonal–metabolic changes increases with increasing age. These include gain in body weight, decrease in glucose tolerance and hypercholesterolaemia, and it suggests a common physiological cause for these hormonal–metabolic derangements. The author believes this cause to be the phenomenon of age-associated elevation of the hypothalamic threshold to homeostatic feedback suppression.

Patients with breast cancer can be divided into two types. One is characterized by elevation of the hypothalamic threshold and is described as the late-onset type. The other, characterized by a predominantly oestrogen dependent tumour, is described as the early-onset type. Although the latter type of hormone-dependent breast cancer is more frequently observed in pre-menopausal woman and the former in post-menopausal women, many patients with breast cancer who are pre-menopausal also tend to show signs of age-associated changes in hormonal homeostasis. These disturbances take the form of failure to inhibit blood GH levels after glucose loading, increased excretion of total gonadotrophins and non-classical phenol-steroids, and increase in blood 17-oxysteroid level. Post-menopausal breast cancer patients show, in addition, more pronounced signs of secondary metabolic disturbances such as obesity, hypercholesterolaemia and diminished tolerance to carbohydrate.

Although elevation of the hypothalamic threshold to feedback is common to all types of specific age pathology, different diseases may have individual features of hormonal disturbance. Thus, patients with endometrial cancer show a lesser degree of reactive hyperinsulinaemia in response to glucose loading, a high level of immunoreactive LH excretion and a lower total gonadotrophin excretion level as compared with breast cancer patients. This is in addition to certain differences in the phenol-steroid pattern.

At present, the following tests for the major homeostatic systems are available. For the evaluation of energy homeostasis: growth hormone level before and after glucose loading; for reproductive homeostasis: level of excretion of total gonadotrophins and total phenol-steroids (or androgens); for the adaptation system: cortisol level and diurnal rhythm and dexamethasone suppression test; for integrity of the hypothalamo-hypophyseal pathway: levodopa inhibition and chlorpromazine stimulation.

Methods currently employed for the treatment of endocrine-dependent types of advanced cancer are mainly aimed at steroid hormone balance. In the author's opinion it is necessary to aim at increasing the hypothalamic sensitivity to regulating homeostatic influences. There are observations suggesting that extracts of the pineal gland may possess such properties. A trial is suggested also of pituitary inhibitors, especially sigetin, phenytoin and eliptene which act as inhibitors of gonadotrophin secretion, although their influence on prolactin secretion is still not determined. Investigations need to be carried out also on the use of dibotin for elimination of hyperinsulinaemia and with eliptene and phenytoin for decreasing phenol-steroid and cortisol production. Finally, it is suggested that anahormones might be studied further with a view to using them to reduce excessive secretion of protein hormones.

## REFERENCES

Adlersberg, D., Schaefer, L. E., Steinberg, A. G. and Chun-I Wang, (1956). 'Age, sex, serum lipids, and coronary atherosclerosis.' *J. Am. med. Ass.* **162**, 619.

Albert, A. (1956). 'Human urinary gonadotropins.' *Recent Progr. Hormone Res.* **12**, 227.

Anisimov, V. N. (1971). 'Blastomogenesis in rats with persistent estrus.' *Vopr. Oncol.* **8**, 68.

— Pavlova, M. V. (1972). 'Hormonal shifts and tumor localization in rats with a persistent estrus.' *Vopr. Oncol.* **5**, 68.

Benjamin, F., Donald, J., Sherman, L. and Kolodny, H. (1969). 'Growth hormone secretion in patients with endometrial carcinoma.' *New Engl. J. Med.* **25**, 1448.

Berstein, L. M. (1973). 'Data on the birth weight of new-born infants in oncological patients.' *Vopr. Oncol.* in patients.' *Vopr. Oncol.* **3**, 48.

— Bochman, J. V., Mandelstam, V. A. and Dilman, V. M. (1969). 'On the origin and action of nonclassical phenolsteroids in cancer of the corpus uteri in menopausal patients.' *Vopr. Oncol.* **4**, 42.

— Remisov, A. L., Sofronov, B. N. and Dilman, V. M. (1972). 'Anahormones— chimeras. Hormonally inactive conjugate of ox ACTH and human somatotrophin preserving antigenic properties of original hormones.' *Rep. Acad. Sci. USSR* **203**, 219.

Bishop, M. C. and Ross, E. J. (1970). 'Adrenocortical activity in disseminated malignant disease in relation to prognosis.' *Br. J. Cancer* **24**, 719.

Blackard, W. G., Boylen, C. T., Hinson, T. C. and Nelson, N. C. (1969). 'Effect of lipid and ketone infusion on insulin-induced growth hormone elevations in rhesus monkeys.' *Endocrinology* **85**, 1180.

Bobrov, Y. F. and Patokin, S. V. (1971). 'Radioimmunoassay of STH with aid of immunosorbent.' *Lab. delo.* **3**, 70.

— Patokin, S. V. and Dilman, V. M. (1971). 'The resistance to inhibition of growth hormone and fatty acids with glucose in patients with cancer of the mammary gland and uterine body.' *Vopr. Oncol.* **17**, 40.

Braun, T. B. and Hechter, O. (1969). 'Insulin-like action of oxytocin.' *Endocrinology* **85**, 1092.

Brown, J. B. (1960). 'The determination and significance of the natural estrogens.' *Adv. clin. Chem.* **3**, 157.

Bulbrook, R. D., Hayward, J. L., Spicer, C. C. and Thomas, B. S. (1962). 'A comparison between the urinary steroid excretion of normal women and women with advanced breast cancer.' *Lancet* **15**, 1235.

—— and Thomas, B. S. (1964). 'The relation between the urinary 17-hydroxycorticosteroids and 11-deoxy-17-oxo-steroids and the fate of patients after mastectomy.' *Lancet* **1**, 945.

—— and Spicer, C. C. (1971). 'Relation between urinary androgen and cortisol excretion and subsequent breast cancer.' *Lancet* **2**, 395.

Bulovskaya, L. N., Prokhudina, E. A., Konstantinov, V. L., Tugunov, S. S. and Dilman, V. M. (1969). 'Reversed action of acetylated corticotrophin: inhibition of adreno-cortical secretion.' *Acta endocr.* **61**, 193.

Chevallier, F. and Lutton, C. (1971). 'Origines du cholesterol de sécrétion interne chez le rat: théorie du renouvellement cellulaire.' *Revue europ. d'etud. clin. biol.* **16**, 16.

Danowski, T. S. (1957). *Diabetes Mellitus with Emphasis on Children and Young Adults.* Baltimore; Williams and Williams.

Davies, B. M. A. (1970). 'Diabetes and growth of tumor transplants.' *J. Cancer* **24**, 364.

De Waard, F., Thyssen, J. H. H., Veeman, W. and Sander, P. C. (1969). 'Steroid hormone excretion pattern in women with endometrial carcinoma.' *Cancer* **22**, 988.

Dicfalusy, E. and Lauritzen, Ch. (1961). *Oestrogens beim Menschen.* Berlin; Springer-Verlag.

Dilman, V. M. (1958). 'About age increase of activity of some hypothalamic centres.' *Trans. Inst. Physiol. USSR (Leningrad)* **7**, 326.

— (1960). 'Increase of gonadotrophin secretion in cancer of the breast as an indication of diencephalohypophysial activity.' *Vopr. Oncol.* **6**, 105.

— (1966). 'Anahormones of growth hormone, exophthalmic factor, melanophore-stimulating hormone, adrenocorticotrophin and gonadotrophin in experimental and clinical endocrinology.' *Int. J. Cancer* **1**, 239.

— (1968). *Ageing, Climacteric and Cancer.* Leningrad; Medizina.

— (1970a). 'Elevation mechanism of ageing and cancer.' *Vopr. Oncol.* **6**, 45.

— (1970b). 'Elevation concept of the ageing mechanism and age pathology. Compensation diseases.' *Kazan. Med. J.* **4**, 3.

— (1971). 'Age-associated elevation of hypothalamic threshold to feedback control, and its role in development, ageing and disease.' *Lancet* **1**, 1211.

— (1972). *Why Do We Die?* Leningrad; Medizina.

— Berstein, L. M., Bobrov, J. F., Bohman, J. V., Kovaleva, I. G. and Krilova, N. V. (1968). 'Hypothalamopituitary hyperactivity and endometrial carcinoma.' *Am. J. Obstet. Gynec.* **102**, 880.

— Elubaeva, G. O., Vishnevsky, A. S., Tsyrlina, E. V., Bulovskaja, L. N. and Lwowitsch, E. G. (1971a). 'The basis for the use of diphenine (diphenyl hydantoin) in oncological practice.' *Vopr. Oncol.* **7**, 70.

— Sofronov, B. N., Golubev, V. N., Krylova, N. V. and Ostroumova, M. N. (1971b). 'Anahormone of sheep luteinizing hormone inducing antibodies against human gonadotrophin.' *Bull. Expl. Biol. Med.* **9**, 69.

— Golubev, V. N. and Kovaleva, I. G. (1971). 'A biological effect of antisera to human somatotropin anahormone.' *Vopr. Oncol.* **11**, 103.

— Krylova, N. V., Tsyrlina, E. V. and Vishnevsky, A. S. (1969). 'The effect of aminoglutethimide on excretion of gonadotrophins and phenolsteroids.' *Vopr. Oncol.* **3**, 94.

Dilman, V. M. and Ostroumova, M. N. (1972). 'The influence of pineal extract on the sensitivity of the hypothalamic threshold to prednisolone suppression.' *Vopr. Oncol.* **11**, 3.

— and Pavlova, M. V. (1963a). 'The secretion of gonadotrophins, oestrogens and 17-ketosteroids in some precancerous and cancer diseases. Breast cancer, dysfunctional uterine haemorrhage.' *Vopr. Oncol.* **9**, 72.

— — (1963b). 'The secretion of gonadotrophins, estrogens and 17-ketosteroids in some pretumorous and tumorous diseases. The influence of age, menopause and radiation castration.' *Vopr. Oncol.* **9**, 75.

— Ryabov, S. I., Tsyrlina, E. V., Kirsanov, A. I., Kovaleva, I. G., Berstein, L. M., Ljvovich, E. G., Buslaeva, V. P. and Golubev, V. N. (1972). 'Reduction of the body weight, cholesterol and blood sugar under the effect of phenformin (phenylbiguanide) in patients with cancer and atherosclerosis.' *Vopr. Oncol.* **2**, 84.

Dole, V. P. (1956). 'A relation between non-esteritied fatty acids in plasma and the metabolism of glucose.' *J. clin. Invest.* **35**, 150.

Donovan, B. T. and Van der Werff ten Bosch, J. J. (1959). 'The hypothalamus and sexual maturation in the rat.' *J. Physiol.* **147**, 78.

Eddy, R. L., Jones, A. L., Chamkajion, L. H. and Silverthorne, M. C. (1971). 'Effect of levodopa on human hypophyseal trophic hormone release.' *J. clin. Endocr.* **33**, 709.

Everitt, A. V. (1970). 'Food intake, endocrines and ageing.' *Proc. Aust. Ass. Geront.* **1**, 65.

Furth, J. (1971). 'Hormones and cancer: historical perspective.' In *Oncology* (Proceedings of the Tenth International Congress), Vol. 1, p. 288. Chicago.

Glick, S. M., Roth, J., Valow, R. S. and Berson, S. A. (1965). 'The regulation of growth hormone secretion.' *Recent Progr. Hormone Res.* **21**, 241.

Golubev, V. N. (1972). 'Immunologic and hormonal activity of gonadotrophins in tumors of the female genitalia.' *Vopr. Oncol.* **2**, 42.

— Dilman, V. M., Kovaleva, I. G., Pavlova, M. V., Remisov, A. L. and Sofronov, B. N. (1969). 'Anahormones of somatotrophin and prolactin with added antigenic capacity.' *Rep. Acad. Sci. USSR* **184**, 966.

Hertig, A. T. and Sommers, S. (1949). 'Genesis of endometrial carcinoma.' *Cancer* **2**, 946.

Howard, B. V. and Kritchevsky, D. (1969). 'The lipids of normal diploid (WS–38) and SV40-transformed human cells.' *Int. J. Cancer* **4**, 393.

Jellinck, P. H. (1966). 'The relation of chemical carcinogens to steroid metabolism.' *Canad. Cancer Conf.* **6**, 124.

Kleinberg, D. L., Noel, G. L. and Frantz, A. G. (1971). 'Chlorpromazine stimulation and L-dopa suppression of plasma prolactin in man.' *J. clin. Endocr.* **33**, 873.

Kovaleva, I. G., Rischka, J. F. and Dilman, V. M. (1972). 'Inhibition of lipolytic activity of human growth hormone with sheep prolactin derivative (anaprolactin).' *Acta endocr.* **69**, 209.

Lawrence, L. H., Conn, J. W. and Appelt, M. M. (1971). 'Induction of hyperinsulinemia and hyperglycemia in dogs by administration of diabetogenic bovine pituitary peptide.' *Metabolism* **20**, 326.

Leathem, J. H. (1949). 'Antihormone problem in endocrine therapy.' *Recent Progr. Hormone Res.* **4**, 115.

Lipschutz, A. (1957). *Steroid Homeostasis; Hypophysis and Tumorigenesis.* Cambridge.

Littman, M. L., Taguchi, T. and Mosbach, E. H. (1966). 'Effect of cholesterol-free, fat-free diet and hypocholesteremic agents on growth of transplantable animal tumors.' *Cancer Chemother. Rep.* **50**, 25.

MacBride, J. M. (1957). 'Estrogen excretion levels in the normal postmenopausal woman.' *J. clin. Endocr.* **17**, 1440.

Mackay, W. D., Edwards, M. H., Bulbrook, R. D. and Wang, D. J. (1971). 'Relations between plasma cortisol, plasma androgen sulphates and immune response in women with breast cancer.' *Lancet* **2**, 1001.

Malarkey, W. B. and Daughaday, W. H. (1971). 'Variable response of plasma GH in acromegalic patients treated with medroxyprogesterone acetate.' *J. clin. Endocr.* **33**, 424.

Mayberry, W. E., Gharib, H., Bilstad, J. M. and Sizemore, G. W. (1971). 'Radioimmunoassay for human thyrotrophin.' *Ann. intern. Med.* **74**, 471.

Meites, J. (1972). 'Hypothalamo-pituitary-ovarian function in old female rats.' In *Proceedings of the Ninth International Congress on Gerontology*, Kiev, Vol. 2, p. 388.

Mølsted-Pedersen, L. (1972). 'Aspects of carbohydrate metabolism in newborn infants of diabetic mothers.' *Acta endocr.* **69**, 174.

Ostroumova, M. N. (1970). 'The peculiarities of chemical content of gonadotrophins in cancer of the uterine body.' *Vopr. Oncol.* **4**, 76.

— (1972). 'The reduced excretion of antigonadotrophic factor in patients with cancer of the endometrium and the mammary gland.' *Vopr. Oncol.* **2**, 38.

Papavasiliou, P. S., Cotzios, G. C., Düly, S. E., Steck, A. J., Fehling, G. and Bell, M. A. (1972). 'Levodopa in parkinsonism: potentiation of central effects with a peripheral inhibitor.' *New Engl. J. Med.* **286**, 8.

Parlow, A. P. (1958). 'A rapid bioassay method for LH and factors stimulating LH secretion.' *Fedn Proc.* **17**, 402.

Pickens, J. M., Burkeholder, J. N. and Womack, W. N. (1967). 'Oral glucose tolerance test in normal children.' *Diabetes* **16**, 11

Randle, P. J. (1965). 'The glucose fatty acid cycle.' In *On the Nature and Treatment of Diabetes*, p. 361, Ed. by B. S. Leibel and G. A. Wrenchall.

Rao, L. G. (1970). 'Discriminant function based on steroid abnormalities in patients with lung cancer.' *Lancet* **2**, 441.

Robinson, D. S., Nies, A., Davis, J. N., Benney, W. E., Davis, J. M., Colburn, R. W., Bourne, H. M., Show, D. M. and Coppen, A. J. (1972). 'Ageing, monoanmines, and monoamine-oxidase levels.' *Lancet* **1**, 290.

Sackett, G. J. (1925). Cited by Kyng, E. G. (1947). *Micro-analysis in Medical Biochemistry*, p. 16. London.

Saez, S. (1971). 'Adrenal function in cancer: relation to its evolution.' *Europ. J. Cancer* **7**, 381.

Schwartz, M. J., Mirsky, S. and Schaefer, L. E. (1966). 'The effect of phenformin hydrochloride on serum cholesterol.' *Metabolism* **15**, 808.

Smyth, D. G. (1967). 'Acetylation of amino- and tyrosine hydroxyl groups.

Preparation of inhibitors of oxytocin with no intrinsic activity on isolated uterus.' *J. biol. Chem.* **242**, 1579.

Sofronov, B. N., Kovaleva, I. G., Golubev, V. N., Chepik, O. F. and Dilman, V. M. (1972). 'A breakdown of immunological tolerance to somatotrophin by anahormone of human somatotropin with additional antigenicity.' *Bull. expl. Biol. Med.* **6**, 52.

Steelman, S. L. and Pohley, F. M. (1953). 'Assay of FSH based on augmentation with HCG.' *Endocrinology* **53**, 604.

Stoll, B. A. (1972). 'Brain catecholamines and breast cancer: a hypothesis.' *Lancet* **1**, 431.

Streeten, D. H. P., Gerstein, M. M., Marmor, B. M. and Doisy, R. J. (1965). 'Reduced glucose tolerance in elderly human subjects.' *Diabetes,* **14**, 579.

Szepsenwol, J. (1966). 'Carcinogenic effect of cholesterol in mice.' *Proc. Soc. expl Biol. Med.* **121**, 168.

Taylor, L. M. and Blackard, W. G. (1971). 'Effect of lipids on growth hormone synthesis by isolated pituitaries.' *Proc. Soc. expl Biol. Med.* **137**, 1026.

Tsai, C. C. and Yen, S. S. C. (1971). 'Acute effects of intravenous infusions of 17β-estradiol on gonadotropin release in pre- and postmenopausal woman.' *J. clin. Endocr.* **32**, 766.

Tzagourhis, M., Seidensticker, J. F. and Hamwi, G. J. (1968). 'Metabolic abnormalities in premature coronary disease: effect of therapy.' *Ann. N.Y. Acad. Sci.* **148**, 945.

Welborn, T. A., Stenhouse, N. S. and Johnstone, C. G. (1969). 'Factors determining serum-insulin response in a population sample.' *Diabetologia* **5**, 263.

Werner, W. (1955). 'Diabetes mellitus und Carcinom. Statistische Untersuchungen an Hand Von 25147 Sektionstallen.' *Z. Krebsforsch.* **60**, 3.

Wexler, B. C. (1971). 'Comparative aspects of hyperadrenocorticism and arteriosclerosis.' *Human Path.* **2**, 180.

Wide, L. and Gemsell, C. (1962). 'Immunological determination of pituitary luteinizing hormone in the urine of fertile and post-menopausal women and adult men.' *Acta Endocr.* **39**, 539.

Wilkins, L., Bongiovanni, A. M., Clayton, G. W., Grumbach, M. M. and Van Wyk, J. (1955). 'Virilising adrenal hyperplasia: its treatment with cortisone and the nature of the steroid abnormalities.' In *Ciba Foundation Symposium on Endocrinology,* Vol. 8, p. 460.

# 11

# Functions of Prolactin in Vertebrates

## Karen C. Swearingen and Charles S. Nicoll

### INTRODUCTION

Prolactin is unique among the pituitary hormones for its number and variety of functions in the vertebrates (Bern and Nicoll, 1968, 1969a, b; Nicoll and Bern, 1972; Nicoll, 1974; Mazzi, 1969). These numerous and diverse effects are listed in Table 11.1. It is apparent that prolactin was not committed early in vertebrate evolution to serve any one function, nor even a group of related physiological actions. Among the functions known to be influenced by the hormone are many related to reproduction, care of the young, osmo-regulation, growth, and the functions of integumentary structures.

In looking for a common denominator of the action of prolactin, it was concluded that at present none is apparent and that prolactin appears to have been available for the regulation of emerging physiological processes important in adapting to new environments and for adaption of new life styles (Nicoll and Bern, 1972). Thus, as examples, prolactin favours aquatic existence in amphibians, is necessary for water and salt balance in some fishes, is essential for egg incubation in birds, and promotes milk secretion in mammals.

Although most studies of the action of prolactin among the vertebrates have used mammalian prolactins, the hormone has been separated from the pituitaries of a variety of non-mammalian species (Nicoll and Nichols, 1971; Nicoll and Licht, 1971). In addition, histological studies have identified prolactin in the adenohypophyses of virtually all of the vertebrate groups (Aler, Bage and Fernholm, 1971; Benoit and DaLage, 1963; Harris and Donovan, 1966).

TABLE 11.1

Comparative Endocrinology of Prolactin. Unabridged List of the Manifold Actions Claimed for Prolactin

CYCLOSTOMES

(1) Electrolyte metabolism in hagfish (ACTH-like)

TELEOSTS

(1) Osmo-regulatory actions including:
- (a) Survival of hypophysectomized euryhaline freshwater species
- (b) Restoration of water turnover in hypophysectomized *Fundulus kansae*
- (c) Restoration of plasma $Na^+$ and $Ca^{++}$ in hypophysectomized eels when given with cortisol
- (d) Skin, buccal and gill mucus secretion
- (e) Reduced gill $Na^+$ efflux (reduced permeability)
- (f) Reduced gill permeability to water
- (g) Inhibition of gill $Na^+$, $K^+$—ATPase
- (h) Renotrophic (glomerular and tubular changes)
- (i) Increased urinary water elimination and decreased salt excretion
- (j) Stimulation of renal $Na^+$, $K^+$—ATPase
- (k) Decreased water absorption and increased $Na^+$ absorption in flounder bladder
- (l) Decreased salt and water absorption from eel gut

(2) Adrenocorticotrophic
(3) Resistance to high temperature stress
(4) Dispersion of pigment in xanthophores of *Gillichthys mirabilis, Arothron hispidus and Gobius minutus*
(5) Melanogenesis and proliferation of melanocytes (synergism with MSH)
(6) Thyroid (TSH?) stimulation
(7) Lipid metabolism
(8) Growth and secretion of seminal vesicles
(9) Reduction of toxic effects of oestrogen

(10) Parental behaviour (nest building, fin fanning, buccal incubation of eggs)
(11) Maintenance of brood pouch in male seahorse
(12) Gonadotrophic (increased 3–β–OH dehydrogenase in cichlid ovaries)

AMPHIBIANS

(1) Water drive, including skin and tail changes
(2) Larval growth [especially tail (including collagen synthesis) and gills]
(3) Somatotrophic in post-metamorphic anurans
(4) Lipid metabolism in anurans
(5) Peripheral thyroxin antagonism (anti-metamorphic)
(6) Goitrogenic-thyrotrophic (TSH release)
(7) Growth of brain in frog tadpoles
(8) Limb regeneration
(9) Decreased urea excretion and suppression of ornithine cycle enzymes in some anuran tadpoles
(10) Increased urea excretion and hepatic arginase activity in other anuran tadpoles secondary to thyroid activation
(11) Hyperglycaemic–diabetogenic
(12) Proliferation of melanophores
(13) Skin yellowing in frogs
(14) Restoration of plasma $Na^+$ levels in hypophysectomized newts
(15) $Na^+$ and water transport across toad bladder
(16) Secretion of oviducal jelly
(17) Spermatogenic and/or anti-spermatogenic
(18) Cloacal gland development (urodele)
(19) Stimulation of ultimobranchial and possible hypercalcaemia (toads)

## REPTILES

(1) Somatic growth
(2) Tail regeneration
(3) Hyperphagia
(4) Epidermal sloughing
(5) Lipid metabolism
(6) Antigonadotrophic
(7) Restoration of plasma sodium levels in hypophysectomized lizard.

## BIRDS

(1) Production of crop 'milk' (columbids)
(2) Formation of brood patch
(3) Stimulation of feather growth
(4) Somatic growth (including splanchnomegaly)
(5) Lipid metabolism
(6) Hyperglycaemic-diabetogenic
(7) Stimulation of nasal (orbital) salt gland secretion
(8) Anti-gonadal (anti-gonadotrophic)
(9) Synergism with steroids on female reproductive tract
(10) Parental behaviour
(11) Suppression of sexual phase of reproductive cycle (including calling and mating in quail)
(12) Pre-migratory restlessness (Zugunruhe)

## MAMMALS

(1) Stimulation of mammary growth and development
(2) Stimulation of milk secretion
(3) Stimulation of sebaceous gland size and activity (including preputial glands)
(4) Hair maturation
(5) Stimulation of somatic growth (including splanchnomegaly)
(6) Lipid metabolism
(7) Hyperglycaemic-diabetyogenic; increased insulin secretion
(8) Erythropoietic
(9) Renotrophic including Na + retention
(10) Increased fertility in male and female dwarf mice
(11) Actions on male reproductive organs including:
   (a) Synergism with androgens on male sex accessory glands
   (b) Increased androgen binding in human prostate
   (c) Increased cholesterol levels in mouse testis
   (d) Stimulation of β-glucuronidase activity in rodent testes
(12) Decreased copulatory activity in male rabbits
(13) Advancement of puberty in rats
(14) Progesterone secretion by rat and mouse ovaries: possible synergism in other species (luteotrophic)
(15) Luteolytic action in rats and mice
(16) Parental behaviour (retrieval of young; nest building)
(17) Vaginal mucification in rats
(18) Altered progesterone metabolism by rat uterus

The functions of prolactin can be classified under several headings: reproduction, nurturing of the young (including parental behaviour), osmo-regulation, somatotrophic effects, and actions on integumentary structures. The first three categories will be given the most emphasis here; in addition, recent evidence concerning prolactin in primates will be discussed briefly. For specific references, the reader is referred to the reviews cited above.

# FUNCTION IN REPRODUCTION

One of the synonyms for prolactin is luteotrophin. This name resulted from the finding by Astwood (1941) and Evans et al. (1941), that prolactin maintained functional corpora lutea in rats. It has since been established that prolactin is necessary for ovarian progesterone synthesis in the rat, mouse and hamster and probably other species. However, the study of prolactin's role in luteal function in these and other species is complicated by several factors. One of these is the presence in many species of a luteolysin of uterine origin. Du Mesnil du Boisson and Denamur (1969) have been able to demonstrate reliably a luteal trophic effect of prolactin in sheep, pigs and cows only after hysterectomy. Another complicating factor is the fact that the gonadotrophic hormones (including prolactin) can be either lytic or trophic, depending on a variety of factors including the physiological status of the animal. A further complication is that maintenance of ovarian progesterone secretion may involve a 'luteotrophic complex' of hormones rather than a single gonadotrophin. This has been shown to be the case in rats, mice, hamsters, rabbits and domestic ungulates.

The mechanism of action of prolactin in those species in which it has been shown to promote progesterone secretion, seems to involve the maintenance of precursor pools (i.e. cholesterol esters) for steroid synthesis. The enzyme sterol acyl transferase is apparently involved in this response to the hormone (Behrman et al., 1970). Thus prolactin may enhance the response of the luteal tissue to gonadotrophins by providing precursors for the synthesis of progesterone. In addition, it has been shown in the rat that prolactin inhibits the production of the enzyme (20-α-hydroxysteroid dehydrogenase) which converts progesterone to an inactive derivative (20-α-hydroxypregn-4-en-3-one). Accordingly, prolactin acts to ensure that steroid biosynthesis will result in the secretion of a progestationally-active hormone. The effects of prolactin on luteal function in rats are summarized in Table 11.2.

Although prolactin has been shown to be luteotrophic in certain circumstances in some species, it has also been reported to be luteolytic. Malven (1969) has shown that prolactin can be luteotrophic on new corpora lutea and lytic on old ones. In rats, there is a sharp increase in serum prolactin levels on the afternoon of pro-oestrus. If this prolactin surge is selectively inhibited for several cycles, the corpora lutea in the ovary accumulate (Billeter

## TABLE 11.2

Effects of Hypophysectomy ($\bar{H}$) and Prolactin Replacement ($\bar{H} + PRI$) on Parameters of Rat Corpus Luteum Function

Percentage Change from Controls

| | $\bar{H}$ | $\bar{H} + PRI$ | | $\bar{H}$ | $\bar{H} + PRI$ |
|---|---|---|---|---|---|
| Steroid synthesis: | | | Acetate — $1^{14}C$ incorporation into: | | |
| progesterone | − 52 | + 112 | Cholesterol | | |
| 20α-OH-pregn-4-en-3-one | + 112 | − 52 | free | − 88 | − 70 |
| | | | ester | − 60 | + 2 |
| 20α-hydroxysteroid dehydrogenase | + 400 | + 12 | Fatty acids | | |
| | | | free | − 12 | + 40 |
| Cholesterol content | | | of sterol esters | + 18 | + 900 |
| free | − 8 | + 20 | of triglyceride | − 14 | + 142 |
| ester | + 4 | + 34 | of phospholipid | + 34 | + 241 |
| Sterol acyl transferase | − 90 | − 36 | | | |

233

and Flückiger, 1971; Wuttke and Meites, 1971). This is apparently due to the absence of the pro-oestrus surge of prolactin which may function to rid the ovary of old corpora.

Other effects of prolactin on female reproduction include synergism with steroid hormones to promote the development of oviducts in several avian species and synergism with oestrogen and progesterone to promote vaginal mucification in rats (Kennedy and Armstrong, 1972). It may also modify progesterone metabolism by the rat uterus (Armstrong and King, 1971).

The role of prolactin in male mammals has puzzled endocrinologists for years. Prolactin is present in significant amounts in the pituitary of many male mammals but its function was not clearly described until recent studies by Bartke and colleagues (Bartke, 1965, 1966a, b, 1969, 1971; Bartke and Lloyd, 1970). They found that infertile male mice, which are deficient in prolactin and growth hormone, could be made fertile by injections of prolactin. The increased spermatogenesis was found to be mediated via an effect on the Leydig cells. Prolactin acts to maintain androgen precursor pools in the Leydig cells, assuring a sufficient supply of cholesterol esters for LH stimulation of androgen synthesis. Thus prolactin's function in the testis is similar to its role in the ovary in maintaining pools of steroid hormone precursors for mobilization by LH.

Prolactin is reported to influence male sex accessory organs, synergizing with androgens to stimulate the development and secretory activity of the rat prostate. It has also been shown in several mammalian species to synergize with androgens to increase the weight and secretory activity of the seminal vesicles, as well as other male sex accessory organs in other mammals and in non-mammalian species. There is some evidence (Farnsworth, 1970) that the mechanism of prolactin's action on male sex accessory organs is to increase the uptake of testosterone by the tissue. Thus prolactin may act to increase the number or activity of androgen receptors in the target organs.

While prolactin is gonadotrophic in many groups of vertebrates, it can be anti-gonadal in some avian species. Prolactin injections into birds with fully developed gonads reduces the gonad weight. Simultaneous injections of FSH tend to counteract this effect, suggesting that prolactin acts by inhibition of gonadotrophin secretion. There is also evidence that it can act additionally at the level of the gonad to block the effect of the gonadotrophic hormones. Whether prolactin exerts gonadotrophic or anti-gonadal effects, or acts to inhibit the secretion of the other gonadotrophins, probably depends upon the overall physiological (especially endocrinological) status of the animal. The latter may vary according to a variety of conditions, including season, nutrition and day length, among others.

The anti-gonadotrophic effects of prolactin may serve to suppress sexual activity during the period when the bird should be incubating eggs or caring for the young. Prolactin may also predispose the birds for incubation of eggs and caring for the young, as well as affecting parental behaviour. These functions will be discussed further below. However, prolactin has also been suggested to play a role in other behaviours. It has been suggested that the hormone predisposes birds for migration and it promotes migration of salamanders from the terrestrial to the aquatic habitat. It may also promote migration of stickleback fish from sea to fresh water. In each of these instances, distinct physiological changes also occur. It is thus difficult to establish if the hormone affected the behaviour by a direct neural action or via the induced physiological changes which in turn evoked the migratory behaviours.

## FUNCTION IN NURTURING OF YOUNG

Prolactin was originally defined and isolated as the adenohypophyseal principal responsible for the induction of lactation in mammals and for the formation of pigeon 'crop milk'. These long-known effects of the hormone have provided the basis for its bioassay as well as alternative names (mammotrophin, lactogenic hormone).

In rats and mice mammary gland growth during pregnancy requires prolactin, a corticosteroid, oestrogen and progesterone. Insulin and growth hormone are probably additional prerequisites for the development from the elementary duct system to the fully differentiated, secretory lobular–alveolar structure. The hormonal requirements for the final developmental stages and functional differentiation of mouse mammary glands have been studied extensively in organ culture using explants from mid-pregnant animals. This development involves the multiplication of the epithelial cells to form the lobular–alveolar structure, in addition to cytological and functional differentiation of the cells. This process includes an increase in rough endoplasmic reticulum, Golgi development, enlarged alveolar lumina and the appearance of secretory granules (Topper, 1970). Prolactin, a corticosteroid and insulin are the minimum hormonal requirements for the *in vitro* response.

Milk contains casein, α-lactalbumin, β-lactoglobulin, lipids, and lactose. Following synthesis on the endoplasmic reticulum, the milk proteins are transferred to the Golgi region where they are packaged into membrane-bound granules. The lactose, which is apparently synthesized in the Golgi, is also packaged with the proteins into the granules. These granules are released from the cells into the alveolar lumen by fusion of the granule membrane with the cell membrane. The esterification of fatty acids to form lipids appears to occur in the endoplasmic reticulum. The lipid droplets lack limiting membranes within the cytoplasm, but become enclosed in cell membrane when they are released into the lumen (Linzell and Peaker, 1971). The release of these secretory products into the mammary gland lumina can be evaluated histologically and has been used as a bioassay for prolactin (Frantz and Kleinberg,

1970; Frantz, Kleinberg and Noel, 1972; Forsyth, 1972; Forsyth and Myres, 1971).

At the biochemical level, the response to prolactin includes increased synthesis of messenger, transfer and ribosomal RNA. A new population of polysomes enters the cytoplasm and the synthesis of enzymes (lactose-synthetase) and specific milk proteins occurs. The responses to prolactin at the biochemical level have also been used as assays for the hormone in mammary gland cultures (Loewenstein et al., 1971; Turkington, 1972b).

The mechanism by which prolactin affects this sequence of biochemical and morphological events has been investigated extensively by Turkington (1972a). He reports that the initial step is the binding of prolactin to a cell membrane receptor. A cyclic AMP binding protein and two protein kinases may then participate in relaying the message from the membrane receptor to the nucleus where increased transcription occurs. Turkington claims that, unlike some other polypeptide hormones, prolactin does not stimulate membrane adenyl cyclase activity, and neither cyclic AMP, nor dibutyryl cyclic AMP can mimic its effects on the mammary cell.

Like the mammary gland, the pigeon crop-sac responds to stimulation by prolactin to produce crop 'milk' which is used to feed the young. The avian crop-sac is an outpocketing of the oesophagus which is used as a food-storage organ. In pigeons and doves, it has acquired a sensitivity to prolactin and responds to the hormone by a proliferation of the mucosal epithelium. This proliferation results in a sloughing off of cells which form a cottage cheese-like crop 'milk'. It is rich in fat, protein and nucleic acids, but contains no casein-like protein or lactose. The young obtain this substance by inserting their beaks down into the parent's throat. The proliferation of the crop sac mucosa in response to prolactin provides the classical bioassay of the hormone.

Another function of prolactin in avian species is promotion of the development of the incubation or brood patch. Prior to, or during the period of egg-laying, prolactin synergizes with gonadal steroids to produce the incubation patch. It is a de-feathered area of the ventral abdominal skin which becomes highly vascularized, ensuring adequate heat transfer to the eggs during incubation. In those avian species in which the female cares for the eggs and young, oestrogen synergizes with prolactin to form the incubation patch. However, in some species both males and females develop it, and in the phalaropes, where the male incubates the eggs, only he develops the incubation patch. In this case, prolactin acts in concert with androgens.

The function of prolactin in stimulating 'milk secretion' is not limited to mammals and some avian species. Certain teleosts also produce a mucous substance from modified skin glands which the young use for nourishment. Prolactin increases the number, size, and secretory activity of these glands.

In addition to eliciting physiological changes involved in nurturing the young of many species, prolactin has been implicated in parental behaviour in teleosts, birds and mammals. Studies by Riddle, Bates and Lahr (1935) first indicated that prolactin was involved in incubation and broody behaviour in hens. Injections of the hormone were later reported to induce parental behaviour in pheasants, turkeys and ring doves. However, prolactin's behavioural effects, especially in pigeons and doves, are controversial. Although Riddle (1963) contends that prolactin is the inducer of the behaviour pattern, Lehrman (1963) advocates that progesterone is the inducer and prolactin is a sustainer of these behaviours. In mammals, pup retrieval by rats and nest building by rabbits have been suggested to rely on prolactin (Zarrow, Gandelman and Denenberg, 1971). In several cichlid fishes, prolactin is reported to increase fin-fanning, which serves to ensure that a constant current of fresh water passes over the eggs, and to decrease fighting behaviour. Other fish behaviours reported to be produced by prolactin include brooding and foam nest building.

## FUNCTION IN OSMO-REGULATION

Those fish which migrate between sea water and fresh water face a profound osmo-regulatory problem which requires numerous physiological adjustments, particularly in the gill, gut and kidney. In the fresh water habitat, the osmo-regulatory problems are those of salt loss to the hypotonic external environment, and water inundation. These are prevented by reduced permeability of the gills to efflux of ions, by increased ion uptake across the gills, and by the excretion of large amounts of dilute urine.

In recent years, the role of prolactin in facilitating osmo-regulatory adjustments at the gill and kidney in certain species has become apparent. If sea water adapted fish are hypophysectomized before being placed in fresh water, they do not survive, due to loss of sodium chloride. Prolactin injections permit survival in fresh water. The hormone reduces NaCl loss primarily by acting on the gills to prevent efflux. This effect is accompanied by a reduction in the levels of a $Na^+$-$K^+$-ATPase which is associated with the active outward pumping of sodium chloride in sea water. In the fresh water environment, prolactin also acts on the kidney to increase water excretion and reduce salt loss. This action is accomplished in some species by increased size of glomeruli, and hypertrophy of renal tubular cells.

The sodium-retaining effect of prolactin has provided another means of bioassay of the hormone. The plasma sodium concentration is linearly related to the log dose of prolactin injected into salt water adapted *Tilapia mossambica* (Clarke, 1971, 1972), or into hypophysectomized *Poecilia latipina* (Ensor and Ball, 1968). These assays should be of particular value in assaying fish prolactins which dō not have full crop-sac stimulating or mammotrophic activity. Prolactin may also be involved in osmo-regulation in amphibians, reptiles and birds (Nicoll, 1974)

The role of prolactin in osmo-regulation in mammals has received little attention; however, there is some evidence to suggest that it may act in mammals to increase sodium retention. Lockett (1965) and Lockett and Nail (1965) reported that prolactin decreased sodium excretion in rats and cats. Human placental lactogen may increase aldosterone secretion (Melby et al., 1966) and ovine prolactin was reported to increase the adrenal responsiveness to ACTH in a single patient (Ingvarsson, 1969). In another study on humans, Horrobin et al. (1971) found that injections of ovine prolactin resulted in decreased excretion of sodium and water. It has also been reported that prolactin accelerated recovery of rat kidneys which were damaged by ischaemia (Köhnlein, Bianchi and Bierman, 1966). Thus it is possible that prolactin has a role in mammalian osmo-regulation. This function may be of significance during lactation, when there is a substantial loss of water and electrolytes into milk (Nicoll, 1971). In this connection, Linzell and Peaker (1971) have speculated that prolactin may act on the apical membrane of the mammary cell to reduce Na-K-ATPase (similar to its action on the fish gill). This action would account for the low levels of this enzyme found on the apical surface, and the lower concentration of Na in milk than in mammary cells.

## SOMATOTROPHIC EFFECTS

Ovine and bovine prolactin have been reported to mimic the effect of growth hormone in promoting body growth in teleosts, amphibians, reptiles, birds and mammals. Prolactin can also have growth hormone-like metabolic effects such as hyperglycaemic and diabetogenic actions, effects on lipid deposition and/or mobilization, and actions in man similar to HGH (effects on BUN, nitrogen balance, blood glucose, fatty acids, and calcium metabolism). However, these effects may be more apparent than real, reflecting the similarity in structure of mammalian growth hormones and prolactins. In some species, the tissue receptors may not discriminate well between the two similarly structured foreign hormones, whereas the animal's endogenous prolactin might not have significant growth hormone-like actions. For example, in sheep, ovine prolactin does not duplicate the effects of sheep growth hormone (Manns and Boda, 1965). Whether a growth hormone-like or prolactin-like response is elicited by prolactin administration may depend on whether certain steroids are available for synergism with prolactin, the general endocrinological state of the animal, and the time of day of administration of the hormone (see below).

One case in which prolactin may be of significance in regulating growth and development is in larval amphibians. The hormone promotes the growth of those structures which are distinctly larval, especially the tail and the tail fin. In addition, prolactin blocks the metamorphosis-inducing effects of thyroxine.

Several species of urodeles undergo a second metamorphosis. After living on land for a period of time, they return to an aquatic environment for breeding. Prolactin stimulates this 'water drive' and the reappearance of a keeled tail, and a smooth mucoid skin. During this second metamorphosis, prolactin blocks the effects of thyroxine, as it does during the first metamorphosis. Thus, in amphibians, prolactin appears to be the hormone which promotes the growth and retention of those structures necessary for an aquatic existence.

## ACTIONS ON INTEGUMENTARY (ECTODERMAL) STRUCTURES

Most actions of prolactin which can be considered under this category have been discussed in previous sections on care of the young, osmo-regulation, and growth. These include effects on the mammary gland, the crop sac, the brood patch, and the skin glands of some fish. Other effects on ectodermal structures include those on the fish gill which facilitate fresh water survival, and the skin changes associated with 'water drive' in certain amphibians. One effect not previously mentioned is the yellowing response in the teleost *Gillichthys mirabillis*. Local prolactin injections cause the pigment in the xanthophores to disperse, which results in yellowing. Other integumentary effects not previously mentioned include epidermal sloughing in reptiles, stimulation of feather growth and nasal gland secretion in birds, and in mammals stimulation of sebaceous and preputial gland size and activity, and of hair maturation.

## DIURNAL VARIATIONS IN PROLACTIN RESPONSIVENESS

In recent years, A. Meier and his colleagues have suggested a new principle in endocrine physiology. They have shown that in several vertebrate species the response to prolactin depends on the time of day the hormone is injected (Meier, 1969). For example, if given early in the photoperiod, the hormone can stimulate lipid mobilization, whereas if given to the same species late in the photoperiod, it will cause fat deposition (Meier et al., 1971). They also found that the responsiveness of the pigeon crop sac varied with the time of day of prolactin injection (Burns and Meier, 1971). This variation is apparently phased by the circadian rhythm of adrenal corticoids. The studies from Meier's laboratory make it apparent that the time of day at which prolactin, and possibly other hormones, is administered may be of critical importance in determining the nature as well as the degree of response to the hormone.

## PRIMATE PROLACTIN

For many years there was some question as to whether the primate pituitary possesses a separate prolactin and growth hormone, since until recently all attempts to chemically isolate prolactin were unsuccessful. However, a number of clinical studies indicated that it was possible to have elevations in

239

the activity of one of the hormones without an increase in the other (Nicoll et al., 1970; Sherwood, 1971). Furthermore, several investigators, taking advantage of the general tendency of mammalian pituitaries to secrete abundant amounts of prolactin in the absence of hypothalamic control (Nicoll, 1971) have shown that monkey (Nicoll, 1972b; Channing et al., 1970; Friesen and Guyda, 1971; Nicoll et al., 1970) and human (Pasteels, Brauman and Brauman, 1963; Pasteels, 1972; Hwang et al., 1971) pituitaries secrete prolactin independently of growth hormone *in vitro*.

Some of these studies (Nicoll et al., 1970; Channing et al., 1970; Pasteels, Brauman and Brauman, 1963; Pasteels, 1972) have used the crop sac bioassay for prolactin and an immunoassay for growth hormone. Others have used immunoprecipitation of labelled hormones with antisera to ovine prolactin and to human growth hormone (Friesen and Guyda, 1971; Hwang et al., 1971) or disc electrophoresis (Nicoll, 1972). The independent secretion of prolactin and growth hormone has also been shown *in vivo* in the monkey, as measured by crop sac bioassay and growth hormone immunoassay of cavernous sinus serum (Nicoll et al., 1972). Several investigators (Forsyth and Myres, 1971; Forsyth, 1972; Turkington, 1972b; Frantz, Kleinberg and Noel, 1972; Frantz and Kleinberg, 1970; Loewenstein et al., 1971) have used sensitive mammary gland bioassays to show the independence of prolactin and growth hormone levels in human sera.

It has thus been unequivocably established that prolactin and growth hormone are separate hormones in the primate. Furthermore, the chemical separation of the two hormones has recently been accomplished from monkey (Peckham and Nicoll, 1971; Guyda and Friesen, 1971) and human (Lewis et al., 1971; Lewis, Singh and Seavey, 1971; Hwang, Guyda and Friesen, 1972) pituitaries. It has thus been possible to develop specific radioimmunoassays for human prolactin and to measure the circulating levels under various conditions.

Friesen and his colleagues (Friesen et al., 1972; Hwang, Guyda and Friesen, 1971) have found prolactin to be detectable by immunoassay in the serum of virtually all subjects, with 'normal' levels found in acromegalics. In patients with galactorrhoea the mean level (100 ng/ml) was approximately ten times the normal (Friesen et al., 1972). In lactating women, suckling (Friesen et al., 1972; Bryant and Greenwood, 1972) increased serum prolactin levels, as did phenothiazine drugs (Bryant and Greenwood, 1972) in non-lactating subjects. These results confirm those found by mammary gland bioassay (Forsyth and Myres, 1971; Forsyth, 1972; Turkington, 1972b; Frantz, Kleinberg and Noel, 1972; Frantz and Kleinberg, 1970; Lowenstein et al., 1971). It has also been shown by bioassay that prolactin levels increase in patients after pituitary-stalk section (Turkington, Underwood and Van Wyk, 1971). Interestingly, Turkington (1971) has reported the production of prolactin by two different ectopic carcinomata.

No significant changes in immunoassayable prolactin levels have been observed during the menstrual cycle (Friesen et al., 1972); however, samples were taken only once a day and prolactin has a short half-life (less than 10 minutes in humans—Bryant and Greenwood, 1972). Thus any surges in prolactin levels which did not occur near the time of sampling would be missed. Friesen and his colleagues (Friesen et al., 1972; Hwang, Guyda and Friesen, 1971) have found that during pregnancy serum prolactin levels are elevated, reaching 20 times normal levels at term (207 ng/ml). They also found the level in foetal serum at birth was equal to that in the mother, declining in the neonate to less than 20 ng/ml by four to six weeks. Surprisingly, they found the concentration of prolactin in the amniotic fluid was ten times higher than in either the mother or the foetus.

At this time it is only possible to speculate on the physiological role of the elevated levels of prolactin observed in the serum of the pregnant woman and foetus and in the amniotic fluid. In the pregnant woman the levels of placental lactogen are also quite high (mean 4 µg/ml—Friesen et al., 1972). It would seem likely that the placental and pituitary prolactins promote the development of a structurally mature secretory mammary gland, and may stimulate the secretion of colostrum. They may in addition decrease the excretion of salt and consequently water. In the foetus, the level of placental lactogen (less than 100 mg/ml) is lower than that of pituitary prolactin (Friesen et al., 1972). One could speculate than in the foetus prolactin functions as a growth hormone, analagous to its larval somatotrophic effects in amphibians. In addition, it may promote kidney development, facilitating the excretion of the amniotic fluid which is reportedly drunk by the foetus. It may also stimulate sebaceous gland secretion, promoting the development of the protective ointment of foetal skin, the vernix caseosa. The prolactin level in amniotic fluid is much higher than the concentration of placental lactogen (Friesen et al., 1972). Perhaps prolactin influences the transfer of salt and water across the placenta. However, these proposed functions of prolactin and placental lactogen in the pregnant woman, foetus, and amniotic fluid are purely speculative at this time.

## CONCLUSIONS

The foregoing speculation on the role of prolactin during pregnancy in humans serves to emphasize the diversity of functions which it is possible to ascribe to prolactin. Since the hormone was apparently not committed to one function early in vertebrate phylogeny, it has been available for the regulation of many emerging functions. As the physiology of prolactin in mammals is more thoroughly investigated its role in functions which hark back to its role in the 'lower' vertebrates may become more obvious. For example, its role in osmo-regulation in mammals, particularly during lactation, may be of greater significance than is presently appreciated. There is also the possibility that additional functions of the hormone emerged with mammals, or perhaps with the primates, other than those which have already been described. Prolactin may thus be viewed as a most unusual hormone, not only for the number and diversity of its actions, but also for the dynamics of its changing functions in vertebrates.

## ACKNOWLEDGMENTS

Work in our laboratory was supported by N.I.H. Grants AM-11161 and AM-13605 and by a Grant from the Population Council, Dr. Swearingen held a post-doctoral fellowship from the N.I.H.

## REFERENCES

Aler, G., Båge, G. and Fernholm, B. (1971). 'On the existence of prolactin in cyclostomes.' *Gen. comp. Endocr.* **16**, 498.

Armstrong, D. T. and King, E. R. (1971). 'Uterine progesterone metabolism and progestational response: effects of estrogens and prolactin.' *Endocrinology* **89**, 191.

Astwood, E. B. (1941). 'The regulation of corpus luteum function by hypophysial luteotropin.' *Endocrinology* **29**, 309.

Bartke, A. (1965). 'Influence of luteotrophin on fertility of dwarf mice.' *J. Reprod. Fert.* **10**, 93.

— (1966a). 'Reproduction of female dwarf mice treated with prolactin.' *J. Reprod. Fert.* **11**, 203.

— (1966b). 'Influence of prolactin on male fertility in dwarf mice.' *J. Endocr.* **35**, 419.

— (1969). 'Prolactin changes cholesterol stores in the mouse testis.' *Nature, Lond.* **224**, 700.

— (1971). 'Effects of prolactin on spermatogenesis in hypophysectomized mice.' *J. Endocr.* **49**, 311.

— and Lloyd, C. W. (1970). 'Influence of prolactin and pituitary isografts on spermatogenesis in dwarf mice and hypophysectomized rats.' *J. Endocr.* **46**, 321.

Behrman, H. R., Orczyk, G. P., MacDonald, G. J. and Greep, R. O. (1970). 'Prolactin induction of enzymes controlling luteal cholesterol ester turnover.' *Endocrinology* **87**, 1251.

Benoit, J. and DaLage, C. (1963). 'Cytologie de l'adenohypophyse.' *CNRS Colloq. Internat.* **128**.

Bern, H. A. and Nicoll, C. S. (1968). 'The comparative endocrinology of prolactin.' *Recent Progr. Hormone Res.* **24**, 681.

— — (1969a). 'The zoological specificity of prolactins.' *CNRS Colloq. Internat.* **177**, 193.

— — (1969b). 'The taxonomic specificity of prolactins.' In *Progress in*

*Endocrinology,* pp. 433–439, Ed. by C. Gual. Amsterdam; Excerpta Medica Foundation.

Billeter, E. and Flückiger, E. (1971). 'Evidence for a luteolytic function of prolactin in the intact cyclic rat using 2-Br-α-ergokryptine (CB154).' *Experientia* **27**, 464.

Bryant, G. D. and Greenwood, F. C. (1972). 'The concentrations of human prolactin in plasma measured by radioimmunoassay: experimental and physiological modifications.' In *Lactogenic Hormones,* pp. 197–206, Ed. by G. E. W. Wolstenholme and J. Knight. Edinburgh; Churchill Livingstone.

Burns, J. T. and Meier, A. (1971). 'Daily variations in pigeon cropsac responses to prolactin.' *Experientia* **27**, 572.

Channing, C. P., Taylor, M., Knobil, E., Nicoll, C. S. and Nichols, C. W. Jnr. (1970). 'Secretion of prolactin and growth hormone by cultures of adult simian pituitaries.' *Proc. Soc. expl Biol. Med.* **135**, 540.

Clarke, C. (1971). 'Bioassay for prolactin using intact *Tilapia mossambica* acclimated to sea water.' *Am. Zool.* **11**, Abstr. No. 124.

— (1972). 'Studies on the role and occurrence of prolactin in fishes.' PhD Dissertation, Department of Zoology, University of California, Berkeley.

Ensor, D. M. and Ball, J. N. (1968). 'Prolactin and freshwater sodium fluxes in Poecilia latipinna (Teleostei).' *J. Endocr.* **41**, 16.

Evans, H. M., Simpson, M. E., Lyons, W. R. and Turpeinen, K. (1941). 'Anterior pituitary hormones which favor the production of traumatic uterine placentomata.' *Endocrinology* **28**, 933.

Farnsworth, W. E. (1970). 'Prolactin and androgen binding by human prostate.' *Program for the Endocrine Society,* Abstr. No. 245, 159.

Forsyth, I. A. (1972). 'Use of a rabbit mammary gland organ culture system to detect lactogenic activity in blood.' In *Lactogenic Hormones,* pp. 151–167, Ed. by G. E. W. Wolstenholme and J. Knight. Edinburgh; Churchill Livingstone.

— and Myres, R. (1971). 'Human prolactin. Evidence obtained by the bioassay of human plasma.' *J. Endocr.* **51**, 157.

Frantz, A. and Kleinberg, D. (1970). 'Prolactin: evidence that it is separate from growth hormone in human blood.' *Science* **170**, 745.

— — and Noel, G. L. (1972). 'Physiological and pathological secretion of human prolactin studied by *in vitro* bioassay.' In *Lactogenic Hormones,* pp. 137–150, Ed. by G. E. W. Wolstenholme and J. Knight. Edinburgh; Churchill Livingstone.

Friesen, H. and Guyda, H. (1971). 'Biosynthesis of monkey growth hormone and prolactin *in vitro.' Endocrinology* **88**, 1353.

— Belanger, C., Guyda, H. and Hwang, P. (1972). 'The synthesis and secretion of placental lactogen and pituitary prolactin.' In *Lactogenic Hormones,* pp. 83–103, Ed. by G. E. W. Wolstenholme and J. Knight. Edinburgh; Churchill Livingstone.

Guyda, H. and Friesen, H. (1971). 'The separation of monkey prolactin from monkey growth hormone by affinity chromatography.' *Biochem. Biophys. Res. Commun.* **42**, 1068.

Harris, G. W. and Donovan, B. J. (Eds.) (1966). *The Pituitary Gland,* Vol. 1. London; Butterworths.

Horrobin, D. F., Curstyn, P. B., Lloyd, I. J., Durkin, N., Lipton, A. and Muiruri, K. L. (1971). 'Actions of prolactin on human renal function.' *Lancet* **2**, 352.

Hwang, P., Friesen, H., Hardy, J. and Wilansky, D. (1971). 'Biosynthesis of human growth hormone and prolactin by normal pituitary glands and pituitary adenomas.' *J. clin. Endocr.* **33**, 1.

Hwang, P., Guyda, H. and Frieses, H. (1971). 'A radioimmunoassay for human prolactin.' *Proc. natn. Acad. Sci.* **68**, 1902.

— — — (1972). 'Purification of human prolactin.' *J. biol. Chem.* **247**, 1955.

Ingvarsson, C. G. (1969). 'The action of prolactin on adrenocortical function.' *Acta rheum. scand.* **15**, 18.

Kennedy, T. G. and Armstrong, D. T. (1972). 'Extra-ovarian effect of prolactin on vaginal mucification in the rat.' *Endocrinology* **90**, 815.

Köhnlein, H. E., Bianchi, L. and Bierman, F. J. (1966). 'Der Einflub von Lacationshorman auf die ischämisierte Rattenniere.' *Arzn.-Forsch.* **16**, 480.

Lehrman, D. S. (1963). 'On the initiation of incubation behavior in doves.' *Anim. Behav.* **11**, 433.

Lewis, U. J., Singh, R. N. P. and Seavey, B. K. (1971). 'Human prolactin: isolation and some properties.' *Biochem. Biophys. Res. Commun.* **44**, 1169.

— — Sinha, Y. N. and VanderLaan, W. P. (1971). 'Electrophoretic evidence for human prolactin.' *J. clin. Endocr.* **33**, 153.

Linzell, J. L. and Peaker, M. (1971). 'The mechanism of milk secretion.' *Physiol. Rev.* **51**, 564.

Lockett, M. F. (1965). 'A comparison of the direct renal actions of pituitary growth and lactogenic hormones.' *J. Physiol.* **181**, 192.

— and Nail, B. (1965). 'A comparative study of the renal actions of growth and lactogenic hormones in rats.' *J. Physiol.* **180**, 147.

Loewenstein, J. E., Mariz, I. K., Peake, G. T. and Daughaday, W. H. (1971). 'Prolactin bioassay by induction of N-acetyllactosamine synthetase in mouse mammary gland explants.' *J. clin. Endocr.* **33**, 217.

Malven, P. V. (1969). 'Hypophysial regulation of luteolysis in the rat.' In *The Gonads*, pp. 367–382, Ed. by K. W. McKerns. New York; Appleton-Century-Crofts.

Manns, J. G. and Boda, J. M. (1965). 'Effects of ovine growth hormone and prolactin on blood glucose, serum insulin, plasma nonesterified fatty acids and amino nitrogen in sheep.' *Endocrinology* **76**, 1109.

Mazzi, V. (1969). 'Biologia della prolattina.' *Boll. Zool.* **36**, 1.

Meier, A. H. (1969). 'Diurnal variations of metabolic responses to prolactin in lower vertebrates.' *Gen. Comp. Endocr.* Suppl. **2**, 55.

— Trobec, T. N., Joseph, M. M. and John, T. M. (1971). 'Temporal synergism of prolactin and adrenal steroids in the regulation of fat stores.' *Proc. Soc. expl Biol. Med.* **137**, 408.

Melby, J. C., Dale, S. L., Wilson, T. E. and Nichols, A. S. (1966). 'Stimulation of aldosterone secretion by human placental lactogen.' *Clin. Res.* **14**, 283 (Abstr.).

duMesnil du Boisson, F. and Denamur, R. (1969). 'Mécanismes de contrôle de la fonction lutéale chez la truie, la brebis et la vache.' In *Progress in Endocrinology*, pp. 927–934, Ed. by C. Gual. Amsterdam; Excerpta Medica Foundation.

Nicoll, C. S. (1971). 'Aspects of the neural control of prolactin secretion.' In *Frontiers in Neuroendocrinology, 1971*, pp. 291–330, Ed. by L. Martini and W. F. Ganong. New York; Oxford University Press.

— (1972). 'Secretion of prolactin and growth hormone by adenohypophyses of rhesus monkeys *in vitro*.' In *Lactogenic Hormones*, pp. 257–268, Ed. by G. E. W.

Wolstenholme and J. Knight. Edinburgh; Churchill Livingstone.

— (1974). 'Physiological actions of prolactin.' In *Handbook of Physiology*, in press.

Nicoll, C. S. and Bern, H. A. (1972). 'On the actions of prolactin among the vertebrates: is there a common denominator?' In *Lactogenic Hormones*, pp. 299–324, Ed. by G. E. W. Wolstenholme and J. Knight. Edinburgh; Churchill Livingstone.

— Blair, S. M., Nichols, C. W. Jnr., Russell, S. M. and Taylor, M. (1972). 'Prolactin and growth hormone levels in serum from the cavernous sinus of rhesus monkeys.' *J. clin. Endocr.* **34**, 167.

— and Licht, P. (1971). 'Evolutionary biology of prolactins and somatotropins. II. Electrophoretic comparison of tetrapod somatotropins.' *Gen. comp. Endocr.* **17**, 490.

— and Nichols, C. W. Jnr. (1971). 'Evolutionary biology of prolactins and somatotropins. I. Electrophoretic comparison of tetrapod prolactins.' *Gen. comp. Endocr.* **17**, 300.

— Parsons, J. A., Fiorindo, R. P., Nichols, C. W. Jnr. and Sakuma, M. (1970). 'Evidence of independent secretion of prolactin and growth hormone *in vitro* by adenohypophyses of rhesus monkeys.' *J. clin. Endocr.* **30**, 512.

Pasteels, J. L. (1972). 'Tissue culture of human hypophyses: evidence of a specific prolactin in man.' In *Lactogenic Hormones*, pp. 269–277, Ed. by G. E. W. Wolstenholme and J. Knight. Edinburgh; Churchill Livingstone.

— Brauman, H. and Brauman, J. (1963). 'Etude comparée de la sécrétion d'hormone somatotrope par l'hypophyse humaine *in vitro* et de son activité lactogénique.' *C.R. Acad. Sci. Paris* **256**, 2031.

Peckham, W. D. and Nicoll, C. S. (1971). 'On the isolation of monkey pituitary prolactin.' *Program of the Endocrine Society*, Abst. No. 123.

Riddle, O. (1963). 'Prolactin or progesterone as key to parental behavior: a review.' *Anim. Behav.* **11**, 419.

— Bates, R. W. and Lahr, E. L. (1935). 'Prolactin induces broodiness in fowl.' *Am. J. Physiol.* **3**, 352.

Sherwood, L. M. (1971). 'Human prolactin.' *New Engl J. Med.* **284**, 774.

Topper, Y. J. (1970). 'Multiple hormone interactions in the development of mammary gland *in vitro*.' *Recent Progr. Hormone Res.* **26**, 287.

Turkington, R. W. (1971). 'Ectopic production of prolactin.' *New Engl J. Med.* **285**, 1455.

— (1972a). 'Molecular biological aspects of prolactin.' In *Lactogenic Hormones*, pp. 111–127, Ed. by G. E. W. Wolstenholme and J. Knight. Edinburgh; Churchill Livingstone.

— (1972b). 'Measurement of prolactin activity in human serum by the induction of specific milk proteins *in vitro*: results in various clinical disorders.' In *Lactogenic Hormones*, pp. 169–184, Ed. by G. E. W. Wolstenholme and J. Knight. Edinburgh; Churchill Livingstone.

— Underwood, L. E. and Van Wyk, J. J. (1971). 'Elevated serum prolactin levels after pituitary-stalk section in man.' *New Engl J. Med.* **285**, 707.

Wuttke, W. and Meites, J. (1971). 'Luteolytic role of prolactin during the estrous cycle of the rat.' *Proc. Soc. expl Biol. Med.* **137**, 988.

Zarrow, M. X., Gandelman, R. and Denenberg, V. H. (1971). 'Prolactin: is it an essential hormone for maternal behavior in the mammal?' *Hormones and Behavior* **2**, 343.

# PART III

# Neuroendocrine Aspects of Breast Cancer Therapy

# 12

# Roles of Steroid and Pituitary Hormones in Tumour Growth

## R. Tchao

## INTRODUCTION

Neoplasms of hormone target tissues retain some of the characteristics, particularly in growth and metabolism, of the normal cells from which they arose. In human mammary cancers hormone dependence, as shown by the results of endocrine ablation therapy, is well established. About 30–40 per cent of pre-menopausal women with breast tumours respond to oophorectomy (Pearson, 1967; Block et al., 1960; Dao, 1962). Bilateral adrenalectomy is reported to lead to response in 39–50 per cent of patients (Dao, Nemoto and Bross, 1967) and hypophysectomy in 35–50 per cent of patients (Pearson and Ray, 1960). On the other hand, it has also been demonstrated that large doses of oestrogen will inhibit the growth of a proportion of breast tumours (AMA Report, 1960; Kennedy, 1962).

There is no doubt that 30–40 per cent of breast cancers show clinical hormone sensitivity and the hormones implicated in the stimulation of the cancer cell are oestrogen and pituitary hormones, of which prolactin seems the most likely candidate. Oestrogen administration will exacerbate the activity of breast cancer regressing after oophorectomy (Pearson et al., 1954), but breast cancer regressing after hypophysectomy is not reactivated by oestrogen administration (Pearson and Ray, 1959). Recently, Salih et al. (1972) demonstrated that 32 per cent of 50 human mammary cancers responded to prolactin *in vitro*. It seems, therefore, that prolactin and oestrogen can be regarded as separate stimulants of growth in their influence on human mammary cancer.

In this chapter the evidence for the participation of oestrogen and especially oestradiol, and of prolactin in the growth of breast cancers will be evaluated. The terms hormone dependent, hormone responsive and hormone independent are used as defined by Furth (1963) to describe the characteristics of endocrine related neoplasms.

## BREAST CANCER AS AN OESTROGEN TARGET TISSUE

It has been established that mammalian tissues which depend on oestrogens for growth and function have a particular affinity for oestradiol. This affinity has been demonstrated by the presence of specific oestradiol-binding protein in the cells of tissues such as the uterus, vagina and anterior pituitary gland. The specificity of this protein is shown by competitive blocking of the oestrogen–protein complex by anti-oestrogenic compounds such as ethamoxyhiphetol (MER-25) and nafoxidine (Upjohn 11,100). The isolation of the oestrogen receptor protein, the mechanism of oestrogen–receptor interaction, and the molecular biology of oestrogen regulation have recently been reviewed extensively (Dao, 1972).

The uptake of oestradiol by the normal mammary gland is lower, but the specificity of the receptor protein has been shown to be similar to that present in the uterus and vagina (Puca and Bresciani, 1969; Sander, 1968a, b; Sander and Attramadal, 1968). In human mammary tissue Deshpande et al. (1967) demonstrated the accumulation of $^3$H-oestradiol, and in human mammary cancer, Demetriou et al. (1964), Braunsberg, Irvine and James (1967) and Pearlman et al. (1969) have shown a higher uptake of oestradiol than in normal breast tissue.

Shortly after the original demonstration by Glascock and Hoekstra (1959) and Burgos-Gonzalez and Glascock (1960) of hexoestrol uptake in oestrogen target tissues, Folca, Glascock and Irvine (1961) reported the retention of $^3$H-hexoestrol after intravenous injection in patients with advanced breast cancer. They found that the patients fell into two groups. In four patients high hexoestrol retention was observed, and they showed clinical improvement after oophorectomy and adrenalectomy. In six patients, the uptake of hexoestrol by the tumour was low and these patients showed no evidence of tumour regression after the operation.

This attempt to predict which patients are potentially responsive to ablation treatment has been adopted by several groups. Jensen and his group (1967, 1971) have developed elegant techniques to study the binding of oestradiol in slices of human breast cancer. In his recent series (1971), he reports a total of 39 cases where endocrine ablation was performed, and the clinical responses evaluated against $^3$H-oestradiol receptor studies. Of 28 patients showing no distinct evidence of oestrogen receptor, only 1 experienced tumour remission after ablation therapy—in this case adrenalectomy. In contrast, 8 out of 11 patients whose cancers contained oestrogen receptor showed objective remission after ablation therapy.

Johansson, Terenius and Thorén (1970) and Korenman and Dukes (1970) have also reported similar findings with smaller series. There was no obvious correlation shown between the oestradiol binding capacity of breast cancer and other factors in the disease such as clinical stage, histopathological classification, differentiation of the tumour and the menopausal state at the time of operation.

These observations suggest that in hormone-dependent human mammary cancer, there exists in the tumour cells a protein which is capable of binding oestradiol specifically. From studies with the oestradiol receptor in the uterus, and the known effect of oestrogen on the growth and function of the uterus, it is logical to conclude that oestradiol must be necessary for the growth of those human mammary cancers which exhibit the presence of oestradiol receptor protein. It is likely that oestrogen administration will exacerbate the growth of breast cancer in patients who have shown tumour regression following oophorectomy.

The role of oestrogen in the growth of experimental mammary tumours has been studied extensively. The induction of a hormone dependent mammary adenocarcinoma in Sprague–Dawley rats with 7-12, dimethylbenzanthracene has been described (Huggins, Briziarelli and Sutton, 1959; Huggins, Grand and Brillantes, 1961; Huggins and Yang, 1962). A large proportion of these tumours are hormone dependent and regress after either ovariectomy or hypophysectomy (Young, Cowan and Sutherland, 1963; Teller 1969). Both *in vivo* and *in vitro* studies with $^3$H-oestradiol have shown that these tumours possess the oestrogen-receptor as do other oestrogen responsive tissues (King, Panattoni and Gordon, 1965; King, 1968; Sander, 1968b).

It has been shown further that tumours which do not respond to ovariectomy have a lower capacity to retain injected oestradiol (Mobbs, 1966; Sander, 1968a; Sander and Attramadal, 1968). It seems that the DMBA-induced rat mammary tumour parallels closely the oestrogen-binding ability of hormone-dependent human mammary cancer. As is the case with human mammary tumours, oestrogen administration to ovariectomized or adrenal-ectomized animals bearing regressing tumours, will reactivate the tumour. However, after hypophysectomy, the tumour cannot be reactivated by oestrogen administration (Sterental et al., 1963), and this applies to the human also.

The oestrogen sensitivity of mammary cancer shows an apparent dichotomy. On the one hand, the withdrawal of oestrogenic hormones by adrenalectomy or ovariectomy can induce regression of some mammary tumours. On the other hand, administration of large doses of oestrogen may also inhibit tumour growth, particularly in post-menopausal women. Kennedy (1962) has induced regression of breast cancer in pre-menopausal women by oral administration of massive doses of oestrogenic hormones, and postulated that oestrogenic hormones may have a dual action; stimulation of cancer growth by small doses and a more potent inhibitory effect on cell growth with large doses. In experimental animals also, Eisen (1941) had observed tumour inhibition associated with secretory changes caused by massive doses of oestrogen, and subsequently Huggins and Yang (1962) and Meites, Cassell and Clark (1971) showed that the growth of DMBA-induced mammary carcinoma is also inhibited by high dosage oestradiol administration.

The R3230AC rat mammary tumour is a transplantable tumour, whose growth is not affected by ovariectomy but, remarkably enough, is inhibited by large doses of oestrogen (Hilf et al., 1965; Hilf, 1971). McGuire, Julian and Chamness (1971) compared the cytoplasmic oestradiol binding of this tumour with that of the DMBA-induced tumour. They found that both tumours have a high affinity for oestradiol in the cytoplasmic binding sites. However, the concentration of these sites in the R3230AC tumour is ten fold less than that in the DMBA-induced tumour. This may account for the ovary-independent growth of R3230AC tumours.

In normal mammary tissue *in vitro*, oestradiol can stimulate or inhibit cells entering DNA synthesis, depending on the concentration of oestradiol. In contrast, it has been shown that a similar oestradiol concentration has no effect in stimulating or inhibiting the entry of R3230AC tumour cells *in vitro* into the DNA synthetic phase of the cell cycle (Turkington and Hilf, 1968). In a similar system Mobbs (1969) reported that spontaneous regression of DMBA-induced tumours was not due to a loss in the ability to bind injected oestradiol but the receptor–protein concentration was not studied in this instance. It has not yet been shown in human mammary cancer whether the concentration of oestradiol receptor sites is related to the extent of oestradiol influence on DNA synthesis of the cell.

If oestradiol does have a role in the growth of mammary cancer, one might consider the effect of naturally occurring competitors of oestradiol, such as oestriol. This is known as an 'impeded' oestrogen (Huggins and Hensen, 1955; Velardo and Sturgis, 1955), and is capable of reducing the activity of oestradiol on the growth of uterus. The binding of oestriol to the receptor protein in the uterus is less than that of oestradiol (Brecher and Wotiz, 1968; Korenman, 1969). In reviewing the epidemiology of human mammary cancer, there appears to be an inverse correlation between the incidence of mammary cancer and known variations of oestriol production in different races, during pregnancy and at the menopause (Cole and MacMahon, 1969; Lemon, Miller and Foley, 1971).

Lemon et al. (1966) reported reduced oestriol excretion in patients with breast cancer, and later (Lemon, 1969; Lemon, Miller and Foley, 1971), in both human mammary cancer and in the DMBA-induced tumour, showed that oestriol competes with oestradiol for the specific receptor. They also showed that oestriol markedly inhibited DMBA carcinogenesis in the rat mammary tumour. It seems that, certainly in cancer induction and probably in cancer growth, oestriol, by being an 'impeded' oestrogen has an inhibitory effect and this evidence indirectly suggests the participation of oestradiol in mammary cancer formation and growth. However, a limited clinical trial of oestriol therapy in eight patients (Lemon, Miller and Foley, 1971) has not indicated any inhibitory effect from exogenous oestriol on the growth of the established tumour. In fact in two patients oestriol caused exacerbation of the disease, apparently acting like oestradiol.

## PROLACTIN ROLE IN MAINTAINING BREAST CANCER GROWTH

It has been shown in breast cancer patients following an oophorectomy-induced remission that oestrogen administration may reactivate tumour growth, but after hypophysectomy-induced remission, oestrogen fails to reactivate the tumour (Pearson et al., 1954; Pearson and Ray, 1959). This suggested that a pituitary factor was necessary for the oestrogen stimulation of tumour growth. The stimulatory effect of the pituitary gland on the growth of rodent mammary tumours has been well established by experiments involving multiple pituitary isografts. In mice Loeb pioneered the studies, and the hormonal changes induced by pituitary isografts were later defined clearly in a series of papers by Boot and Mühlbock. They arrived at the conclusion that a pituitary factor rather than oestrone is involved in the induction and growth of mammary tumours (Mühlbock and Boot, 1959; Boot et al., 1962; Boot, 1970).

In the rat, similar results have been obtained. Sterental et al. (1963) showed that in the DMBA-induced mammary tumour, oestrogen stimulated the growth of the regressing tumour in adrenalectomized–ovariectomized animals, but was ineffective in hypophysectomized animals. Kim, Furth and Yannapoulos (1963) demonstrated that the stimulation of the female rat mammary gland and of a transplantable mammary tumour MTW9A in the rat, by small doses of oestrogen, is indirect and results from specific stimulation of prolactin release in the animal. Pearson et al. (1969) confirmed the findings of Sterental and demonstrated the direct relation of prolactin to the induction and growth of DMBA-induced rat mammary tumours.

A similar conclusion was reached by Talwalker, Meites and Mizuno (1964) who reported an increased incidence of DMBA-induced tumours in animals treated with prolactin and growth hormone. Kim (1965) observed resumption of DMBA-induced tumour growth after regression from adrenalectomy–ovariectomy, by grafting of a pituitary tumour known to secrete prolactin and growth hormone. The incidence and growth of DMBA-induced tumours is increased in rats bearing hypothalamic lesions (Clemens, Welsch and Meites, 1968; Kleiber et al., 1969; Welsch, Clemens and Meites, 1969). Recently

Nagasawa and Yanai (1970) studied the effect of exogenous administration of bovine prolactin and bovine growth hormone on regressing DMBA-induced tumour in adrenal–ovariectomized rats. They found that growth hormone had no effect on mammary tumour growth, although it stimulated the growth of normal mammary gland and increased the body weight. Prolactin, on the other hand, markedly stimulated the growth of mammary tumours.

The possible role of prolactin in relation to the growth of human breast cancer has been emphasized by a number of workers (Pearson, 1967; Stoll, 1956, 1958; Furth and Clifton, 1958, Kim, Furth and Yannapoulis, 1963). Clinically, Hadfield (1957) observed that a mammotrophic agent, probably prolactin, was present in the urine of pre-menopausal and some post-menopausal women with breast cancer, and favourable response of the tumour to hypophysectomy was associated with the disappearance of the mammotrophic agent from the urine. McCalister and Welbourn (1962) reported that after provocative injection of ovine prolactin in patients with bone metastases from breast cancer, an increase in calcium excretion may predict the likelihood of tumour responsiveness to hypophysectomy. Lipsett and Bergenstal (1960), however, could not demonstrate any effect from short-term administration of ovine prolactin and human growth hormone on the growth of breast cancer as measured by urinary calcium excretion. They confirmed the observation of Pearson and Ray (1959) that, following hypophysectomy, further remission of breast cancer cannot be obtained with oestrogen, and oestrogen administration does not exacerbate the disease in those patients who are in remission. It was suggested by Segaloff et al. (1954) that the presence in patients of breast cancer regressing after treatment with high doses of oestrogen, is associated with a decrease in urinary prolactin level. With the development of a bioassay and radioimmunoassay for human prolactin, we look forward to more definite information on the prolactin level in patients with regressing breast cancer.

It was mentioned earlier that large doses of oestrogen will inhibit the growth of established mammary tumours in animals (Gropper and Shimkin, 1967; Teller, 1969; Kim, Furth and Yannapoulis, 1963) but the mechanism is not clear. Kim, Furth and Yannapoulis suggested that after large doses of oestrogen, inhibition of prolactin release precedes inhibition of prolactin production. However, Chen and Meites (1970) and Pearson et al. (1969) could find no evidence that large doses of oestrogen can inhibit prolactin release, although small doses of oestrogen are potent stimulators of prolactin release in rats.

The relationship between prolactin and oestrogen in their effects on mammary tissue in rats have been reviewed recently (Meites et al., 1972). Meites and Sgouris (1953) suggested that large doses of oestrogen can inhibit the peripheral action of prolactin on the mammary gland. Recently, Meites, Cassell and Clark (1971) found that by injecting 20 µg of oestradiol into ovariectomized rats bearing DMBA-induced mammary carcinoma, tumour regression is obtained, although the serum prolactin level is raised. The tumour regression in such cases can be prevented by injection of prolactin. They suggested, therefore, that oestrogen may retard entry of prolactin into the mammary tumour cells or otherwise interfere with the ability of prolactin to stimulate tumour growth.

It has been mentioned earlier that oestrogen acts directly on target tissues to stimulate cells proliferation. Pettersson (1962) found that while a small dose of oestradiol increased the mitotic index of the uterine epithelium and bone marrow of the mouse both *in vivo* and *in vitro*, a large dose of oestrogen inhibited their growth *in vitro* by blocking cell division in metaphase. Prolactin, on the other hand, has been shown to be mitogenic in mammary epithelial cells *in vivo* (Lyons, Li and Johnson, 1958; Meites and Nicoll, 1966; Baldwin and Martin, 1968). However, the mitogenic effect of prolactin has not been demonstrated *in vitro* in the mouse or the rat (Stockdale and Topper, 1966; Dilley, 1971a, b).

Mayne and Barry (1970) have reported that prolactin may prolong the effect of insulin *in vitro*, and it is well recognized that insulin will stimulate mammary epithelial cells to proliferate *in vitro*, although not *in vivo* (Stockdale and Topper, 1966; Prop, 1961; Elias, 1959; Friedberg, Oka and Topper, 1970). In the case of DMBA-induced mammary tumours, insulin not only stimulates growth *in vitro* (Heuson, Conne and Heimann, 1966; Heuson and Legros, 1971) but also *in vivo*. Heuson, Legros and Heimann (1972) have shown that it has an unequivocal intrinsic growth-stimulating effect on mammary tumour in rats which have been hypophysectomized. It seems, therefore, that there is a distinct contrast between mammary tumour cells and normal mammary epithelial cells with respect to the response to insulin.

Recently, Oka and Topper (1972) have related the insulin sensitivity of mammary epithelial cells to the presence of prolactin. It appears that prolactin itself is not mitogenic, but it renders mammary epithelial cells sensitive to the mitogenic effect of insulin. It is very likely that in mammary tumours such as the DMBA-induced mammary tumour studied by Heuson, the tumour cells have already been primed by prolactin and the agent stimulating cell proliferation is, in fact, insulin.

This introduces the interesting concept that one hormone may prime cells to become sensitive to another hormone. Thus, for example, it has been shown that hydrocortisone can sensitize fat cells to the action of ACTH in the rat (Braum and Hechter, 1970). It is tempting to suggest that the difference between hormone-sensitive and hormone-insensitive mammary tumours is not their dependence on a direct action of hormones to stimulate growth, but a difference in the degree to which the tumour cells have to be primed by prolactin or oestradiol in order to render them sensitive to a mitogen such as insulin.

It should be emphasized that the influence of prolactin on the growth of established mammary tumours may be quite distinct from that on the induction of the tumour. It has been mentioned earlier that prolactin will enhance tumour growth in established DMBA-induced mammary tumour in rats and counteract the regressing effect of high dosage of oestradiol (Meites, Cassell and Clark, 1971; Nagasawa and Yanai, 1970). In the induction of tumours by DMBA, on the other hand, prolactin will inhibit tumorigenesis (Welsch, Clemens and Meites, 1968; Meites, 1972). Since prolactin treatment before the administration of a carcinogen stimulates the growth of normal mammary epithelium, Meites (1972) suggested that this renders the mammary tissue refractory to the action of the carcinogen.

The role of prolactin on mammary tumour growth has been further demonstrated in studies on the effect of ergocornine or 2-bromo-α-ergocryptine. These ergot alkaloids have been shown to inhibit directly the pituitary secretion of prolactin (Lu, Koch and Meites, 1971; Wuttke, Cassell and Meites, 1971; Nagasawa and Meites, 1970; Hökfelt and Fuxe, 1972), and there is no evidence that the drugs affect the secretion of other pituitary hormones. Their administration inhibits the growth of DMBA-induced mammary tumours (Nagasawa and Meites, 1970; Cassell, Meites and Welsch, 1971), and also causes regression of spontaneous mammary tumours in old rats (Quadri and Meites, 1971). Recently, Besser et al. (1972) reported that in patients with inappropriate lactation and amenorrhoea brom-ergocryptine was found to suppress the lactation and to diminish the raised plasma prolactin levels. This agent has shown no benefit in human mammary tumours and this is discussed in Chapter 17.

## EFFECTS OF HORMONES ON HUMAN MAMMARY CANCER IN VITRO

To obtain epithelial cell lines from breast tumours is especially difficult because of the dense fibrous stroma characteristic of most carcinomas. A trypsinization procedure releases both epithelial cells and an abundance of fibroblasts which usually become prevalent in the cell culture (Whitescarver et al., 1968), but a successful method was developed by Lasfargues and Ozzello (1958). By using the 'spilling' technique, they obtained a cell line BT-20 which was isolated from an intraductal comedo-carcinoma. Although it has been growing as a monolayer culture since 1958, it still has the same histological appearance when transplanted on the chorioallantoic membrane of the chick (Tchao et al., 1973). The cell line BT-20 is dependent upon insulin for growth but is not sensitive to other hormones (Lasfargues, personal communication). Recently Sykes et al. (1970) have reported the separation of mammary epithelial tumour cells from fibroblasts by using gradient centrifugation and this technique may lead to the establishment of more breast tumour cell lines.

There are few reports of the effects of hormones on human mammary cancer *in vitro*. Rienits (1959) described a series of 24 human breast cancer explants, the growth rate being assessed by the oxygen consumption of the cells. He observed that the addition of stilboestrol decreased the growth rate in eight cultures, Burstein et al. (1971) have used the 'spilling' technique and studied the influence of various hormones on the incorporation of $^3$H-thymidine into the tumour cells over the 48 hour culture period following dispersion of cells from the clinical specimen. They found some tumours to be oestradiol sensitive but prolactin was without effect.

In another system, the organ culture, the effect of hormones on rodent mammary tissue *in vitro* has been well studied (Prop, 1961; Rivera, 1971). Recently Welsch and Rivera (1972) showed that in organ culture of DMBA-induced rat mammary tumour, DNA synthesis is stimulated by prolactin. Oestradiol added at physiological doses is without effect, but at high dose level it is inhibitory to DNA synthesis. These observations clearly parallel the growth response to hormones *in vivo* of the DMBA-induced tumour in the rat.

Human mammary gland has also been cultured in organ culture (Barker, Fanger and Farnes, 1964; Flaxman and van Scott, 1972) and maintenance of tissue was achieved in the absence of hormones. Prop (1969) reported that the addition of human placental lactogen encouraged cultures of human mammary ductal epithelium to proliferate over the surface of the explant. This observation was confirmed recently by Geriani, Contesso and Nataf (1972), who found that some specimens showed response to oestradiol and prolactin. Ovine prolactin in the presence of insulin, induced epithelial cell growth, and the lobulo-alveolar development was maintained by oestradiol.

It appears that organ culture observations may possibly reflect the expected response of the tissue to hormones *in vivo*. Several workers have reported hormone responsiveness of human breast carcinoma in organ culture. Chayen, Altman and Bitensky (1970) reported that oestradiol improved the survival rate of some fragments of breast cancer in organ culture and this effect may be inhibited by testosterone or dromostanolone. Stoll (1970) studied the activation of lysosomal acid phosphatase and iso-enzymes of lactic acid dehydrogenase in organ culture of breast cancer, and reported hormone effects on these enzyme activities.

Mioduszewska, Koszarowski and Gorski (1968) reported that ovine prolactin and various steroids altered the growth rate in some breast cancer organ cultures. They found some correlation between the *in vitro* observations of hormone effect, with those of clinical hormone responsiveness of the cancer. Barker and Richmond (1971) also studied the effect of prolactin and stilboestrol on explant cultures of breast cancer. They observed a decreased rate of growth from prolactin in only one tumour out of eight cultured, while stilboestrol had either stimulating or inhibitory effects. The different results obtained by different groups of investigators may be due to differences in culture systems and different methods of assaying the growth rate of tumour cells.

Recently, Salih, Flax and Hobbs (1972) and Salih et al. (1972) used a short-term organ culture technique and the pentose-shunt activity to measure the viability of the culture. They demonstrated that, over 48 hours, the growth of some breast cancers *in vitro* can be enhanced by oestradiol as well as by prolactin. To sum up, therefore, it appears that *in vitro* studies on human mammary tissue have been successful in demonstrating the responsiveness of the tissue to oestrogen and prolactin. So far, however, they have failed to establish the clinical correlation which is necessary if one is to show that for a particular tumour, prolactin or oestrogen is growth promoting or is inhibitory.

## CONCLUSIONS

There is enough evidence to support the hypothesis that both oestradiol and prolactin at suitable concentrations can enhance the growth of experimental as well as human mammary cancer. At high concentrations of oestradiol, however, inhibition of mammary tumour growth is observed in some cases, and this inhibition may be counteracted by administration of prolactin. Tissue culture studies of experimental mammary tumour and normal mammary tissue have shown the important role of insulin in the growth of the mammary cell. It is suggested that stimulation of mammary growth by prolactin may not be by a direct effect on the cells, but that priming of the mammary cells by the hormone may render the cells sensitive to insulin.

By analogy with other oestrogen target tissues, the mechanism of oestrogen activation of mammary cells is assumed to be via the oestrogen–receptor in the cytoplasm of the cell. It must be pointed out that organ culture media usually contains insulin and a direct action by oestradiol alone, to enhance mammary cell proliferation, has not yet been demonstrated. Although it appears from *in vivo* studies that prolactin is the more important factor in affecting the growth of mammary carcinoma, the interaction of both oestradiol and prolactin with human mammary carcinoma in the presence of insulin should be elucidated by more studies on the tissue culture system.

## REFERENCES

A.M.A. Council on Drugs (Subcommittee on Breast and Genital Cancer, Committee on Research). (1960). 'Androgens and oestrogens in treatment of disseminated mammary carcinoma: retrospective study of 944 patients.' *J. Am. med Ass.* **172**, 1271.

Baldwin, R. L. and Martin, R. J. (1968). 'Protein and nucleic acid synthesis in rat mammary glands during early lactation.' *Endocrinology* **82**, 1209.

Barker, B. E., Fanger, H. and Farnes, P. (1964). 'Human mammary slices in organ culture.' *Expl Cell Res.* **35**, 437.

Barker, J. R. and Richmond, C. (1971). 'Human breast carcinoma culture: the effect of hormones.' *Br. J. Surg.* **58**, 732.

Besser, G. M., Parke, L., Edwards, C. R. W., Forsyth, I. A. and McNeilly, A. S. (1972). 'Galactorrhoea: successful treatment with reduction of plasma prolactin levels by brom-ergocryptine.' *Br. med. J.* **3**, 669.

Block, G. E., Lampe, I., Vial, A. B. and Coller, F. A. (1960). 'Therapeutic castration for advanced mammary cancer.' *Surgery* **47**, 877.

Boot, L. M. (1970). 'Prolactin and mammary gland carcinogensis. The problem of human prolactin.' *Int. J. Cancer* **5**, 167.

— Mühlbock, O., Röpcke, G. and Van Ebberhorst Tengberger, W. (1962). 'Further investigation on induction of mammary cancer in mice by isografts of hypophyseal tissue.' *Cancer Res.* **22**, 713.

Braum, T. and Hechter, O. (1970). 'Glucocorticoid regulation of ACTH sensitivity of adenyl cylase in rat fat cell membranes.' *Proc. natn Acad. Sci. (U.S.A.)* **66**, 995.

Braunsberg, H., Irvine, W. T. and James, V. H. (1967). 'A comparison of steroid hormone concentrations in human tissues including breast cancer.' *Br. J. Cancer* **21**, 714.

Brecher, P. I. and Wotiz, H. H. (1968). 'Stereospecificity of the uterine nuclear hormone receptors.' *Proc. Soc. expl Biol. Med.* **128**, 470.

Burgos-Gonzalez, J. and Glascock, R. F. (1960). 'Identity of the metabolites of hexoestral accumulated by the genital organs of sheep.' *Biochem. J.* **74**, 33p.

Burstein, N. A., Kjellberg, R. N., Raker, J. W. and Schonidek, H. H. (1971). 'Human carcinoma of the breast in-vitro: the effect of hormone. A preliminary report.' *Cancer (Phil.)* **27**, 1112.

Cassell, E., Meites, J. and Welsch, G. W. (1971). 'Effects of ergocormine and ergocryptine on growth of 7,12-dimethyl benz (a) anthracene-induced mammary tumours in rats.' *Cancer Res.* **31**, 1051.

Ceriani, R. L., Contesso, G. P. and Nataf, B. M. (1972). 'Hormone requirement for growth and differentiation of the human mammary gland in organ culture.' *Cancer Res.* **32**, 2190.

Chayen, J., Altman, F. P. and Bitensky, L. (70). 'Response of human breast cancer tissue to steroid hormones in-vitro.' *Lancet* **1**, 868.

Chen, C. L. and Meites, J. (1970). 'Effects of oestrogen and progesterone on serum and pituitary prolactin levels in ovariectomized rats.' *Endocrinology* **86**, 503.

Clemens, J. A., Welsch, W. C. and Meites, J. (1968). 'Effects of hypothalamic lesions on incidence and growth of mammary tumors in carcinogen-treated rats.' *Proc. Soc. expl. Biol. Med.* **137**, 969.

Cole, P. and MacMahon, B. (1969). 'Oestrogen fractions during early reproductive life in the aetiology of breast cancer.' *Lancet* **1**, 604.

Dao, T. L. (1962). 'Site of metastases and response to therapy in women with cancer of the breast.' *Acta Unio Int. Contra. Canc.* **18**, 928.

— (1972). 'Ablation therapy for hormone-dependent 7026 tumours.' *Ann. Rev. Med.* **23**, 1.

— Nemoto, T. and Bross, I. D. (1967). 'A controlled randomised comparative study of early and late adrenalectomy in women with advanced breast cancer.' In *Prognostic Factors in Breast Cancer*, p. 177, Ed. by A. P. M. Forrest and P. B. Kunkler. Baltimore; Williams and Wilkins.

Demetriou, J. A. Crowley, L. G., Kushinsky, S., Donovan, A. J., Kotin, P. and

MacDonald, I. (1964). 'Radioactive oestrogens in tissues of postmenopausal women with breast neoplasms.' *Cancer Res.* **24**, 926.

Deshpande, N., Jensen, V., Bulbrook, R. D., Berne, T. and Ellis, F. (1967). 'Accumulation of tritiated oestradiol by human breast tissue.' *Steroids* **10**, 219.

Dilley, W. G. (1971a). 'Morphogenic and mitogenic effects of prolactin on rat mammary gland in vitro.' *Endocrinology* **88**, 514.

— (1971b). 'Relationship of mitosis to alveolar development in the rat mammary gland.' *J. Endocr.* **50**, 501.

Eisen, M. J. (1941). 'Tumor inhibition associated with secretory changes produced by oestrogen in a transplanted mammary adenocarcinoma of the rat.' *Cancer Res.* **1**, 457.

Elias, J. J. (1959). 'Effect of insulin and cortisol on organ cultures of adult mouse mammary gland.' *Proc. Soc. expl Biol.* **101**, 500.

Flaxman, B. A. and Van Scott, E. J. (1972). 'Growth of normal human mammary gland epithelium in vitro.' *Cancer Res.* **32**, 2407.

Folca, P. J., Glascock, R. F. and Irvine, W. T. (1961). 'Studies with tritium-labelled hexoeatrol in advanced breast cancer. Comparison of tissue accumulation of hexoestrol with response to bilateral adrenalectomy and oophorectomy.' *Lancet* **2**, 796.

Friedberg, S. H., Oka, T. and Topper, Y. J. (1970). 'Development of insulin-sensitivity by mouse mammary gland in vitro.' *Proc. natn Acad. Sci. (U.S.A.)* **67**, 1493.

Furth, J. (1963). 'Influence of host factors on the growth of neoplastic cells. *Cancer Res.* **23**, 21.

— and Clifton, K. H. (1958). 'Experimental observations on mammatropes and the mammary gland.' In *Endocrine Aspects of Breast Cancer,* p. 276, Ed. by A. R. Currie and C. F. W. Illingworth. Edinburgh; Livingstone.

Glascock, R. F. and Hoekstra, W. G. (1959). 'Selective accumulation of titrium-labelled hexoestrol by the reproductive organs of immature female goats and sheep.' *Biochem. J.* **72**, 673.

Gropper, L. and Shimkin, M. B. (1967). 'Combination therapy of 3-methyl-cholanthrene induced mammary carcinoma in rats; effect of chemotherapy, ovariectomy and food restrictions.' *Cancer Res.* **27**, 26.

Hadfield, G. (1957). 'The nature and origin of the mamaotropin agent present in human female urine.' *Lancet* **1**, 1058.

Heuson, J. C., Legros, N. and Heimann, R. (1972). 'Influence of insulin administration on growth of the 7,12-dimethyl benz (a) anthracene-induced mammary carcinoma in intact, oophorectomized and hypophysectomized rats.' *Cancer Res.* **32**, 233.

— Conne, A. and Heimann, R. (1966). 'Cell proliferation induced by insulin in organ cultures of rat mammary carcinoma.' *Expl Cell Res.* **45**, 351.

— and Legros, N. (1971). 'Effect of insulin on DNA synthesis and DNA polymerase activity in organ culture of rat mammary carcinoma and the influence of insulin pretreatment and of alloxan diabetes.' *Cancer Res.* **31**, 59.

Hilf, R. (1971). 'Will the best model of breast cancer please come forward?' In *Prediction of Response in Cancer Therapy.* National Cancer Institute Monograph No. 34, p. 43.

— Michel, I., Bell, C., Freeman, J. J. and Borman, A. (1965). 'Biochemical and morphological properties of a new lactating mammary tumour line in the rat.' *Cancer Res.* **25**, 286.

Hökfelt, T. and Fuxe, K. (1972). *Neuroendocrinology* **9**, 100.

Huggins, C. and Jensen, E. V. (1955). 'The depression of oestrone-induced uterine growth by phenolic oestrogens with oxygenated functions at position 6 or 16; the impeded oestrogens.' *J. expl Med.* **102**, 335.

— Briziarelli, G. and Sutton, H. (1959). 'Rapid induction of mammary carcinoma in the rat and the influence of hormones on the tumours.' *J. expl Med.* **109**, 25.

— Grand, L. C. and Brillantes, F. P. (1961). 'Mammary cancer induced by a single feeding of polynuclear hydrocarbons and its suppression.' *Nature, Lond.* **189**, 204.

— and Yang, N. C. (1962). 'Induction and extinction of mammary cancer.' *Science* **137**, 257.

Jensen, E. V., DeSombre, E. R. and Jungblut, P. W. (1967). 'Oestrogen receptors in hormone-responsive tissues and tumours.' In *Endogenous Factors Influencing Host–Tumour Balance*, Ed. by R. W. Wissler, T. L. Dao, and S. Wood Jnr. University of Chicago.

— Block, G. E., Smith, S., Kyser, K. and DeSombre, E. R. (1971). 'Oestrogen receptors and breast cancer response to adrenalectomy.' In *Prediction of Response in Cancer Therapy*. National Cancer Institute Monograph No. 34, p. 55.

Johansson, J., Terenius, L. and Thorén, L. (1970). 'The binding of oestradial-17β to human breast cancers and other tissues in-vitro.' *Cancer Res.* **30**, 692.

Kennedy, B. J. (1962). 'Massive oestrogen administration in premenopausal women with metastatic breast cancer.' *Cancer (Phil.)* **15**, 641.

Kim, U. (1965). 'Pituitary function and hormonal therapy of experimental breast cancer.' *Cancer Res.* **25**, 1146.

— Furth, J. and Yannopoulos, K. (1963). 'Observations on hormonal control of mammary cancer. I. Oestrogen and mammotropes.' *J. natn Cancer Inst.* **31**, 233.

King, R. J. B. (1968). 'The uptake of (6,7-3H) oestradiol by dimethyl benzanthracene-induced rat mammary tumours.' In *Prognostic Factors in Breast Cancer*, p. 354, Ed. by A. P. Forrest and P. B. Kimkler. Edinburgh; Livingstone.

— Panattoni, M. and Gordon, J. (1965). 'The metabolism of steroids by tissue from normal and neoplastic rat breast.' *J. Endocr.* **33**, 127.

Kleiber, M. S., Gruenstein, M., Meranze, D. R. and Shimkin, M. B. (1969). 'Influence of hypothalamic lesions on the induction and growth of mammary cancers in Sprague-Dawley rats receiving 7, 12-dimethylbenz (a) anthracene.' *Cancer Res.* **29**, 999.

Korenman, S. G. (1969). 'Comparative binding affinity of oestrogens and its relation to oestrogenic potency.' *Steroids* **13**, 163.

— and Dukes, B. A. (1970). 'Specific oestrogen binding by the cytoplasm of human breast carcinoma.' *J. clin. Endocr.* **30**, 639.

Lasfargues, E. Y. and Ozzello, L. (1958). 'Cultivation of human breast carcinomas.' *J. natn Cancer Inst.* **21**, 1131.

Lemon, H. M. (1969). 'Endocrine influence on human mammary cancer formation.' *Cancer (Phil.)* **23**, 781.

— Wotiz, H. H., Parson, L. and Mozden, P. J. (1966). 'Reduced oestriol excretion in patients with breast cancer prior to endocrine therapy.' *J. Am. med. Ass.* **196**, 1128.

— Miller, D. M. and Foley, J. F. (1971). 'Competition between steroids for hormonal receptor.' In *Prediction of Response in Cancer Therapy*. National Cancer Institute Monograph No. 34, p. 77.

Lipsett, M. B. and Bergenstal, D. M. (1960). 'Lack of effect of human growth hormone and ovine prolactin on cancer in women.' *Cancer Res.* **20**, 1172.

Lu, K. H., Koch, Y. and Meites, J. (1971). 'Direct inhibition by ergocormine of pituitary prolactin release.' *Endocrinology* **89**, 229.

Lyons, W. R., Li, C. H. and Johnson, R. E. (1958). 'The hormonal control of mammary growth and lactation.' *Recent Progr. Hormone Res.* **14**, 219.

McCalister, A. and Welbourn, R. B. (1962). 'Stimulation of mammary cancer by prolactin and the clinical response to hypophysectomy.' *Br. med. J.* **1**, 1669.

McGuire, W. L., Julian, J. A. and Chamness, G. C. (1971). 'A dissociation between ovarian dependent growth and oesteogen sensitivity in mammary carcinoma.' *Endocrinology* **89**, 969.

Mayne, R. and Barry, J. M. (1970). 'Biochemical changes during development of mouse mammary tissue in organ culture.' *J. Endocr.* **46**, 61.

Meites, J. (1972). 'Relation of prolactin and oestrogen to mammary tumourigenesis in the rat.' *J. natn Cancer Inst.* **48**, 1217.

— and Nicoll, C. S. (1966). 'Adenohypophysis: Prolactin.' *Ann. Rev. Physiol.* **28**, 57.

— and Sgouris, J. T. (1953). 'Can the ovarian hormones inhibit the mammary response to prolactin?' *Endocrinology* **53**, 17.

— Cassell, E. and Clark, J. (1971). 'Oestrogen inhibition of mammary tumour growth in rats: counteraction by prolactin:' *Proc. Soc. expl Biol. Med.* **137**, 1225.

— Lu, K. H., Wuttke, W., Welsch, C. W., Nagasawa, H. and Quadri, S. K. (1972). 'Recent studies on function and control of prolactin secretion in rats.' *Recent Progr Hormone Res.* **28**, 471.

Mioduszewska, O., Koszarowski, T. and Gorski, C. (1968). 'The influence of hormones on breast cancer in-vitro in relation to the clinical course of the disease.' In *Prognostic Factors in Breast Cancer*, p. 347, Ed. by A. R. Forrest and P. B. Kunkler, Baltimore; Williams and Wilkins.

Mobbs, B. G. (1966). 'The uptake of tritiated oestradiol by dimethylbenzanthracene-induced mammary tumours of the rat.' *J. Endocr.* **36**, 409.

— (1969). 'Uptake of $^3$H-oestradiol by dimethylbenzanthracene induced rat mammary tumours regressing spontaneously or after ovariectomy.' *J. Endocr.* **44**, 463.

Mühlbock, D. and Boot, L. M. (1959). 'Induction of mammary cancer in mice without the mammary tumor's agent by isografts of hypophysis.' *Cancer Res.* **19**, 402.

Nagasawa, H. and Meites, J. (1970). 'Suppression by ergocornine and iproniazid of carcinogen-induced mammary tumours in rats. Effect on serum and pituitary prolactin.' *Proc. Soc. expl Biol. Med.* **135**, 469.

— and Yanai, R. (1970). 'Effects of prolactin or growth hormone on growth of carcinogen-induced mammary tumours of adreno-ovariectomized rats.' *Int. J. Cancer* **6**, 488.

Oka, T. and Topper, Y. J. (1972). 'Is prolactin mitogenic for mammary eipthelium?' *Proc. natn Acad. Sci. (U.S.A.)* **69**, 1693.

Pearlman, W. H., deHertogh, R., Laumas, K. R., Pearlman, M. R. J. (1969). 'Metabolism and tissue uptake of oestrogen in women with advanced carcinoma of the breast.' *J. clin. Endocr.* **29**, 707.

Pearson, O. H. (1967). 'Hormone dependence of tumours in man.' In *Modern Trends in Endocrinology*—3, p. 242, Ed. by H. Gardiner-Hill, London; Butterworths.

— West, C. S., Hollander, V. P. and Trevers, N. E. (1954). 'Evaluation of endocrine therapy of advanced breast cancer.' *J. Am. med. Ass.* **154**, 234.

— and Ray, B. S. (1959). 'Results of hypophysectomy in the treatment of metastatic mammary carcinoma.' *Cancer (Phil.)* **12**, 85.

— — (1960). 'Hypophysectomy in the treatment of metastatic mammary cancer.' *Am. J. Surg.* **99**, 544.

— Llerena, O., Llerena, L., Molina, A. and Butler, T. (1969). 'Prolactin-dependent rat mammary cancer: a model for man.' *Trans. Ass. Am. Phys.* **82**, 225.

Pettersson, I. (1962). 'The effect of oestrogenic hormones on cell division and growth in some tissue of mice.' *Acta physiol. scand.* **55**, 1.

Prop, F. J. A. (1961). 'Effects of hormones on mouse mammary glands in-vitro, analysis of the factors that cause lobulo-alveolar development.' *Path. Biol. (Paris)* **9**, 640.

— (1969). 'Action of prolactin and human placental lactogen on human mammary gland in-vitro.' In *Proteins and Polypeptide Hormones*, p. 508, Ed. by Margoulies.

Puca, G. A. and Bresciani, F. (1969). 'Interaction of 6, 7 $^3$H-17-β-oestradiol with mammary gland and other organs of the C3H mouse in-vitro.' *Endocrinology* **85**, 1.

Quadri, S. K. and Meites, J. (1971). 'Regression of spontaneous mammary tumours in rats by ergot drugs.' *Proc. Soc. expl Biol. Med.* **138**, 999.

Rienits, K. G. (1959). 'The effects of oestrogen and testosterone on respiration of human mammary cancer in-vitro.' *Cancer (Phil.)* **12**, 958.

Rivera, E. M. (1971). In *Methods in Mammalian Embryology*, p. 442, Ed. by J. C. Daniel. Freeman.

Salih, H., Flax, H. and Hobbs, J. R. (1972). 'Oestrogen sensitivity of breast carcinomas in-vitro.' *Lancet* **1**, 1198.

— Brander, W., Flax, H. and Hobbs, J. R. (1972). 'Prolactin dependence in human breast cancers.' *Lancet* **2**, 1103.

Sander, S. (1968a). 'The uptake of 17-β-oestradiol in breast tissue of female rats.' *Acta endocr. (Kobenhavn)* **58**, 49.

— (1968b). 'In-vitro uptake of oestradiol in DMBA-induced breast tumours of the rat.' *Acta path. microbiol. scand.* **75**, 520.

— and Attramadal, A. (1968). 'An autoradiographic study of oestrodiol incorporation in the breast tissue of female rats.' *Acta endocr. (Kobenhavn)* **58**, 235.

Segaloff, A., Gordon, D., Carabasi, R. A., Horwitt, B. N., Schlosser, J. V. and Murison, P. J. (1954). 'Hormone therapy in cancer of the breast. VII. Effect of conjugated oestrogens (equine) on clinical course and hormonal excretion.' *Cancer (Phil.)* **7**, 758.

Sterental, A., Dominquez, J. M., Weissman, C. and Pearson, O. H. (1963). 'Pituitary role in the oestrogen dependency of experimental mammary cancer.' *Cancer Res.* **23**, 481.

Stockdale, F. E. and Topper, Y. J. (1966). 'The role of DNA synthesis and mitosis in hormone-dependent differentiation.' *Proc. natn Acad. Sci. (U.S.A.)* **56**, 1283.

Stoll, B. A. (1956). 'P-hydroxypropiophenone for advanced breast cancer.' *Med. J. Aust.* **2**, 181.

— (1958). 'Endocrine factors in the aetiology and treatment of cancer of the breast and prostate.' In *Modern Trends in Endocrinology*—p. 212, Ed. by H. Gardiner-Hill. London; Butterworths.

Stoll, B. A. (1970). 'Investigation of organ culture as an aid to the hormonal management of breast cancer.' *Cancer (Phil.)* **25**, 1228.

Sykes, J. A., Whitescarver, J., Brigg, L. and Anson, J. H. (1970). 'Separation of tissue cells from fibroblasts with use of discontinuous density gradients.' *J. natn Cancer Inst.* **44**, 855.

Talwalker, P. K., Meites, J. and Mizuno, H. (1964). 'Mammary tumour induction by oestrogen or anterior pituitary hormones in ovariectomized rats given 7, 12-dimethylbenz(a) anthracene.' *Proc. Soc. expl Biol. (N.Y.)* **116**, 531.

Tchao, R., Justh, G., Mansukhani, S., Leighton, J. and Lasfargues, E. (1973). 'Histopathologic comparison of cell line B 7-20 in matrix culture and on CAM with the surgical specimen of breast cancer from which the line was derived.' American Tissue Culture Association Meeting. *In Vitro* **8**, 423.

Teller, M. N. (1969). 'Influence of oestrogens and endocrine ablation on duration of remission produced by ovariectomy or androgen treatment of 7, 12-dimethylbenz(a) anthracene-induced mammary tumours.' *Cancer (Phil.)* **29**, 349

Turkington, R. W. and Hilf, R. (1968). 'Hormonal dependence of DNA synthesis in mammary carcinoma cells in-vitro.' *Science* **160**, 1457.

Velardo, J. T. and Sturgis, S. H. (1955). 'Interaction of 16 epi-estriol and oestradiol 17β on uterine growth.' *Proc. Soc. expl. Biol. Med.* **90**, 609.

Welsch, C. W., Clemens, J. A. and Meites, J. (1968). 'Effects of multiple pituitary homographs or progesterone on 7, 12-dimethylbenz(a) anthracene-induced mammary tumours in-vitro.' *J. natn Cancer Inst.* **41**, 465.

— — — (1969). 'Effects of hypothalamic and amygdaloid lesions on development and growth of carcinogen induced mammary tumours in-female rats.' *Cancer Res.* **29**, 1541.

— and Rivera, E. M. (1972). 'Differential effects of estrogen and prolactin on DNA synthesis in organ cultures of DMBA induced rat mammary carcinoma.' *Proc. Soc. expl Biol. Med.* **139**, 623.

Whitescarver, J., Recher, L., Sykes, J. A. and Briggs, L. (1968). 'Problems involved in culturing human breast tissue.' *Texas Rep. Biol. Med.* **26**, 613.

Wuttke, W., Cassell, E. and Meites, J. (1971). 'Effect of ergocormine on serum prolactin and LH, and on hypothalamic content of PIF and LRF.' *Endocrinology* **88**, 737.

Young, S., Cowan, D. M. and Sutherland, L. E. (1963). 'The histology of induced mammary tumours in rats.' *J. Path. Bact.* **85**, 331.

# 13

# Treatment by Progestin–Oestrogen–Corticosteroid Combinations

## R. Chemama*, M. F. Jayle and A. Ennuyer

The concept of inhibiting specific functions of the hypothalamohypophyseal centre in patients with advanced breast cancer springs from two basic considerations.

In the first place, the effects of endocrine surgery—ovariectomy, adrenalectomy, hypophysectomy—on breast cancer metastases are well established. The work of Beatson (1896) opened up the era of endocrine surgery with his observations on the beneficial effects of bilateral ovariectomy on the progress of breast cancer, and was followed by that of Lacassagne (1932), who demonstrated the influence of high doses of oestrogens on the development of mammary cancer in male mice. Ablation of the adrenals was advocated by Huggins and Bergenstal (1951), while Perrault (1952, 1953) and Luft, Olivecrona and Sjogren (1952) simultaneously suggested destruction of the pituitary gland. The aim of this surgery was to arrest the body's secretion of oestrogen, and the hypothesis underlying endocrine surgery places the entire responsibility for the evolution and even for the production of breast cancer on the oestrogens. We need not deal at length with this hypothesis for the moment but can merely accept the fact that surgical ablation of the ovaries, adrenals and pituitary is capable of restraining and even of causing regression of metastasizing breast cancer which is beyond any other therapeutic control.

## RATIONALE OF METHOD

Advances in pharmacology, in their turn, have made available several groups of steroids which act specifically upon certain hypophyseal trophic hormones and can thereby suppress ovarian and adrenal function. These are the

* Now deceased.

oestrogens, the progestins and the glucocorticosteroids, three classes of synthetic steroids whose action on the hypothalamohypophyseal centre differs one from the other. The oestrogens have a powerful anti-FSH effect in hemi-castrated female rats or in parabionts associating a castrated male with an intact female. The C-21 progestins such as chlormadinone have only a weak suppressant action on the over-secretion of gonadotrophins in the castrated or hemi-castrated animal. However, unlike the oestrogens, in minimal doses they suppress the peak of LH production in the female rabbit in oestrus in coitus with the male (Jayle, 1968). On the other hand, the C-18 progestins like norethindrone, ethynodiol acetate, ethinyl-oestrenol and norethynodrel are partly metabolized by the body into oestrogens, and this endows them with an anti-gonadotrophic (anti-FSH) action in addition to their anti-ovulatory (anti-LH) effect. Finally, a corticosteroid such as dexamethasone is a powerful hypothalamo-hypophyseal inhibitor which, even in low doses, suppresses the production of corticotrophin-releasing factor and ACTH.

Thus, the combination of a progestin, an oestrogen and a glucocortico-steroid in low doses will suppress the function not only of the ovaries but also of the adrenals. It therefore seemed rational to test it in cases of advanced breast cancer.

It may seem somewhat paradoxical to administer oestrogens to breast cancer patients especially before the menopause, considering that earlier studies postulated the harmful role of this group of steroids in such patients. But several arguments influenced us:

First, endocrine surgery does not remove all the body's oestrogen sources. This is well established, and suggests that the beneficial effects of such surgery are due not only to a depression of oestrogen levels. In this connection it is important to emphasize that the ovaries of post-menopausal females do not secrete appreciable quantities of the classical oestrogens. Schenker, Polishuk and Eckstein (1971) incubated six homogenized ovaries with $7\alpha$-$^3$H-pregnenolone and produced evidence of radioactive androstenedione and testosterone. In another experiment the homogenate was separated into three parts and incubated with $7\alpha$-$^3$H-pregnenolone, $14$-$^{14}$C-progesterone, and $4$-$^{14}$C-testosterone respectively. As in the previous experiment, the first steroid led to tritiated androstenedione and testosterone, whereas the two latter steroids were not metabolized. These results as a whole led the authors to conclude that the ovaries of post-menopausal women produced C-19 steroids but are unable to aromatize them into oestrogens. This conclusion is consistent with the very low levels of classical oestrogens ($E_1$, $E_2$, $E_3$) which Brown (1966) estimated in the urine of post-menopausal females. Brown's results were later confirmed by gas-phase chromatography (Hans et al., 1972).

We ourselves (Tsyrlina et al., 1970), using 2 mg of $\beta^{1-24}$ corticotrophin-retard, stimulated the adrenals of healthy or breast tumour-bearing post-menopausal females and measured the urinary oestrogens by fluorescence reactions and gas chromatography. Our results showed that oestrogen levels were very low, identical in normal and in cancerous women, and not affected by adrenocortical stimulation. More recently, the level of plasma oestradiol was determined by radioimmunological measurement in five women with breast cancer, before and after prolonged stimulation by means of 4 mg of $\beta^{1-24}$ corticotrophin-retard; no response was noted (Table 13.1).

TABLE 13.1

Values for Plasma Oestradiol and Cortisol Before and After Stimulation by 4 mg of $\beta^{1-24}$ Corticotrophin-retard in 5 Patients with Breast Cancer

| Patient | Oestradiol* (pg/ml) | | Cortisol (μg/100 ml) | |
|---|---|---|---|---|
| | Before | After | Before | After |
| Se | ⩽30 | ⩽30 | 18 | 69 |
| Li | ⩽30 | ⩽30 | 16·5 | 33 |
| Le | ⩽30 | ⩽30 | 16 | 38 |
| Fo | ⩽30 | ⩽30 | 21 | 66 |
| Nu | ⩽30 | ⩽30 | 28 | 21 |

* Values recorded are at the limit of sensitivity of the method of measurement used. It is important to note that they do not increase after stimulation.

In an experiment we are currently conducting with Morin and Engelman, the same method is being used to measure the level of oestradiol in the lumbo-ovarian vein of post-menopausal women during hysterectomy. Stimulation with 15,000 i.u. of HCG has produced no change in the oestrogen level. Overall, it would appear unlikely, at least in so far as post-menopausal women are concerned, that endocrine surgery exerts its effect via a depression of oestrogen levels.

Another well-established fact is that breast cancer occurring after the menopause may be improved by prolonged treatment with oestrogens at high doses. Furthermore, the anabolizing norsteroids such as norandrostenolone phenylpropionate, which are employed with occasional success in the treatment of bone metastases in breast cancer, are partly converted into oestrogens in the course of their metabolism.

There were two last arguments which were particularly convincing. First, the work of Huggins and Yang (1962) had proved that mammary tumours in rats induced by polycyclics such as 7,12-dimethylbenzanthracene regress when treated with a combination of ethinyl-oestradiol and progesterone, whereas progesterone alone stimulates tumour growth. Since mammary cancer of the rat represents an experimental model that is very close to human breast cancer, this finding was crucial. Second, the important observation that in the presence of progestins, natural or synthetic oestrogens do not provoke their typical changes in the utero-vaginal receptors of normal women, and the combination of progestin and oestrogen, given over long periods to young women, produces an endometrial and vaginal hypoplasia (Jayle, personal observation). In other words, a progestin–oestrogen combination can be considered as having essentially an inhibitory effect on the gonadotrophic functions of the hypothalamo-hypophyseal centre.

We had no hesitation, therefore, in administering oestrogens to all our patients whether post- or pre-menopausal.

## REPORT OF CLINICAL TRIAL

Upon this basis we conducted a clinical trial in 26 patients (Jayle et al., 1967). Two years later, we reported the results of this treatment in a group of 70 patients (Jayle et al., 1969). They can be summarized as follows:

All patients received daily combined therapy of:

|  |  |
|---|---|
| Lynestrenol | 10 mg |
| Mestranol | 0·3 mg |
| Dexamethasone | 1 mg |

or of

|  |  |
|---|---|
| Chlormadinone | 4 mg |
| Ethinyl oestradiol | 0·1 mg |
| Dexamethasone | 1 mg |

In a few cases, the dose of Lynestrenol was increased to 30 mg and that of Mestranol to 0·9 mg per 24 hours. Dexamethasone was usually cut to 0·5 mg daily after a few months.

Table 13.2 shows the distribution of patients according to the stage of the

TABLE 13.2

Distribution of Cases According to Stage of Disease, Pre- or Post-menopausal, With or Without Previous Treatment

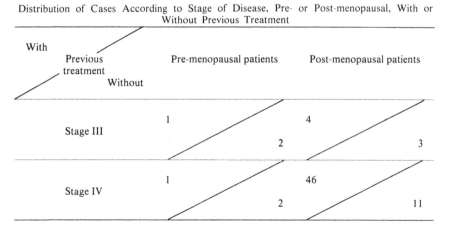

|  | Pre-menopausal patients | | Post-menopausal patients | |
|---|---|---|---|---|
| With / Without Previous treatment | With | Without | With | Without |
| Stage III | 1 | 2 | 4 | 3 |
| Stage IV | 1 | 2 | 46 | 11 |

disease, whether they were pre- or post-menopausal, and the existence or absence of previous treatment.

TABLE 13.3

Results of Hormonal Therapy

| | Pre-menopausal | Menopause | | | | Total |
|---|---|---|---|---|---|---|
| | | < 1 year | 1–5 years | 5–10 years | > 10 years | |
| Regression | 3 | 1 | 5 | 7 | 7 | 23 |
| Stationary | 1 | 1 | 5 | 5 | | 12 |
| Total number of cases treated | 6 | 6 | 15 | 22 | 21 | 70 |

TABLE 13.4

Frequency of Improvement According to Site

| | |
|---|---|
| Disappearance of lung metastases | 40% |
| Regression of tumours | 37% |
| Regression or stabilization of bone metastases | 32% |
| Regression or stabilization of skin metastases | 17% |
| Regression or stabilization of liver metastases | 8% |

Table 13.3 records the results of the treatment, and Table 13.4 the frequency of improvement according to the site of the lesions. Table 13.5 lists the duration of responses, and Table 13.6 relates response to the length of the recurrence-free intervals in the same patients. Taken as a whole, these results indicate that 50 per cent of patients benefited from the treatment, of which 32 per cent showed objective improvement and 18 per cent showed non-progression, and that the beneficial effects were noted in both post- and pre-menopausal cases. The sole parameter which seemed to influence response

TABLE 13.5

Duration of Regression or Stabilization

| | 3–6 months | 7–12 months | 13–18 months | 19–24 months | 24 months |
|---|---|---|---|---|---|
| Regression | 4 | 13 | 3 | 2 | 1 |
| Stabilization | 7 | 5 | | | |
| | | 29 | | 6 | |

TABLE 13.6

Response Related to Length of Free Interval

| Duration | < 1 year | 1–2 years | 3–5 years | > 5 years |
|---|---|---|---|---|
| Improved cases | 6 | 1 | 5 | 4 |
| Stationary states | 2 | 3 | 5 | 2 |

*In 7 cases we were unable to establish the duration of free interval.

was the existence or absence of previous treatment (Table 13.7). This is discussed further later.

TABLE 13.7

Influence of Previous Treatment on Effects of Hypophyseal Inhibition

| | Previous treatment | |
|---|---|---|
| | With | Without |
| Number of cases treated | 52 | 18 |
| Number of regressions | 12 | 11 |
| Number of stabilizations | 12 | — |
| % {Regression | 23 | 61 |
| {Stabilization | 23 | — |

## Effect of treatment on the hypothalamo–hypophyseo–ovarian axis

The effect of treatment on the hypothalamo–hypophyseo–ovarian axis was assessed by estimations of urinary metabolites of the ovarian hormones, and by measurements of total urinary gonadotrophin (TUG) or of human menopausal gonadotrophin (HMG) in post-menopausal patients. Table 13.8 records for both pre- and post-menopausal patients the marked fall in total urinary pregnanediol and oestrogen values. The values for TUG or for HMG fell to a level lower than 5 and even 3 MU per 24 hours (Table 13.9).

We did not perform radio-immunological measurements of serum FSH and LH, which would have made it possible to differentiate the effect of the treatment on each of the two gonadotrophins, but a recently published work (Franchimont, 1971) shows that under the influence of oestrogen–progestin therapy FSH secretion is depressed and the inter-menstrual peak of LH is suppressed. Even more recently Morcos, Crockford and Beck (1972) recorded that the basal levels of LH in young women are considerably lowered or even

TABLE 13.8

Effects of Ovarian Blockade

|  | Oestrogens (µg/24 hours) | Pregnanediol* (mg/24 hours) |
|---|---|---|
| *Patient pre-menopausal before treatment* | | |
| *Case No. 11:* | | |
| Before treatment | 35 | 4 |
| After 3 months' treatment | 5 | Trace |
| | | |
| *Post-menopausal patients* | | |
| *Case No. 2, 5 < M < 10 years:* | | |
| Before treatment | 10 | 1 |
| After 3 months' treatment | 5 | 0·1 |
| | | |
| *Case No. 3, 5 < M < 10 years:* | | |
| Before treatment | 10 | 0·5 |
| After 3 months' treatment | 5 | Trace |
| *Case No. 8, i M > 10 years:* | | |
| Before treatment | 1·5 | 1 |
| After 3 months' treatment | 10 | 0·5 |

*Measurement of pregnanediol complex by method of Crepy, Meslin and Jayle (1956).

TABLE 13.9

Inhibition of Hypophyseal Gonadotrophin after Hormonal Treatment, in Improved Patients

| Case No. | Age | Years since menopause or patient pre-menopausal | HMG in MU/24 hours | |
|---|---|---|---|---|
| | | | Before treatment | After 3 months' treatment |
| 1 | 72 | > 10 years | 40–80 | < 5 |
| 2 | 64 | 5–10 years | 40–80 | < 3 |
| 3 | 63 | 5–10 years | > 80 | < 5 |
| 4 | 51 | Pre-menopausal | < 40 | n.m.* |
| 5 | 62 | > 10 years | n.m. | = 3 |
| 6 | 57 | 1–5 years | 40–80 | < 5 |
| 7 | 57 | 1–5 years | 40–80 | < 3 |
| 8 | 70 | > 10 years | > 80 | < 5 |
| 9 | 63 | > 10 years | 40–80 | < 5 |
| 10 | 42 | 5–10 years | > 80 | < 5 |
| 11 | 37 | Pre-menopausal | < 40 | < 3 |

*n.m. = no measurement.

suppressed under the influence of a contraceptive combination containing 2 mg of norethindrone and 100 µg of Mestranol.

## Effect of the hypothalamo–hypophyseo–adrenal axis

This was evaluated by measurements of urinary metabolites of the adrenal hormones. As seen in Table 13.10, levels of 17-ketosteroids and of 170H-

TABLE 13.10

*Effects of Adrenal Blockade*

|  | 17–KS*<br>(mg/24 hours) | 17–OHCS<br>(mg/24 hours) |
|---|---|---|
| *Case No. 2* | | |
| Before treatment | 5 | 4·5 |
| After 3 months' treatment | 0·2 | 0·5 |
| *Case No. 11* | | |
| Before treatment | 5 | 6 |
| After 3 months' treatment | Traces | 0·4 |

* 17–KS = 17-ketosteroids; 17-OHCS = 17-hydroxycorticosteroids (Porter and Silber).

corticosteroids fall drastically after a few months' treatment, despite the minimal doses of dexamethasone employed (1 mg daily, cut to 0·5 mg after a few months).

## Effect on growth hormone (HGH) and other hypophyseal hormones

In a few of our patients, we carried out measurements of serum HGH, before and after insulin stimulation.* Table 13.11 shows the values obtained in

TABLE 13.11

HGH Level in ng/ml Plasma in 7 Patients with Stage IV Breast Cancer Before Treatment

| Patient | Age | Basal level | 1 hour<br>after insulin |
|---|---|---|---|
| B.O. | 47 | 1 | 80 |
| C.A. | 50 | 1 | 67 |
| D.U. | 55 | 3·5 | 62·5 |
| M.A. | 45 | 4 | 21·5 |
| S.M. | 55 | 6 | 77 |
| H.I. | 70 | 2 | 21 |

* Thanks to the courtesy of Dr. Rosselin.

seven patients with stage IV breast cancer. The HGH levels are normal both before and after insulin hypoglycaemia. In one case where we performed these measurements before and after three months of treatment, the basal levels of HGH were unchanged, but response to the insulin hypoglycaemia was markedly diminished (see *Figure 13.1*).

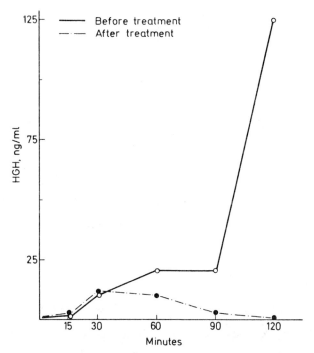

*Figure 13.1. Test of stimulation under insulin hypoglycaemia Before and after hormonal therapy in patient aged 70. Bone metastases treated by Lyndiol, two tablets per 24 hours, and Dexamethasone, 1 mg per 24 hours*

It may be advisable, therefore, to investigate further whether the progestin–oestrogen–corticosteroid combination has an effect on HGH production. This is all the more important in view of the report that oestrogen–progestin combinations act as growth hormone promoters (Spellacy, 1967).

Experiments in rats and mice during the past few years have demonstrated the role of prolactin in mammary tumour growth, but biological and radioimmunological assays of human prolactin are not yet entirely reliable. We have no data on prolactin levels or on the thyroid function during the treatment, but, in addition to the progestin–oestrogen–corticosteroid combination, a few of our patients were given L-tri-iodothyronine with the aim of restraining production of pituitary TSH. The dose employed was 50 μg daily. The inhibition of TSH secretion, far from improving clinical benefit, seemed rather to exert a contrary effect, and so we ceased prescribing L-tri-iodothyronine after a few cases.

## SPECIAL CASE REPORTS

It may be useful to give details of the response to treatment particularly in women with normal ovarian activity, suffering from advanced breast cancer. Among the six pre-menopausal patients in our series, we observed three cases of tumour regression and one case of non-progression of the lesions. Our patients were aged 27, 37, 45, 46, 46, and 51 years respectively. The following are detailed observations on two of them, one of whom responded to the treatment while the other failed to respond.

*Case No. 1.* N.R., aged 27. Patient presented with a tumour invading the whole of the left breast and measuring 15 × 15 cm. There was homolateral axillary adenopathy, 4 cm in diameter (Stage III). No previous treatment had been given to the tumour.

On 31.3.1966, treatment was begun with a daily dosage of:

| | |
|---|---|
| Lynestrenol: | 15 mg |
| Mestranol: | 450 μg |
| Dexamethasone: | 1 mg |

There was no response, and six months later, still under treatment, widespread ulceration of the tumour had appeared. When pulmonary metastases appeared, anti-mitotic agents were administered but without result. The patient died on 16.1.1967.

Urinary hormone measurements were performed before and after three months of treatment. Results were as follows:

| | Pregnanediol mg/24 hours | Oestrogens μg/24 hours | 17-KS mg/24 hours | 17-OHCS mg/24 hours | TUG MU/24 hours |
|---|---|---|---|---|---|
| Before | 5·5 | 30 | 20·5 | 6 | < 40 |
| After | trace | 5 | 1 | 0·4 | < 3 |

*Case No. 2.* L.B., aged 37. Patient presented with a tumour of the left breast invading almost the entire gland, and measuring 10 × 8 cm. There was retraction of the nipple and of the gland as a whole, and cutaneous infiltration over a surface of 2 sq. cm with threatened ulceration. There was also homolateral axillary adenopathy of 1 cm diameter (Stage III). She gave a history of having been treated daily for the past three years with androgens (Glossosterandryl 10) for mastalgia.

On 24.6.1965, treatment was begun with a daily dosage of:

Lynestrenol: 10 mg
Mestranol: 300 µg
Dexamethasone: 1 mg

By five months later, there was considerable regression of the tumour. The tumour then remained stationary for over one year, but in January 1967 it resumed its progression although there was still no sign of distant metastasis. The lesion and draining node areas were then submitted to radiotherapy and this was followed by clinical disappearance of the tumour and adenopathy. This patient survived until 1972 (February).

Hormone measurements before and during treatment are as follows:

|  | Pregnanediol mg/24 hours | Oestrogens µg/24 hours | 17-KS mg/24 hours | 17-OHCS mg/24 hours | TUG MU/24 hours |
|---|---|---|---|---|---|
| Before | 4 | 35 | 5 | 6 | < 40 |
| After 3 months' treatment | trace | 20 | 1 | 1 | < 3 |
| After 6 months' treatment | trace | trace | trace | 0·4 | < 3 |

## DISCUSSION

The unexpected results we obtained in young women with advanced breast cancer encouraged us to make an attempt at prophylactic treatment of metastases of breast cancer in young patients, by the use of an oestrogen–progestin combination (Chlormadinone, 4 mg, with ethinyl oestradiol, 100 µg) administered daily shortly after radical treatment of the primary tumour and draining node areas.

In 1970 we published the case histories of the first six patients submitted to this treatment and showed that the oestrogen–progestin combination employed had produced no untoward effects (Chemama et al., 1970). At the present time we are undertaking regular supervision of 23 patients treated for from six months to over seven years with the chlormadinone–ethinyl oestradiol combination and 33 patients serving as the control group. The selection of patients for the treated or for the control group was on a random basis. Table 13.12 summarizes the present status of this experiment. Whilst it is still too early to pronounce on the preventive effects, it is clear that the chlormadinone–ethinyl oestradiol combination is not harmful in young patients, whether pre-menopausal or castrated.

Thus the low doses of oestrogens present in the oestrogen–progestin combination we used (whether or not combined with corticoids) have had a favourable effect in some young women with advanced breast cancer, and have produced no untoward effects when employed in young women as a preventive treatment after radical therapy. These preliminary results may provide the beginning of a reply to the question raised by Stoll (1967). He

TABLE 13.12

Preliminary Results of an Attempt at Prevention of Metastases of Breast Cancers in Young Patients Treated with the Combination Chlormadinone 4 mg, with Ethinyl Oestradiol 100 µg

|  | Control group* | Treated group† |
|---|---|---|
| Total number of cases | 33 | 23 |
| Patients { pre-menopausal | 10 | 19 |
| castrated | 23 | 4 |
| Number of patients having presented metastases | 2 | 5 |
| Number of patients deceased | 5 | 0 |

* Average period of observation: 2·7 years.

† Average period of observation: 2·9 years.

noted remission of breast cancer in post-menopausal patients following therapy with usual doses of oral contraceptives, and asks whether similar results might not be achieved in pre-menopausal patients.

We observe no evidence of hypothalamo-hypophyseal stimulation in the course of the treatment, at the low doses of oestrogen we used. It could be objected that such stimulation might be found in non-responsive cases and could indeed be the cause of failure. Table 13.13, which gives examples of hormonal measurement in some non-responsive patients, shows clearly that in post-menopausal cases hypothalamo-hypophyseal inhibition similar to that observed in the responsive cases was obtained in four patients out of five. In one of the two young patients who showed no benefit from the treatment and in whom the same measurements were performed (Case No. 1), hypothalamo-hypophyseal inhibition of the same order was achieved.

We mentioned earlier that the only criterion influencing response to hypothalamo-hypophyseal inhibition of gonadotrophin and corticotrophin was the existence or the absence of previous treatment. We had expected to find a reduction of favourable responses in cases subjected to other hormone therapy previously. This was not so, and in the 23 improved or stabilized patients there was a record of hormonal pre-treatment in 11 cases, whilst in the 28 patients who showed no response to the progestin–oestrogen–corticosteroid combination there was a similar pre-treatment in 12 cases. In point of fact, the likelihood of a favourable response is correlated with only one criterion: whether the patient has undergone pre-treatment by surgery, radiotherapy, anti-mitotic drugs, or hormones. In such cases, the chances of response to the inhibitory treatment are diminished, whereas if the patient has received no pre-treatment, a favourable response will be more frequent by far.

This is difficult to explain at the present stage of our knowledge. One could perhaps envisage that the stress experienced by a woman after amputation of

## TABLE 13.13

### Urinary Hormone Estimations in Non-responding Patients

| Age of patient | Treatment | | HMG (MU/24 hours) | Pregnanediol (mg/24 hours) | Oestrogens (μg/24 hours) | | 17-KS* (mg/24 hours) | 17-OHCS (mg/24 hours) |
|---|---|---|---|---|---|---|---|---|
| | | | | | Oestriol | Oestrone + oestradiol | | |
| 62 | *Before treatment* | Lyndiol | >80 | 0·5 | 5 | 5 | 5·5 | 5 |
| | After 2 months' treatment | Dectancyl† | =3 | Trace | 5 | 5 | 1·5 | 1·5 |
| 69 | *Before* | Lyndiol | | | | | | |
| | After 3 days' treatment | Dectancyl | <3 | Trace | Trace | Trace | 0·5 | |
| 53 | *Before* | Lyndiol | 3–40 | Trace | Trace | Trace | 1·5 | 3·5 |
| | After 3 months' treatment | Dectancyl | <3 | Trace | 5 | 5 | 1 | 2 |
| 49 | *Before* | Lyndiol | >80 | 0·5 | 5 | 5 | 12 | 4·5 |
| | After 6 months' treatment | Dectancyl | <3 | Trace | 5 | 5 | 1·5 | 1·5 |
| 60 | *Before* | Lyndiol | 5–40 | Trace | 10 | 10 | 10·5 | 6 |
| | After 4 months' treatment | Dectancyl | 40–80 | 0·5 | Trace | Trace | 0·6 | 0·7 |

*17–KS = 17-ketosteroids; 17–OHCS = 17-hydroxycorticosteroids.
† Dectancyl = Dexamethasone.

the breast or radiotherapy for breast tumour could bring about changes in the catecholamine content of brain tissue, including that of the hypothalamus. This might affect the response to hormonal therapy in accordance with a hypothesis recently advanced by Stoll (1972).

It is interesting to examine what points there are in common between hypophysectomy, either surgical or by yttrium-90 implant, and hypothalamo-hypophyseal inhibition of gonadotrophin and corticotrophin. The results of either type of technique are fairly similar, bearing in mind that the contra-indications of hypophysectomy—liver metastases, brain metastases, free interval of less than one year—do not extend to the pharmacological method. Furthermore, it must not be overlooked that some form of hormone replacement therapy—hydrocortisone, thyroid extract, or pitressin—are essential after hypophysectomy, since hypophysectomy suppresses all the hypophyseal secretions, whether anterior or posterior pituitary.

Treatment by progestin–oestrogen–corticosteroid combinations inhibits LH and ACTH secretion, and may possibly depress that of HGH. These trophic hormones do not appear to be of themselves carcinogenic. In a young woman who has undergone bilateral ovariectomy as the initial therapy for breast cancer, there often follows stabilization or even regression of the lesions, even though FSH and LH are being secreted at a higher level because of the suppression of the hypothalamo–hypophyseo–ovarian feedback. There is a similar considerable increase of ACTH secretion in adrenalectomized patients, and we need not emphasize the beneficial effect of ablation of the adrenals on breast cancer. If medical treatment directed to an inhibition of the gonadotrophic and corticotrophic function of the hypothalamo-hypophyseal centre has the beneficial effects we have reported, it suggests that one of the factors mainly responsible for the growth of the tumour must be peripheral—adrenal and/or ovarian.

How can we reconcile this possible mechanism with the observations of Kennedy (1965), of Landau, Ehrlich and Huggins (1962), and of other investigators, which show that oestrogen–progestin combinations can cause tumour regression even after complete hypophysectomy? Two hypotheses could be invoked to account for this apparent contradiction. First, the progestin–oestrogen–corticoid combination could have a direct restraining effect on the tumour and its metastases. In support of this hypothesis is the variation of the response rate with the site of the metastases, which suggests that uptake of the hormones differs according to the type of metastases.

However, in a recent publication (Chemama et al., 1972a) we examined the uptake of chlormadinone-$^3$H in tumours and in the intact mammary glands of mice bearing spontaneous mammary cancer. We demonstrated that the incorporation of the tritiated steroid at the level of the tumour was of a very low order compared with that measured in the intact mammary glands, although chlormadinone exerts a certain restraining influence on tumours. If the local effect of a steroid is correlated with its uptake in a tumour, it is difficult to incriminate a local action of the steroid in our series.

The second hypothesis would be that the point of impact of the progestin–oestrogen–corticoid combination is primarily hypothalamic and only secondarily hypophyseal. Hypophysectomy suppresses the pituitary secretions but does not affect the hypothalamic hormones, which remain accessible to medical treatment. Is it possible that certain hypothalamic neurohormones possess of themselves a stimulating effect on mammary carcinogenesis? This hypothesis would resolve the contradiction.

Recent experiments (Heuson and Legros, 1972a, b) have demonstrated the role of insulin in the growth of mammary tumours. Alloxan-diabetes produces a reduction of 7,12-DMBA-induced tumours in the rat whilst insulin stimulates their growth. As we have already mentioned, the progestin–oestrogen–corticosteroid combination may possibly depress the secretion of HGH, and we also noticed that certain of our patients showed a tendency to hyperglycaemia. These two observations might imply that production of insulin is reduced during the combination treatment, which could cause a restraining effect on the growth of human breast cancer and their metastases.

Experiments in animals, both in female rats treated by 7,12-DMBA (Nagasawa and Yanai, 1970; Welsch, Nagasawa and Meites, 1970) and in strains of mice with a high incidence of spontaneous mammary cancer, have brought to light the major influence of prolactin secretion on tumour growth. One cannot systematically extrapolate to man mechanisms which are observed in animals; but this is fully discussed in other chapters.

Lastly, certain experiments seem to implicate the secretion of anti-diuretic hormone from the posterior pituitary as a factor of tumour growth. It would have been interesting to carry out free water clearance estimations in our patients before and during treatment, for as Bernard-Weill (1965) has shown, this parameter is lowered in cancer patients. This test is an indirect reflection of the slowing down of water metabolism in cancer cases, and by administering tritiated water to breast cancer-refractory and -predisposed strains of mice we have shown that this metabolism is indeed slowed down in cancerous mice (Chemama et al., 1972b). This observation would support changes in ADH secretion in mice bearing malignant mammary tumours.

## CONCLUSION

A combination of progestin, oestrogen and corticosteroid was administered to patients suffering from advanced breast cancer, at dose levels necessary for inhibiting the gonadotrophic and corticotrophic functions of the hypothalamo-hypophyseal axis.

The results, although short-lived, were favourable and occasionally striking in half of the patients, regardless of their age and endocrine status. These

279

results are comparable to those obtained with hypophysectomy or with adrenalectomy and ovariectomy.

In 23 pre-menopausal or castrated young women who had had breast cancer treated by surgery and/or radiotherapy, we administered the progestin–oestrogen combination in doses twice as high as the oral contraceptive dose. The frequency of subsequent metastases was no greater than in a control group of 33 patients of the same category, untreated and selected at random. While we can affirm that the treatment was not harmful, it is too early to pronounce on its value for the prevention of recurrences of breast cancer.

It is the general opinion that endocrine surgery suppresses the sources of oestrogens responsible for activation of cancerous disease. In our paper we suggest that the level of ovarian oestrogen production in a post-menopausal woman is not appreciable and that adrenocortical oestrogen is minimal even after prolonged stimulation by $\beta^{1-24}$ corticotrophin.

The fact that ethinyl oestradiol in doses of 100–150 µg/24 hours combined with a progestin is devoid of harmful effects in pre-menopausal women calls, in our view, for a reconsideration of the classical viewpoint on hormone-dependent breast cancer. All the evidence indicates that pharmacological depression of the hypothalamo-hypophyseal axis has a beneficial effect on the evolution of breast tumours, by suppressing the secretion of neutral steroids of adrenocortical or ovarian origin, the nature of which is still obscure. We can also conclude that there is no evidence that oral contraceptive therapy is likely to activate the growth of existing cancer of the mammary gland in the pre-menopausal patient.

## REFERENCES

Beatson, G. T. (1896). 'On treatment of inoperable carcinoma of the mamma; suggestions for a new method of treatment, with illustrative cases.' *Lancet* **2**, 104.

Bernard-Weill, E. (1965). 'Variations de la clearance de l'eau libre après surcharge hydrique chez les cancéreux. Corrélations clinico-biologiques.' *An. Endocr.* **25**, 768.

Brown, J. (1966). *Hormone Assays and Their Clinical Application*, p. 262. Edinburgh; Livingstone.

Chemama, R., Jayle, M. F., Ennuyer, A., Bataini, P. and Dhermain, P. (1970). 'Remarques au sujet de quelques malades encore jeunes soumises à l'association gestagène-oestrogène immédiatement après traitement radical de tumeurs malignes du sein.' *Bull. Cancer*, **57**, 239.

— Apelgot, S., Rudali, G., Frilley, M. and Coezy, E. (1972a). 'Courbes d'épuration de la radioactivité de divers tissus de souris réfractaires ou prédisposées au cancer de la mamelle. I. Après administration de chlormadinone tritiée.' *Bull. Cancer* **59**, 187.

— — — — (1972b). 'Courbes d'épuration de la radioactivité de divers tissus de souris réfractaires ou prédisposées au cancer de la mamelle. II. Après administration d'eau tritiée.' *Bull. Cancer* **59**, 207.

Crepy, O., Meslin, F. and Jayle, M. F. (1956). 'Dosage du Pregnandiol urinaire.' *Bull. Soc. Chim. Biol.* **38**, 555.

Franchimont, P. (1971). *Sécrétion Normale et Pathologique de la Somatotrophine et des Gonadotrophines Humaines.* Paris; Masson.

Hans, G., Kaplan, M. D., Myroslaw, M. and Hreshchyshyn, M. D. (1972). 'Gas-liquid chromatographic quantitations of urinary estrogens in non-pregnant women, post-menopausal women and men.' *Am. J. Obstet. Gynec.* **111**, 386.

Heuson, J. C. and Legros, N. (1972a). 'Influence of insulin deprivation on growth of the 7,12-DMBA-induced mammary carcinoma in rats subjected to alloxan diabetes and food restriction.' *Cancer Res.* **32**, 226.

— — (1972b). 'Influence of insulin administration on growth of the 7,12-DMBA-induced mammary carcinoma in intact, oophorectomized and hypophysectomized rats.' *Cancer Res.* **32**, 233.

Huggins, C. and Bergenstal, D. M. (1951). 'Surgery of adrenals.' *J. Am. med. Ass.,* **147**, 101.

— and Yang, N. C. (1962). 'Induction and extinction of mammary cancer.' *Science* **137**, 257.

Jayle, M. F. (1968). 'Influence de la structure des steroides sur leur activité antiovulatoire, antigonadotrope et progestative.' *Thérapie,* **23**, 201.

— Chemama, R., Ennuyer, A. and Bataini, P. (1967). 'L'intérêt de l'inhibition hypophysaire pharmacologique dans le traitement du cancer du sein.' *Bull. Acad. Méd.,* **151**, 66.

— — — (1969). 'L'inhibition pharmacologique du centre hypothalamo-hypophysaire par l'association gestagène-oestrogène-corticostéroïde dans le traitement des cancers mammaires avancés.' In *Cancer et les Glandes Endocrines.* Paris; L'Expansion Scientifique.

Kennedy, B. J. (1965). 'Hormone therapy for advanced breast cancer.' *Cancer* **18**, 1551.

Lacassagne, A. (1932). 'Apparition de cancers de la mamelle chez la souris mâle soumise à des injections de folliculine.' *C. R. Acad. Sci.,* **195**, 630.

Landau, R. L., Ehrlich, E. N. and Huggins, C. (1962). 'Estradiol benzoate and progesterone in advanced human breast cancer.' *J. Am. med. Ass.* **182**, 632.

Luft, R., Olivecrona, H. and Sjogren, B. J. (1952). 'Hypophysektomie pa mannika.' *Nord. Med.* **47**, 351.

Morcos, F., Crockford, P. M. and Beck, R. P. (1972). 'The effect of norethindrone with and without estrogen on serum immunoreactive luteinizing hormone secretion.' *Am. J. Obstet. Gynec.,* **112**, 358.

Nagasawa, H. and Yanai, R. (1970). 'Effects of prolactin or growth hormone on growth of carcinogen-induced mammary tumor of adreno-ovariectomized rats.' *Int. J. Cancer,* **6**, 488.

Perrault, M. (1952). 'Discussion.' *Bull. Mém. Soc. Méd. Hôp. Paris,* **76**, 209.

— (1953). 'Hypophysectomie et cancer du sein.' *Presse Méd.* **61**, 1639.

Schenker, J. G., Polishuk, W. Z. and Eckstein, B. (1971). 'Pathways of the biosynthesis of androgens in the post-menopausal ovary in vitro.' *Acta endocr.* **66**, 325.

Spellacy, W. N. (1967). 'Human growth hormone levels in normal subjects receiving an oral contraceptive.' *J. Am. med. Ass.* **202**, 451.

Stoll, B. A. (1967). 'Effect of lyndiol, an oral contraceptive, on breast cancer.' *Br. med. J.* **1**, 150.

— (1972). 'Brain catecholamines and breast cancer: a hypothesis.' *Lancet* **1**, 431.

Tsyrlina, E., Chemama, R., Ennuyer, A. and Jayle, M. F. (1970). 'Excrétion des stéroïdes urinaires avant et après administration de $\beta^{1-24}$corticotropine chez des patientes atteintes de cancer du sein.' *Path. Biol.*, **18**, 669.

Welsch, C. W., Nagasawa and Meites, J. (1970). 'Increased incidence of spontaneous mammary tumors in female rats with induced hypothalamic lesions.' *Cancer Res.* **30**, 2310.

# 14

# Pituitary Ablation in the Treatment of Breast Cancer

## P. Juret and M. Hayem

The basis for this paper is the data collected in 350 hypophyseolyses (radio-isotope pituitary implantations) performed in 13 years at Institut Gustave-Roussy in Villejuif, and at Centre François-Baclesse in Caen. Physiological or speculative problems are considered secondarily, and only insofar as they are not discussed in the other chapters of this book.

### HISTORICAL BACKGROUND AND RATIONALE

Major endocrine surgery in the treatment of advanced breast cancer—adrenalectomy and hypophysectomy—was born in 1951 and 1952. The possibility that the adrenals and hypophysis might play a role in the growth of certain cancers had been speculated upon for some years, but, if sporadic and unsuccessful previous attempts are excluded, it was not until cortisone became available (in 1949) that removal of these glands seemed to be a reasonable procedure to undertake in man.

The work of the early investigators led to the two following conclusions:

(1) Hypophysectomy can bring about a non-specific anti-neoplastic effect. Suppression of pituitary secretion inhibits the growth of most experimental tumours, whether spontaneous, chemically induced or grafted. When performed before appearance of the tumour, hypophysectomy usually delays its appearance or reduces the number of tumours. When performed after appearance of the tumour, it usually inhibits or slows down tumour growth. More often than not, subsequent administration of growth hormone restores the normal growth rate of the tumour (Loeb, 1940; Lacassagne, 1939; Gardner, 1953; Hertz, 1951; Kirschbaum, 1957; Lipschutz, 1950). Thus, there

were good reasons to think that growth hormone exerts a general control of neoplastic activity, and that it was reasonable to try to obtain regression of all types of human cancer by suppression of growth hormone through hypophysectomy.

(2) Hypophysectomy can bring about an anti-cancer effect in certain cancers by specific mechanisms. The main tumours which were treated by pituitary removal based on such principles were: *(a)* melanomas, as one might suppose that their growth was controlled by the pars intermedia (Shimkin et al., 1952); *(b)* thyroid cancers, as one might expect a therapeutic effect from suppression of T.S.H. (Pearson et al., 1955); *(c)* prostatic cancers, as it was hoped that inhibition of adrenal androgenic corticoids in addition to orchidectomy might result in regression of the malignant lesion (Scott and Walker, 1952); *(d)* mammary cancers in women, and where this malignancy is concerned, hypophysectomy was undertaken with two different specific aims. Some physiologists suggested that prolactin withdrawal might be followed by inhibition of growth in mammary lesions. Others had suppression of oestrogenic hormones in view, as their production is stimulated in the adrenals by corticotrophin and in the ovaries by gonadotrophin. A combination of both aims was postulated later when it appeared that prolactin secretion was controlled by circulating oestrogens.

The first report of removal of an apparently healthy pituitary in a patient with advanced breast cancer was published by Perrault et al. (1952). The therapeutic effect of hypophysectomy, its various operative techniques and the physiological sequelae of pituitary suppression were the main subjects of three international meetings held in New York in 1956 (Pearson, 1957), Glasgow in 1957 (Currie, 1958) and Lyon in 1966 (Dargent and Romieu, 1967). An important part of this paper is based upon their proceedings.

## METHODS OF PITUITARY ABLATION

Removal or ablative irradiation of a healthy pituitary gland are difficult procedures and the difficulties are increased because the surgeon or radiotherapist cannot be satisfied with incomplete destruction of the organ. A large residual pituitary remnant does not inevitably lead to failure but objective remissions are certainly more frequent after complete hypophysectomy (see Table 14.8). It has been demonstrated that the hypopituitary syndrome arises only when more than 85 per cent of anterior pituitary tissue has been destroyed (Sheehan and Summers, 1949), and most authors agree that hypophysectomy is 'functionally complete' when the pituitary remnant amounts to less than 5 per cent of the original volume of the gland.

The principal anatomical points to consider in the different procedures of hypophyseal inhibitions are the following.

Two groups of important nerve structures lie in relation to the sella turcica.

Through the sphenoidal sinus or its fibrous walls pass the third, fourth, and sixth cranial nerves, and above the sella lies the optic chiasma. In consequence of their proximity, the third cranial nerve and the chiasma are particularly endangered by surgical and radiational procedures.

Protrusion of arachnoid is possible into the sella turcica although some anatomists have claimed that this extension is not embryologically feasible (Wilslocki, 1937). When one considers that the cerebrospinal fluid often flows up to the external end of the intra-turcical cannula during stereotactic hypophyseolyses, as well as the incidence of cerebrospinal leakage when the drilled openings of the turcical floor have not been perfectly sealed, one may justifiably suggest that an extension of the subarachnoid surrounding the pituitary is not only possible but almost normal.

Defined as centrifugal by Wilslocki and King (1936) and described in detail by Xuereb, Prichard and Daniel (1954), the hypophyseal portal system originates within the median eminence of the hypothalamus and runs down the infundibular stalk to the pituitary. Its functional role is double—ensuring vascularization of the anterior pituitary, and supplying it with hypothalamic hormones which activate the secretion of pituitary hormones. As a consequence, interruption of the portal vessels results in both necrosis of glandular tissue and decrease or cessation of hormonal release from any hypophyseal islets surviving this necrotic process. This constitutes the therapeutic rationale of stalk section.

Important anatomical variations can be observed in the pituitary and its relation to adjacent structures. These include variations in intrinsic dimensions, ratio of length to width of the sella, diaphragm less or more ossified, diaphragm less or more closed, intra-cavernous nerves and carotid siphon in a less or more anterior position. These individual variations are described in many publications (Bergland, Ray and Torack, 1958; Bull and Schunk, 1962; Busch, 1951; Chiro, 1960; Mahmoud, 1958; Schaeffer, 1924).

X-ray films cannot give accurate information concerning the dimensions of the sella turcica. This does not apply to sagittal films which give a correct appraisal of the pituitary profile, but to transverse films. The fibrous walls separating the sella from the cavernous sinus are radiologically invisible and sometimes the hypophysis balloons into the sinus. If the antero-posterior clinoid axis is taken to represent the pituitary margin, there is a risk of faulty positioning of sources in hypophyseolysis. Some authors utilize intra-sellar Lipiodol injection in order to avoid this possible error (Dutou and Colon, 1967).

Three principal methods have been used in the ablation of pituitary gland activity in advanced breast cancer: surgery, radiation and combined 'radio-surgical' procedures.

## Surgical methods

### Trans-frontal hypophysectomy

The first to be employed (Kennedy, 1957; Le Beau, 1960; Matson, 1957; Ray, 1957), this method deserves to be considered as the reference method in comparison with which the advantages and disadvantages of the other procedures may be evaluated.

The pituitary gland is exposed by a right frontal craniotomy followed by elevation and retraction of the right frontal lobe. The stalk is divided close to the diaphragm sellae. The gland is curetted out and the sella is swabbed with Zenker's solution.

Many neurosurgeons have retained, with small operative differences, this original technique, as the one giving the best opportunity to curette the sella thoroughly and thus perform a complete pituitary ablation. This approach to the hypophysis, however, is not always easy. Occasionally the optic nerves are abnormally short, necessitating removal of the tuberculum sellae to expose the gland and avoid traumatizing the nerves.

When the operation is performed by experienced teams, mortality and morbidity rates are low. In the first patients of their series, Pearson and Ray (1960) reported 6·6 per cent of deaths occurring during the first 30 post-operative days, and less than 10 per cent of complications including visual field defects, wound infection, intracranial thrombosis and rhinorrhoea.

In our personal experience, the main drawback of transfrontal hypophysectomy is psychological. Women with advanced breast cancer have often already been heavily traumatized by mastectomy, radiation therapy, hormonal or chemotherapeutic agents, each associated with unpleasant side-effects. Each of these steps has undermined their moral resources and they are inclined to resist a new aggressive measure. In spite of the low mortality of the operation, the prospect of a craniotomy whose benefit cannot be guaranteed is hardly encouraging. It was logical that surgeons and radiologists should attempt to develop less unattractive methods of pituitary ablation.

### Trans-sphenoidal, trans-ethmoidal hypophysectomy

Under this heading are included several techniques with one common characteristic—the pituitary gland is exposed through the anterior wall or the floor of the sella. Various routes have been advocated including the trans-cutaneous approach between eye and nose, the rhino-septal paragingival approach, and the trans-oral approach (Escher, Roth and Cottier, 1957; Hardy, 1967; Hamberger et al., 1961; Noguera and Haase, 1961; Riskaer, Munthe and Hommelgaard, 1961).

The principal advantage of these methods is that they do not involve a craniotomy, but on the other hand a complete hypophysectomy seems to be more difficult than with the trans-frontal route. Moreover most series of these trans-spheno-ethmoidal hypophysectomies report a substantial frequency of complications, particularly wound infection and meningitis.

## Pituitary stalk section

As mentioned above, stalk section can bring about an indirect hypophysectomy and several groups have attempted to utilize it in patients with advanced breast cancer (Dugger, Van Wyk and Newsome, 1958; Ehni and Eckles, 1959). The operative approach is trans-frontal, the stalk is divided as low as possible and an impervious tantalum or polyethylene plate is inserted to prevent the re-establishment of the hypothalamo-hypophyseal portal system.

This operation has led to valuable physiological findings (which will be reviewed later), concerning the role of this portal system and the control of anterior pituitary functions by hypothalamic secretion. It will be seen also that its anti-cancer effect is beyond doubt, although it is uncertain whether stalk section has the same therapeutic value as trans-frontal hypophysectomy. In Newsome's series one third of patients subjected to stalk section suffered complications, especially wound infections, thrombosis and visual defects, and autopsy frequently showed incomplete infarction of the adenohypophysis (Newsome et al., 1971). It is our opinion that once a trans-frontal approach has been decided and performed, curetting the sella turcica gives the best opportunity to obtain complete ablation of pituitary function.

## Radiational hypophysectomy

### Conventional external irradiation

Destroying the pituitary by external irradiation without surgical trauma appears to present an attractive prospect but two facts make this attempt difficult. First, as seen above, the pituitary gland lies in close apposition to nervous structures which must be spared, whereas complete destruction of the gland is required. Secondly, adeno-hypophyseal tissue is highly radiation-resistant and, whereas the range of dose necessary for complete necrosis is estimated at between 50,000 and 100,000 rads, the maximum tolerated by the hypothalamus or cranial nerves is only 5–10 per cent of these doses. These anatomical and radiobiological considerations account for the rarity of attempts at conventional radiotherapy for pituitary ablation (Kaplan, 1961). Telecobalt therapy (Plunkett, 1957) and electron therapy by a 22 MeV betatron (Nickson, 1957) have hardly improved the results, all attempts so far resulting in a high proportion of severe visual disorders.

## Heavy particle irradiation

The only satisfactory series of pituitary ablation achieved by external irradiation was that reported by the group utilizing the 184 inch cyclotron in Berkeley (Tobias, 1958). With this cyclotron, used either as a 34 MeV proton or as a 910 MeV alpha particle emitter, Lawrence (1967) claimed that by delivering 17,000 rads to the gland they could depress pituitary function, with relatively little damage to the surrounding structures. However satisfactory the Berkeley results may be, a source such as the one utilized by this group is too rarely available to be taken into consideration by most practitioners dealing with breast cancer.

## Combination of radio-isotopes and surgery

The rationale of isotopic irradiation of the pituitary arose from the very causes making external irradiation unsuitable. It seemed likely that the gland could be destroyed without damaging the adjacent nervous structures if judiciously chosen isotopes were introduced into the sella.

## Radio-isotopes as supplement to trans-frontal hypophysectomy

Some neurosurgeons have tried to complete curettage of the pituitary gland by introducing fibrin paste or wax containing radioactive material into the sella. Gold-198 (Greening, 1956) and yttrium-90 (Edelstyn et al., 1958) were utilized with this objective but there is inadequate evidence that this combination is more useful than surgery alone.

## Radio-isotope pituitary implantation (hypophyseolysis)

First attempts to destroy the hypophysis by implantation of radioactive substances into sella turcica date from 1954 (Yuhl et al., 1955). The aim of the operators was to obtain pituitary destruction at the price of minor surgical traumatization and these attempts involved either β-γ emitters such as radon (Forrest et al., 1956) or gold-198 (Greening, 1956), or pure β emitters such as phosphorus-32 (Rothenberg et al., 1955) or yttrium-90 (Forrest, 1958). It rapidly became obvious that β-γ emitters were not suitable, as γ-radiation brought about visual disorders similar to those induced by external radiation. Phosphorus was not utilized for very long either, because, in its colloidal form, it tended to diffuse dangerously, and yttrium-90 was rapidly adopted by most operators. Numerous technical variations were proposed concerning:

(1) The approach—trans-frontal (Yuhl et al., 1955), trans-ethmoidal (Bauer, 1956), bilateral (Forrest, 1958) or unilateral (Juret, Hayem and Flaisler, 1964), trans-nasal route.

(2) The shape of the radioactive sources—spheres (Notter, 1959), cylinders (Forrest, 1958; Juret, Hayem and Flaisler, 1964).

(3) The positioning of the sources into the sella—two cylinders accurately implanted (Forrest, 1958), seeds randomly distributed throughout the pituitary (Juret, Hayem and Flaisler, 1964; Notter, 1959; Yuhl et al., 1955), systematic positioning of the seeds (Juret et al., 1969).

Technical improvements have been discussed by us in other papers (Hayem and Juret, 1962; Juret, 1966, 1971; Juret, Hayem and Flaisler, 1964; Juret et al., 1969), but in spite of these developments many still consider it very difficult to obtain complete ablation by using isotopic implants. Others report that severe complications are not uncommon, including cranial nerve palsies and cerebral fluid leakages often followed by meningeal infections. Nonetheless, our group has, since 1958, regarded radioactive implant of the pituitary as the most suitable method of pituitary destruction. If strict precautions are taken and the operators are experienced, the complication rate is very low (see below).

The main principles of our technique are as follows:

(1) Operating under the control of two image intensifiers.

(2) Using a stereotactic system (Talairach's apparatus) in such a way that the axis of the trephines and cannulae reaches the centre of the sella.

(3) Positioning the yttrium seeds, according to the size of the sella, on one, two or three planes along the radii of a twelve-pointed star, in order that no part of the sella escapes the irradiation. This positioning is obtained after approach through one nostril, by means of a split cannula along which a flexible trocar draws the cylinders.

(4) Implanting inactive seeds in all directions prior to the active seeds so that, in case of poor positioning, the distribution of the active seeds can be corrected before irreparable damage has been caused.

(5) Injecting hot paraffin wax into the sella after yttrium implantation in order to seal the screw into the drilled floor.

In our series severe complications have now become very rare and, in a total of 300 patients, rhinorrhoea was seen only in 24 (8 per cent) and meningitis in 11 (3·6 per cent). Out of these 11 patients, 5 died from infection, in 4 cases as a consequence of delayed treatment. As for the completeness of pituitary ablation evaluated by gonadotrophin excretion or iodine-131 thyroid uptake measurements, it rose from 55 per cent in the first 150 patients to 75 per cent in the second 150 patient series. These results indicate that the above mentioned technical improvements were proving efficacious.

The principal advantage of this technique of pituitary implantation is that it involves only mild physical and psychological trauma. Sellar or major cervical bone metastases are the only local contra-indications to this operation.

## Miscellaneous methods of pituitary ablation

These include attempts at trans-ethmoidal electrocoagulation (Bauer, 1956) intra-hypophyseal alcohol injection (Greco, Sbaragli and Cammilli, 1957), ultrasound pituitary destruction (Hickey et al., 1961) and cryo-pituitary destruction (Abbes, 1971; Bleasel and Lazarus, 1965; Wilson et al., 1966). The literature to date is inadequate to assess the value and drawbacks of these procedures.

# PHYSIOLOGICAL CONSEQUENCES

As the biological disturbances resulting from hypophysectomy embrace almost the entire field of endocrinology, only a general outline of this subject can be referred to. Minor differences will, however, be mentioned according to whether sellar curettage, stalk section or hypophyseolysis has been carried out.

## Sellar curettage

After sellar curettage, pituitary destruction reaches its maximum effects immediately.

### Suppression of gonadotrophin

In the pre-menopausal patient, this usually results in menopause, although menstruation may recur if the operation is performed in the luteal phase. Hypophysectomy is more usually performed after a natural or artificial menopause and since hot flushes do not always disappear completely immediately after the operation, this casts doubt on the role attributed to gonadotrophins in the genesis of menopausal vasomotor phenomena. A decrease in libido usually follows the operation but can be restored by administration of small doses of androgens.

### Suppression of thyrotrophin

Hypothyroidism appears gradually during the two months following hypophysectomy. Dryness of the skin and obesity are the first clinical manifestations of this dysfunction. If replacement therapy is not given, myxoedema gradually becomes complete with cold intolerance, lassitude, mental apathy, constipation and decrease in the growth of axillary and pubic hair.

Biological changes resulting from the suppression of TSH are of particular interest, as some authors judge the completeness of hypophyseal ablation by this means. A fall of basal metabolic rate as low as $-36$ per cent and a fall of

PBI below 3μg/100 ml are the usual features of hypothyroidism induced by hypophysectomy, but they are poor parameters for evaluation of completeness of pituitary inhibition. The thyroid uptake of iodine-131 is more suitable for this purpose and most endocrinologists agree that complete inhibition of pituitary activity may be assumed when the 24-hour iodine-131 thyroid uptake falls below 10 per cent. In French patients a level of 15 per cent is admitted as the upper limit of hypopituitarism, possibly owing to the fact that in France the food is not overloaded with iodine as it is in many countries.

Occasionally, and in spite of an anatomically complete hypophysectomy, one may observe persistence of unaltered thyroid function. This abnormality is rare, being seen in only 8 cases in 400 patients of Pearson (1960), and occurs usually, but not always, in the presence of an autonomous adenoma of the thyroid.

## Suppression of corticotrophin

When the adrenals of hypophysectomized patients are studied at autopsy, it is usual to find atrophied fasciculata and reticulosa zones but a normal glomerulosa. Hormonal production is consistent with this finding, as aldosterone secretion appears to be only slightly affected by pituitary destruction. On the other hand, hormonal production of the central and inner zones is profoundly depressed by hypophysectomy. Androgens and oestrogens disappear from the urine or fall to a very low level.

If corticoid maintenance is withdrawn, urinary 17-ketosteroids and blood and urinary 17-hydroxycorticosteroids reach low values, while clinical signs of adrenal insufficiency develop promptly, including vomiting, weakness and hypotension. However, these symptoms do not appear as fast and dramatically following hypophysectomy as following corticoid withdrawal in an adrenalectomized patient. In several cases we have seen patients whose pituitary function was completely inhibited, survive without hormonal maintenance for 3–5 days. This presumably results from the continuation of aldosterone secretion after hypophysectomy.

The hypophysectomized patient usually requires replacement therapy of 25–50 mg of cortisone acetate by mouth daily. In case of stress of any sort, these doses must be increased by two to ten times and eventually need to be given by injection. Another difference from adrenalectomized patients is that, after hypophysectomy, a satisfactory equilibrium can be obtained with cortisone substitutes such as prednisone 10–15 mg daily.

## Suppression of pitressin

Following hypophysectomy, the development of diabetes insipidus is usual, being more severe when the stalk is cut at a higher level than when cut close to the diaphragma sellae. As described in animals (Fisher, Ingram and Ransom,

1935; Heinbecker and White, 1941), it sometimes assumes a triphasic evolution. The first polyuric phase appears immediately after the operation, in relation to sudden interruption of the anti-diuretic hormone release following pituitary excision; the second phase of diuresis normalization occurs when the anti-diuretic principle is secreted in sufficient amount from the cut stalk; the third phase consists of a secondary polydipso-polyuric syndrome which appears between 5 and 15 days after the operation and is a consequence of a retrograde degeneration of the hypothalamic neurones (Ikkos, Luft and Olivecrona, 1955; Lipsett et al., 1956). If no hormone replacement therapy is given, the polyuria can reach 7–15 litres daily, with a fall in the urinary specific gravity below 1·008. A spontaneous improvement of this syndrome is frequent after several months, but in any case it is usually easily controlled by means of snuff or injections of posterior pituitary extracts.

## Miscellaneous effects

Alterations in carbohydrate metabolism in non-diabetic subjects are minimal. With cortisone maintenance, the fasting blood sugar is unchanged. The oral glucose tolerance test is either normal or presents a slight exaggeration of the late hypoglycaemic phase (Pearson, 1960).

Blood volume and total haemoglobin are usually slightly diminished (Falkheden, Sjogren and Westling, 1963). The glomerular filtration rate decreases for some weeks and then returns slowly to normal (Falkheden, 1963).

No pigmentary disturbance is noted and the skin of hypophysectomized patients tans normally when exposed to sunlight.

Pregnancy diagnosed after hypophysectomy can be maintained and parturition follows its normal course with an increased dosage of cortisone (Kaplan, 1961; Little et al., 1958).

## Stalk section

The physiological rationale of stalk section has been discussed above. Its main biological consequences are identical with those following sellar curettage, but one specific consequence of stalk secretion deserves particular attention. Some groups performing this operation have reported the induction of milk secretion (Dugge, Van Wyk and Newsome, 1958; Ehni and Eckles, 1959). The secreted milk does not flow spontaneously nor by suction but only with strong compression of the mammary tissue. The mechanism of this phenomenon is not clear but the absence of natural milk evacuation suggests that it is a result of the diminution of oxytocin secretion due to degeneration of hypothalamo-neurohypophyseal neurones. The mechanism for the lacto-genesis is more conjectural but it has been hypothesized that the inhibition of FSH, LH and TSH might stimulate prolactin synthesis.

## Hypophyseolysis

A most important distinctive biological change resulting from isotopic implantation is a transient phase of hyperpituitarism or, more exactly, of pituitary hyperhormonaemia, first noted by Notter (1959). It is a consequence of the operative procedure, because when the radioactive seeds are introduced into the sella turcica they tear hypophyseal tissue so that the hormone secretion accumulated in the gland is over-released. Usually the blood hormonal concentration returns to its normal level between the fourth and eighth post-operative days and the maximal definitive inhibition is delayed until after two weeks.

This distinctive feature of pituitary damage after hypophyseolysis permits a delay in hormonal replacement therapy but, more than that, this observation permits speculation concerning the mechanism of subjective improvement after implants. The immediate relief of pain which follows hypophyseolysis in patients with bone metastases cannot be ascribed to the hormonal deprivation, since this subjective improvement occurs at the very time when the blood stream is overloaded with pituitary secretion.

## CLINICAL RESULTS

The anti-cancer effects of hypophysectomy have to be evaluated according to whether subjective or objective response is being considered.

Subjective responses are by no means negligible. Relief of pain, diminution of dyspnoea or cough, recovery of appetite and strength and improvement in the general condition resulting from hypophysectomy are often achieved well before any other benefit. Nevertheless, the subjective results of ablative procedures are unsuitable for accurate evaluation of the response because they depend, in part, on the personality of the patient.

To determine the anti-cancer value of pituitary ablation, it is preferable to take into account only objective results at clinical or radiographic examination, comparing successive post-operative with pre-operative data. An anti-cancer effect from pituitary inhibition may be claimed when objective regression or extended stabilization of metastatic foci is demonstrated. Aggravation of metastatic growth or tumour regression in one site with progression in others are considered as objective failures. According to the rules proposed by the Joint Committee on Endocrine Procedures in Disseminated Mammary Carcinoma, a response should not be considered an objective success if it does not persist longer than six months (MacDonald, 1957).

Some British authors have proposed evaluating the clinical results of endocrine surgery by the mean clinical value (MCV) (Walpole and Paterson,

1949; Atkins, 1958). The method involves giving a mark, denoting activity, to a number of metastatic lesions and calculating the average of these marks. The variations of this index provide information of the therapeutic effect—success when MCV increases, failure when it decreases from pre-operative levels. Assessment of MCV is undoubtedly a precise method, but in our experience it appears to be an unnecessarily tedious practice.

In reviewing the reports of hypophysectomy we found a range of success, according to the authors, of between 36 and 64 per cent (Juret, 1966). It would be of little purpose to repeat this review, as the different authors did not operate on patients selected by the same criteria, nor evaluate their results on the same basis.

More significant is the survey from the literature of 390 cases of hypophysectomy analysed in 1962 by Taylor (1962). He concluded that the average proportion of objective remissions lasting longer than six months was about 30 per cent. The success rate has increased since, owing to the fact that indications and contradictions are now better known and, in recent reports, the proportion of objective remissions is about 40 per cent after sellar curettage as well as after stalk section.

In our personal series of hypophysiolyses, objective improvement lasting longer than three months was obtained in 31 per cent, and longer than six months in 26 per cent of patients. These figures, which seem less favourable than those of other authors, result from our particular method of selecting patients for operation. As the analgesic effect of hypophyseolysis is remarkable in most cases of bone metastases and the operative trauma is slight, a number of patients were operated upon with the main intention of relieving the patient's pain. Our selection of patients was not influenced by data predicting an unfavourable objective result, such as a short recurrence-free interval. This may account for the smaller percentage of objective responses in our series.

Between 1955 and 1960, it was thought that, because of some long remissions, hypophysectomy might be able to induce definitive cures in advanced breast cancer. Now it is universally agreed that a relapse occurs inevitably even after the longest and most complete remission. The longest remissions reported in the literature are about ten years and, in our first 150 patients, we have 2 eight-year, 1 six-year, 1 five-year, 2 four-year, and 7 three-year remissions. The average length of objective remissions is much shorter and about 50 per cent of them do not exceed 18 months. On that score, there is good agreement between the results of hypophysectomies at the Memorial Center (Fracchia et al., 1971) and our personal series of hypophyseolyses (Table 14.1).

According to metastatic location, the principal clinical, radiological and biochemical features of remissions are as follows.

TABLE 14.1

Length of Remission after Hypophysectomy (Memorial Center Series) and Hypophyseolysis (Personal Series)

| Length of remission | 6 months | 9 months | 12 months | 18 months | 24 months |
|---|---|---|---|---|---|
| 203 hypophysectomies (Fracchia et al. 1971) | 68 33% | 59 29% | 50 24% | 32 15% | 25 12% |
| First 150 hypophyseolyses of our series | 39 26% | 37 24% | 33 22% | 22 14% | 18 12% |

## Bone metastases

In osteolytic lesions, progressive healing may appear but is rarely apparent before two to three months. The recalcification process frequently exceeds normal calcification, and in metastatic areas a greater density than in the adjacent healthy bones is finally seen. In patients whose serum and urinary calcium levels had risen abnormally before the operation, a return to normal level is noted and urinary calcium excretion may even fall to subnormal levels (less than 5 mg daily in one of our patients). Alkaline phosphatase levels in the serum tend to rise simultaneously.

Following hypophyseolysis, recovery is often preceded by a short period of aggravation with a higher level of calcium in the urine, a consequence of the transitory hyperhormonaemia mentioned above (Juret and Hayem, 1967). This period is never longer than five days. Subjective improvement is usually dramatic and patients who demanded repeated doses of analgesic drugs are often able to do without them in the days immediately following operation. The pathogenesis of this analgesia will be referred to later. With osteoblastic lesions, the same analgesic effects are observed, but it is exceptional to observe a return to normal calcification.

## Pleural and pulmonary metastases

Pleural effusions diminish and malignant cells disappear from the fluid. Lung lesions cease to grow and begin to decrease in size and dyspnoea tends to improve.

## Soft tissue metastases

Regression of metastases may involve either their complete disappearance or only shrinkage with loss of malignant histological characteristics in the remnant. Swollen lymphoedematous arms may regress if due to vascular compression by neoplastic tissue. Primary breast cancer also may shrink up to the point of complete disappearance.

### Other metastases

Hepatic, peritoneal, ovarian or cerebral metastases may occasionally decrease in size and their symptoms may be improved but, as will be seen later, this is rare.

As mentioned above, remissions resulting from hypophysectomy are always temporary and the cancerous process resumes its growth sooner or later, sometimes after several years. In our experience, it is frequently noted that recurrence often involves new areas which were apparently not involved prior to endocrine surgery, while the metastatic lesions responding to hypophysectomy remain under control, sometimes up to the time of the patient's death.

## PREDICTIVE FACTORS

Any technique of pituitary ablation involves some operative risks, even less traumatizing operations such as hypophyseolysis. On the other hand, it has been seen that all these procedures fail to yield an objective response in more than 50 per cent of cases. It is essential, therefore, to examine factors which may predict the chances of success when the operation is under consideration. Pre-operative predictive factors can be classified as clinical and biological.

### Clinical pre-operative predictive factors

#### Age of the patient

There is some disagreement on this point as some authors obtain a greater percentage of success in young patients while others claim greater success in post-menopausal patients. Our results are consistent with this second opinion (Table 14.2) and show increasing response rate with age.

TABLE 14.2
Age of Patient as a Predictive Factor in 265 Hypophyseolyses

| Age | Number of patients | Number and percentage of objective remissions | |
|---|---|---|---|
| < 40 years | 29 | 6 | 20% |
| 49–49 years | 73 | 19 | 26% |
| 50–59 years | 100 | 29 | 29% |
| 60–73 years | 63 | 21 | 33% |

## Location of metastases

In relation to the site of the lesion, the results of our first 269 hypophyseolyses (involving 357 lesion sites) are as follows (Table 14.3).

TABLE 14.3

Location of Metastases as a Predictive Factor (357 Locations in 269 Patients Submitted to Hypophyseolysis)

| Location | Number of patients | Number and percentage of remissions | |
|---|---|---|---|
| Bone metastases | 199 | 97 | 48% |
| Nodular cutaneous metastases | 41 | 11 | 26% |
| Lymphatic cutaneous metastases | 18 | 0 | 0% |
| Pleural metastases | 20 | 5 | 25% |
| Pulmonary metastases | 21 | 5 | 24% |
| Pleuro-pulmonary metastases | 13 | 5 | 30% |
| Inflammatory primary tumours | 10 | 0 | 0% |
| Swollen arms | 14 | 4 | 21% |
| Liver metastases | 7 | 2 | |
| Brain metastases | 7 | 1 | |
| Peritoneal metastases | 4 | 0 | |
| Choroid metastases | 3 | 2 | |

These results are in good agreement with those in the literature. Bone metastases carry the greatest chance of objective response and this, as well as the frequent analgesic effect obtained in bone metastases, unquestionably make this site the major indication for hypophyseal ablation. It must be added that localized bone lesions respond more often than do generalized metastases in the skeleton.

## Results of previous hormonal therapy

It is generally agreed that a history of previous objective response to a hormonal procedure is a factor favouring response to hypophysectomy. On this point, the previous effect of a therapeutic castration is of particular value. In the series reported by the Memorial Center, out of 21 patients who previously benefited by castration, 19 responded favourably to hypophysectomy, whereas out of 23 patients who did not benefit by castration only 1 was objectively improved by hypophysectomy (Pearson and Ray, 1960). These authors report that success or failure of previous treatment by oestrogens, androgens and corticoids may also provide prognostic information on hormonal dependence. Some authors suggest observing the effect of pre-operative administration of oestrogen (Pearson et al., 1955) or of corticoids

(Emerson and Jessiman, 1956) as a means of predicting response to a future endocrine ablative procedure.

### Recurrence-free interval

The longer the time elapsed between primary surgery and the first evidence of metastasis, the greater the likelihood of obtaining an objective response from hypophysectomy. In 182 patients of our series, the relationship between the free interval and objective response was as follows (Table 14.4).

TABLE 14.4

Free Interval as a Predictive Factor in 180 Hypophyseolyses

| Length of free interval | < 1 year | 1–2 years | 2–5 years | > 5 years |
|---|---|---|---|---|
| Total number of patients | 29 | 38 | 75 | 38 |
| Number and percentage of remissions | 3 9% | 10 26% | 30 40% | 18 47% |

These findings agree with the conclusions of other authors and it can even be said that no clinical factor has a better predictive value than this one. Unfortunately, the recurrence-free interval applies only in the case of patients operated upon soon after tumour detection. A patient presenting with metastases whose primary tumour has existed for some years previously but was neglected, should not, of course, be considered as having no free interval.

## Biological pre-operative predictive factors

### Urinary oestrogens

In 133 patients of our series, urinary oestrogens were measured chemically before hypophyseolysis. Results in Table 14.5 show no correlation between the

TABLE 14.5

Daily Pre-operative Excretion of Oestrogens as a Predictive Factor in 133 Hypophyseolyses

| Daily pre-operative excretion of oestrogens | Total number of patients | Number and percentage of remissions |
|---|---|---|
| $\geqslant 10\,\gamma$ | 62 | 14 22% |
| $< 10\,\gamma$ measurable | 48 | 14 29% |
| Not measurable | 23 | 7 30% |

pre-operative oestrogen excretion and the likelihood of remission. These findings are in agreement with those reported by British authors (Bulbrook et al., 1958) that biochemical estimation of oestrogen excretion is unable to supply valuable predictive information.

## Urinary androgens

Bulbrook's group have pointed out the predictive value of aetiocholanolone excretion (Bulbrook, Greenwood and Hayward, 1960). Our group came to the same conclusion after measuring the daily pre-operative aetiocholanolone + androsterone excretion (Table 14.6). High androgen excretion is a favourable predictive factor.

TABLE 14.6

Daily Pre-operative Excretion of Androgens as a Predictive Factor in 121 Hypophyseolyses

| Daily pre-operative excretion of androsterone + aetiocholanolone | Total number of patients | Number and percentage of remissions | |
|---|---|---|---|
| > 2 mg | 26 | 12 | 46% |
| 1·1–2 mg | 40 | 13 | 32% |
| ⩽ 1 mg | 55 | 13 | 23% |

## 17-Hydroxycorticosteroid excretion

Our conclusions also confirm the predictive value of 17-hydroxycortico-steroid excretion (Bulbrook, Greenwood and Hayward, 1960). The higher this hormonal excretion, the lower the likelihood of tumour remission (Table 14.7).

TABLE 14.7

Daily Excretion of 17-hydroxycorticosteroids as a Predictive Factor in 147 Hypophyseolyses

| Daily excretion of 17-OHCS | Total number of patients | Number and percentage of remissions | |
|---|---|---|---|
| ⩾ 6 mg | 51 | 8 | 15% |
| < 6 mg | 96 | 32 | 33% |

## Gonadotrophin excretion

Contradictory results have been reported concerning the predictive value of gonadotrophin excretion (Chow, Coleman and Lederis, 1967; Colon, Dutou and Motamedi, 1967).

## Other biological predictive factors

Other prognostic factors have been· reported and it is suggested that a greater likelihood of remissions would be obtained in patients: *(a)* with positive sex-chromatin in the tumour cells (Wense, 1969); *(b)* with an O blood group as compared with A (Juret and Hayem, 1968); *(c)* with a low level of plasma glucuronidase (Whitaker, 1961); or *(d)* with a high uptake of tritium-labelled hexoestrol by malignant tissue (Folca, Glascock and Irvine, 1961). The value of all these data is still to be confirmed.

An overall assessment of these factors in hormonal dependency is interesting. Hypophysectomies were first undertaken with the aim of inducing cancer remission through oestrogen suppression, and one might expect particularly favourable results in very young patients as well as in patients excreting high amounts of oestrogens. In fact, these expectations did not prove correct; on the contrary it was androgen excretion which was found of prognostic value.

## Post-operative predictive factor

## Completeness of pituitary destruction

Objective remissions can unquestionably be obtained after incomplete pituitary destruction (Boesen and Radley Smith, 1967; Luft, 1957). In our personal series, one of the two patients whose remission lasted eight years retained thyroid function at a normal level (iodine-131 24-hour uptake of 34 per cent) without evidence of autonomous adenoma of the thyroid. In general, more favourable responses occur in patients whose pituitary function is completely suppressed (Table 14.8).

TABLE 14.8

Completeness of Pituitary Destruction as a Predictive Factor in 165 Hypophyseolyses

|  | Total number of patients | Number and percentage of remissions |
|---|---|---|
| Incomplete destruction of hypophysis | 66 | 11 |
|  |  | 17% |
| Complete destruction of hypophysis | 99 | 34 |
|  |  | 34% |

## SELECTION OF PATIENTS

This problem is actually a double one which can be expressed as follows: In what cases should the surgeon reject pituitary ablation because of the operative or post-operative risks? In what cases should he reject it because the chances of objective remission are too poor? In point of fact, both questions are connected as one is justified in running greater risks in patients whose predictive factors are particularly favourable with regard to hormonal dependency of their cancer.

With regard to the first problem, surgeons are unanimous that hypophysectomy is inadvisable in patients whose general condition is poor, or in patients with serious disturbance in their cardio-renal or hepatic function. Then again it is reasonable not to operate on patients in such a mental state that they cannot understand the necessity for hormonal replacement. As far as hypophyseolysis is concerned, however, one can be less rigid with regard to the general condition of the patient, because the operative trauma is less severe.

With regard to the likelihood of an objective remission, it must be emphasized that there is no criterion whose predictive value is certain. It is easy to schematize an ideal picture of a patient whose chances of remission are optimal: a long recurrence-free interval, limited osseous metastases, a high level of urinary androgens and a history of efficacy of previous hormonal treatment. Also the features of a patient whose chances of remissions are minimal: a short recurrence-free interval, liver or brain involvement, a low level of urinary androgens and inefficacy of previous hormonal treatment. The trouble is that, in most cases, predictive data are not so obvious.

It is even exceptional to find a patient whose predictive factors are in complete agreement. One woman may have a ten-year recurrence-free interval and bone metastases but a cerebral lesion is suspected. Another excretes high amounts of androgenic catabolites but the first recurrence was noted less than one year after primary treatment. A decision on operability therefore entails a synthetic process, in the course of which the respective weights of the predictive factors have to be evaluated. Final decisions resulting from this synthesis may owe more to clinical impressions than to rational arguments!

Some authors have suggested an index of hormonal sensitivity of the cancer (expressing its likelihood of favourable response to ablative procedures), by adding marks obtained in evaluating several clinical or biological aspects of the disease. In this way, Polish authors use five factors marked from 2 to 8, the final 'index of clinical prognostic value' varying from 10 points in the best to 40 points in the worst cases (Koszarowski and Gorski, 1967). We have decided in favour of a simplified index which fits in with the results of our personal series (Juret, 1971), and three predictive factors are taken into account:

|  | Yes | No |
|---|---|---|
| Metastases only in bone | 1 | 0 |
| Androsterone + aetiocholanolone > 1 mg daily | 1 | 0 |
| Free interval longer than two years | 1 | 0 |

Addition of these marks leads to an index ranging from 3 to 0. In the first 149 patients in which this index of hormonal dependency could be evaluated, clinical results were as shown in Table 14.9.

Another problem is the optimal time for pituitary inhibition. In most series, pituitary destruction appears to have been performed as an ultimate measure against cancer when all other therapeutic possibilities of hormonal agents and chemotherapy were exhausted. Carried out earlier, is hypophysectomy better able to benefit the patient?

Pearson and Ray (1960) reported a short series of patients who were subjected to hypophysectomy at the time of their primary treatment because massive node involvement or rapid growth of the tumour suggested the likelihood of early recurrence. No precise conclusion could be drawn from this 'prophylactic' trial because of the small number of patients and the absence of controls.

In patients with recurrent cancer, it could be asked whether hypophysectomy would yield a greater response if performed before other endocrine or chemotherapeutic treatments. A trial conducted by Stewart and Forrest (1969) provides an answer to this question. The chances of remission and overall survival were not statistically different between early and late hypophysectomy. Thus, early hypophysectomy does not appear to be justified and, because of its operative risks, even if they are small, it remains reasonable to undertake this procedure only after attempts at medical treatment have failed. It must not be deduced from this that the road to this decision is perfectly clear because, by waiting too long, the risk is run of massive liver or brain metastases suddenly appearing, meaning that the opportunity for major endocrine procedures has gone.

## MISCELLANEOUS QUESTIONS

### Hypophysectomy versus bilateral ovaro-adrenalectomy

As mentioned above, the original intent of major endocrine procedures was the suppression of oestrogenic sources in the body. This aim could be achieved by two methods—suppressing the hypophysis which stimulates oestrogen production in the gonads and adrenals, or suppressing those targets themselves by performing bilateral ovaro-adrenalectomy.

From the theoretical point of view, the superiority of hypophysectomy is clear. This procedure achieves inhibition, not only of both adrenals but also of ectopic adrenal tissue which exists in more than 50 per cent of subjects, and

## TABLE 14.9

Cumulative Predictive Value of Three Factors in 149 Hypophyseolyses

(Free Interval > 2 years; Androsterone + Aetiocholanolone > 1 mg daily; Metastases only in Bones)

| No favourable factor | | 1 favourable factor | | 2 favourable factors | | 3 favourable factors | |
| --- | --- | --- | --- | --- | --- | --- | --- |
| 23 patients | | 45 patients | | 37 patients | | 44 patients | |
| Success | Failure | Success | Failure | Success | Failure | Success | Failure |
| 0 patient | 23 patients | 6 patients | 39 patients | 13 patients | 24 patients | 31 patients | 13 patients |
| 0% | 100% | 14% | 86% | 36% | 64% | 70% | 30% |

which usually even the most careful bilateral adrenalectomy cannot suppress. Moreover, according to recent investigations, hormonal dependency appears to involve the action of prolactin whose secretion can be stimulated by oestrogens. In that case, hypophysectomy would appear more rational than ovaro-adrenalectomy. But do the facts confirm the theory?

A randomized trial conducted by Atkins' group concludes in favour of hypophysectomy (Atkins, 1958) and this applies as well to a comparison of non-randomized series of both operations at the Memorial Center (Fracchia et al., 1971), although the differences were not statistically significant in either of them. In favour of hypophysectomy would appear to be the second remissions induced by this operation after previous remission obtained by ovaro-adrenalectomy has ceased (Pearson and Ray, 1960). In actual fact, these second remissions are too rare and too short to favour the advocacy of this double ablative procedure, but they do provide confirmation of the above mentioned theoretical consideration.

In conclusion, the superiority of hypophysectomy over adrenalectomy may be more apparent than real. Performed by equally experienced groups, both operations induce not very different degrees of remission.

## Treatment after hypophysectomy

For some time it was asserted that no new remissions could be expected by any treatment whatever, after the control of metastatic growth by pituitary ablation had been lost. Among others, investigators at the Memorial Center reported that, after hypophysectomy, treatment by androgens, oestrogens or high dosage of corticoids as well as by chemotherapy was poorly rewarding (Pearson and Ray, 1960). These findings supported the common belief that hormonal stimulation or inhibition of breast cancer occurs through pituitary mediation.

This opinion has not been confirmed. In Greenberg and Pazianos' series (1967) are quoted 10 objective remissions out of 75 patients treated with androgens, 1 out of 16 with oestrogens, 6 out of 27 with 5-fluorouracil and 3 out of 12 with chlorambucil in the treatment of recurrence following hypophysectomy. In some patients, remission lasted longer than six months and beneficial effects of androgens or chemotherapy were noted both in patients who previously responded to hypophysectomy and in those who did not. In our series we have obtained remissions both by cyclophosphamide and 5-fluorouracil after hypophysectomy.

## The mechanism of pain relief

Since 1954 it has been clear that, in a number of cases, hypophysectomy could achieve relief of symptoms, especially of pain in osseous lesions when, at the same time, there was no evidence of shrinkage, arrest or even slowing of the growth of metastases. However, as this analgesic effect was noted after pituitary removal, it was tacitly admitted that it was a result of the destruction of hypophyseal tissue acting through an unknown mechanism.

Investigations conducted in patients undergoing radioactive seed implants have revealed two observations which make this hypothesis untenable.

(1) After yttrium implants, hypopituitarism was never evident in our series before the sixth to seventh days, nor complete before the fourteenth to sixteenth days. During the first to fifth post-operative days, there was hyper-release of pituitary secretion as a consequence of the pituitary tearing, and this is likely to be the cause of the transient recrudescence of hypercalciuria usually noted at this time (Juret and Hayem, 1967).

(2) The improvement, and often the complete relief, in pain usually occurs the day after operation, and is obvious by the second day in 85 per cent of cases, i.e. at the very time when hyper-release of pituitary secretion reaches its maximum. It cannot, therefore, be ascribed to the actual pituitary destruction.

A fully satisfactory explanation of this phenomenon is not available. One point should, however, be emphasized—this analgesic effect applies almost exclusively to bone metastases. One case of our series is particularly instructive: a patient whose pains were derived from bone metastases and thoracic zoster at the same time. Relief of pain was complete in the bones but not perceptible in the zoster area. Such an observation fits in with the hypothesis that the analgesic process could result from a decrease of the fluid tension in or around the malignant foci. This decrease in tissue tension might be perceived in bone tissue because of the rigidity of this structure but not in soft tissue because of its elasticity, but this is purely conjectural.

There is no more certainty concerning a pain-inhibiting effect which could result from action upon a specific nervous pathway. Hypothala-mo-retropituitary neurons are commonly considered as centrifugal. Is it possible that the occasional centripetal fibres described by some pathologists (Cajal, 1909; Hagen, 1950; Vasquez-Lopez, 1953) may have a functional significance in conducting a stimulus for pain inhibition to the thalamic centres? Such a hypothesis cannot be absolutely excluded as it has been shown that injury to the superior cervical ganglion can induce microscopic morphological changes in hypothalamic structures (Popjak, 1940).

With regard, therefore, to the mechanism of analgesia following pituitary surgery, only one conclusion is established—the impossibility of linking up this early subjective response with hormonal dependency (Juret, 1960). This being so, one might expect to induce the same analgesic effect in osseous metastases associated with non-hormonal-dependent cancers. This suggestion has been confirmed and we have obtained valuable subjective remissions in four out of six cases of bone metastases from such tumours, i.e. two cervical and two rectal cancers (Juret, Hayem and Thomas, 1962). Of course, no objective tumour regression followed this pain relief. In our opinion, these observations warrant a larger study in the field of osseous disease, cancerous or otherwise.

## CONCLUSION

Thirty years ago, one believed that the hypophysis was the indispensable conductor of the endocrine orchestra, and in most minds the thought of undertaking its removal would have been regarded as fantasy. Thousands of people since have lost their pituitary gland either by the surgeon's curette or by isotopic radiation, with subsequent benefit in many cases.

Physiologically, these procedures have accumulated valuable information in many fields of endocrinology. As the principal consequence, the pituitary has lost a fraction of its leading role and has itself become a target gland executing the orders given by higher centres in the diencephalon.

With regard to its therapeutic value, hypophysectomy does not appear as the panacea that physicians of 1952 had hoped for, and breast cancer is almost the only malignancy showing proven regression after pituitary ablation. However, the length and quality of the regressions noted in a number of cases, as well as the remarkable analgesic effects resulting from these procedures, justify the view of pituitary ablation as a major achievement in anti-cancer therapy.

## REFERENCES

Abbes, M. (1971). 'Hypophysiolyse par Yttrium ou azote liquide—Confrontation à propos de 105 cas.' *Marseille Chir.* **2**, 193.

Atkins, H. J. B. (1958). 'Comparisons and results of adrenalectomy and hypophysectomy.' In *Endocrine Aspects of Breast Cancer,* p. 69, Ed. by A. R. Currie and C. F. W. Illingworth. Edinburgh; Livingstone.

Baron, D. N., Gurling, K. J. and Radley Smith, E. J. (1958). 'The effect of hypophysectomy in advanced carcinoma of the breast.' *Br. J. Surg.* **45**, 593.

Bauer, K. H. (1956). 'Ueber die Hypophysenausschaltung bei inkurablen Krebsfällen mit Hilfe perkutaner intrasellärer Implantation von radioaktivem Gold.' *Langenbeck's Arch. Klin. Chir.* **284**, 438.

Bergland, R. M., Ray, B. S. and Torack, R. M. (1958). 'Anatomical variations in the pituitary gland and adjacent structures in 225 human autopsy cases.' *J. Neurosurg.* **28**, 93.

Blease, L. K. and Lazarus, L. (1965). 'Cryogenic hypophysectomy.' *Med. J. Aust.* **2**, 148.

Boesen, E. and Radley Smith, E. J. (1967). 'Pituitary ablation for patients with disseminated breast cancer.' In *Major Endocrine Surgery for the Treatment of Cancer of the Breast in Advanced Stages,* p. 85, Ed. by M. Dargent and C. Romieu. Lyon; Simep.

Bulbrook, R. D. et al. (1958). 'Hypophysectomy in breast cancer—an attempt to correlate clinical results with oestrogen production.' *Br. J. Cancer* **2**, 15.

— Greenwood, F. G. and Hayward, J. L. (1960). 'Selection of breast cancer patients for adrenalectomy by determination of urinary 17 OHCS and aetiocholanolone.' *Lancet* **1**, 1154.

Bull, J. W. D. and Schunk, H. (1962). 'The significance of displacement of the cavernous portion of the internal carotid artery.' *Br. J. Radiol.* **35**, 801.

Busch, W. (1951). 'Die Morphologie der Sellar turcica und ihre Beziehungen zur Hypophyse.' *Arch. Path. Anat.* **320**, 427.

Cajal, S. R. (1909). *Histologie du Système Nerveux de l'Homme et des Vertébrés.* Paris; Maloine.

Chiro, G. di (1960). 'The width (third dimension) of the sella turcica.' *Am. J. Roentg.* **84**, 26.

Chow, Y. F., Coleman, J. R. and Lederis, K. (1967). 'Urinary gonadotropins in metastatic breast cancer.' In *Major Endocrine Surgery for the Treatment of Cancer of the Breast in Advanced Stages,* p. 193, Ed. by M. Dargent and C. Romieu. Lyon; Simep.

Colon, J., Dutou, L. and Motamedi, G. (1967). 'Hypophysiolyse par Yttrium radioactif—Eléments de pronostic clinique et biologique.' In *Major Endocrine Surgery for the Treatment of Cancer of the Breast in Advanced Stages,* p. 139, Ed. by M. Dargent and C. Romieu. Lyon; Simep.

Currie, A. R. (1958). *Endocrine Aspects of Breast Cancer.* Edinburgh; Livingstone.

Dargent, M. and Romieu, C. (1967). *Major Endocrine Surgery for the Treatment of Cancer of the Breast in Advanced Stages.* Lyon; Simep.

Dugger, G. S., Van Wyk, J. and Newsome, J. F. (1958). 'Transection of the hypophyseal stalk in the management of metastatic mammary carcinoma.' *Am. Surg.* **24**, 603.

Dutou, L. and Colon, J. (1967). 'Incidence de la technique d'implantation hypophysaire d'Yttrium 90 sur les résultats cliniques—Apport de l'injection intrasellaire d'une substance de contraste.' In *Major Endocrine Surgery for the Treatment of Cancer of the Breast in Advanced Stages,* p. 131, Ed. by M. Dargent and C. Romieu. Lyon; Simep.

Edelstyn, G. A., Gleadhill, C. A., Lyons, A. R., Rodgers, H. W., Taylor, A. R. and Welbourn, R. B. (1958). 'Hypophysectomy combined with intraseller irradiation with yttrium 90.' *Lancet* **1**, 462.

Ehni, G. and Eckles, N. E. (1959). 'Interruption of the pituitary stalk in patients with mammary cancer.' *J. Neurosurg.* **16**, 628.

Emerson, K. and Jessiman, A. G. (1956). 'Hormonal influences on the growth and progression of cancer. Tests for hormone dependency in mammary and prostatic cancer.' *New Engl. J. Med.* **254**, 252.

Escher, F., Roth, F. and Cottier, H. (1957). 'Paranasal trasethmoido-sphenoidal hypophysectomy in cases of metastatic breast cancer.' *Ann. Otol.* **66**, 1009.

Falkheden, T. (1963). 'Renal function following hypophysectomy in man.' *Acta endocr.* **42**, 57.

— Sjogren, B. and Westling, H. (1963). 'Studies of the blood volume following hypophysectomy in man.' *Acta endocr.* **42**, 552.

Fisher, C., Ingram, W. R. and Ransom, S. W. (1935). 'Relation of hypothalamico-hypophyseal system to diabetes insipidus.' *Arch Neurol. Psychiat.* **34**, 124.

Folca, P. J., Glascock, R. G. and Irvine, W. T. (1961). 'Studies with tritium-labeled hexoestrol with response to bilateral adrenalectomy and oophorectomy.' *Lancet* **2**, 796.

Forrest, A. P. M. (1958). 'Screw implantation pituitary with Yttrium 90.' *Lancet* **2**, 192.

— Peebles Brown, D. A., Morris, S. R. and Illingworth, C. F. W. (1956). 'Pituitary radon implant for advanced cancer.' *Lancet* **1**, 399.

Fracchia, A., Farrow, J. H., Miller, T. R., Tollefsen, R. H., Lindberg, E. J. and Knapper, W. H. (1971). 'Hypophysectomy as compared with adrenalectomy in the treatment of advanced carcinoma of the breast.' *Surg. Gynec. Obstet.* **133**, 241.

Gardner, W. U. (1953). 'Hormonal aspects of experimental tumorigenesis.' In *Advances in Cancer Research,* Vol. 1, p. 173, Ed. by J. P. Greenstein and A. Haddow. New York; Academic Press.

Greco, I., Sbaragli, G. F. and Cammilli, L. (1957). 'L'alcolizzazione della ipofisi per via transfenoidale nella terapia di particolari tumori maligni.' *Settim. médic.* **45**, 355.

Greenberg, E. and Pazianos, A. (1967). 'Treatment of progressive metastatic breast cancer after hypophysectomy.' In *Major Endocrine Surgery for the Treatment of Cancer of the Breast in Advanced Stages,* p. 267, Ed. by M. Dargent and C. Romieu. Lyon; Simep.

Greening, W. P. (1956). 'Irradiation of pituitary for advanced mammary cancer.' *Lancet* **1**, 728.

Hagen, E. (1950). 'Neurohistologische Untersuchungen an der menschichen Hypophyse.' *Z. Anat.* **114**, 640.

Hamberger, C. A., Hammer, G., Norlen, G. and Sjögren, B. (1961). 'Transphenoidal hypophysectomy.' *Archs Otolaryng.* **74**, 2.

Hardy, J. (1967). 'Hypophysectomie transphenoïdale.' In *Major Endocrine Surgery for the Treatment of Cancer of the Breast in Advanced Stages,* p. 97. Lyon; Simep.

Hayem, M. and Juret, P. (1962). 'Prophylaxie des fistules consecutives aux implantations d'Yttrium intra-hypophysaire par mise en place d'un écran paraffiné dans la selle turcique.' *Presse Méd.* **70**, 323.

Heinbecker, P. and White, H. L. (1941). 'Hypothalamico-hypophyseal system and its relation to water balance in the dog.' *Am. J. Physiol.* **135**, 582.

Hertz, R. (1951). 'The relationship between hormone induced tissue growth and neoplasia: a review.' *Cancer Res.* **11**, 393.

Hickey, C. R., Fry, W. J., Meyers, R., Fry, F. J. and Bradbury, J. T. (1961). 'Human pituitary irradiation with focused ultra-sound. An initial report on effect in advanced breast cancer.' *Archs Surg.* **82**, 620.

Ikkos, D., Luft, R. and Olivecrona, H. (1955). 'Hypophysectomy in man; effect on water excretion during the first two post-operative months.' *J. clin. Endocr.* **15**, 553.

Joplin, G. F. and Fraser, R. (1960). 'The radiological anatomy of the human pituitary. In *Ciba Foundation Colloquia on Endocrinology,* Vol. 13, Ed. by G. E. W. Wolstenholme and M. O'Connor. London; Churchill.

Juret, P. (1960). 'A propos de l'action analgésique de l'hypophysectomie vis à vis des cancers métastatiques.' *Presse Méd.* **68**, 1044.

— (1966). *Endocrine Surgery in Human Cancers.* Springfield, Ill.; Thomas.

— (1971). 'Indications and results of hypophysectomy in the treatment of breast cancer.' In *Corso superiore sul trattamanto dei tumori cella mammella.* (Casa editrice ambrosiane, Milano), p. 481.

— and Hayem, M. (1967). 'Données biologiques relatives à l'implantation d'Yttrium intra-hypophysaire dans les cancers du sein métastatique.' In *Major Endocrine*

*Surgery for the Treatment of the Cancer of the Breast in Advanced Stages,* p. 181, Ed. by M. Dargent and C. Romieu. Lyon; Simep.

Juret, P. and Hayem, M. (1968). 'Données biologiques nouvelles concernant l'hormonodépendance des cancers mammaires.' *Rev. Fr. Clin. Biol.* **13**, 884.

— — and Thomas, M. (1962). 'Action analgésique de l'hypophysectomie sur les métastases osseuses des cancers non hormono-dépendants.' *Press Méd.* **70**, 323.

— — and Flaisler, A. (1964). 'About 150 implantations of radio-active Yttrium intra-hypophysaire in the treatment of breast cancer in advanced stage.' *J. Chir.* **87**, 409.

— et al. (1969). 'Implantation of intra-hypophysaire Yttrium 90 in the treatment of breast cancer in advanced stage.' *J. Rad. Electrol.* **50**, 645.

Kaplan, N. M. (1961). 'Successful pregnancy following hypophysectomy during the twelfth week of gestation.' *J. clin. Endocr.* **21**, 1139.

Kelly, D. H. et al. (1951). 'Irradiation of the normal hypophysis in malignancy; report of 3 cases receiving 8 000–10 000 r tissue dose to the pituitary gland.' *J. natn. Cancer. Inst.* **11**, 967.

Kennedy, B. J. (1957). 'Surgical hypophysectomy in patients with cancer.' In *Hypophysectomy,* Ed. by O. H. Pearson, p. 25. Springfield, Ill.; Thomas.

Kirschbaum, A. (1957). 'The role of hormones in cancer; laboratory animals.' *Cancer Res.* **17**, 432.

Koszarowski, I. and Gorski, G. (1967). 'Results of endocrine ablative surgery for mammary carcinoma in women.' In *Major Endocrine Surgery for the Treatment of Cancer of the Breast in Advanced Stages,* p. 247, Ed. by M. Dargent and C. Romieu. Lyon; Simep.

Lacassagne, A. (1939). 'Les rapports entre les hormones sexuelles et la formation du cancer.' *Ergebn. Vitam. Hormonforsch* **2**, 259.

Lawrence, J. H. (1967). 'Heavy particle irradiation to the pituitary in metastatic carcinoma of the breast.' In *Major Endocrine Surgery for the Treatment of Cancer of the Breast in Advanced Stages,* p. 173, Ed. by M. Dargent and C. Romieu. Lyon; Simep.

Le Beau, J. (1960). *L'hypophysectomie dans le Traitement du Cancer du Sein.* Paris; Doin.

Lipschutz, A. (1950). *Steroid Hormones and Tumors.* Philadelphia; Williams and Wilkins.

Lipsett, M. B., MacLean, J. P., West, G. D., Li, M. C. and Pearson, O. H. (1956). 'An analysis of the polyuria induced by hypophysectomy in man.' *J. clin. Endocr.* **16**, 183.

Little, B. et al. (1958). 'Hypophysectomy during pregnancy in a patient with cancer of the breast: case report with hormone studies.' *J. clin. Endocr.* **18**, 425.

Loeb, L. (1940). 'The significance of hormones in the origin of cancer.' *J. natn Cancer Inst.* **1**, 169.

Luft, R. (1957). 'Surgical hypophysectomy in patients with cancer.' In *Hypophysectomy,* p. 3, Ed. by O. H. Pearson. Springfield, Ill.; Thomas.

MacDonald, I. (1957). 'The role of extirpative procedures in cancer of the breast.' *Cancer* **10**, 805.

— (1962). 'Endocrine ablation in disseminated mammary carcinoma.' *Surgery Gynec. Obstet.* **115**, 315.

Mahmoud, M. El S. (1958). 'The sella in health and disease: the value of the radiographic study of the sella turcica in the morbid anatomical and topographic diagnosis of intracranial tumors.' *Br. J. Radiol.* Suppl. **8**, 1.

Matson, D. D. (1957). 'Surgical hypophysectomy in patients with cancer.' In *Hypophysectomy*, p. 14, Ed. by O. H. Pearson. Springfield, Ill.; Thomas.

Newsome, J. F. et al. (1971). 'Pituitary stalk section for metastatic carcinoma of the breast.' *Ann. Surg.* **174**, 769.

Nickson, J. J. (1957). 'Radiation hypophysectomy. In *Hypophysectomy*, p. 127, Ed. by O. H. Pearson. Springfield, Ill.; Thomas.

Noguera, J. T. and Haase, F. R. (1961). 'Transseptal transsphenoïdal route in hypophysectomy.' *Archs. Otol.* **74**, 652.

Notter, G. (1959). 'A technique for destruction of the hypophysis using Y 90 spheres.' *Acta radiol.* Suppl. **184**, 1.

Pearson, O. H. (1957). *Hypophysectomy*. Springfield, Ill.; Thomas.

— (1960). 'Endocrine consequences of hypophysectomy in man.' In *Clinical Endocrinology*, p. 49, Ed. by E. B. Astwood. New York; Grune and Stratton.

— and Ray, B. S. (1960). 'Hypophysectomy in the treatment of metastatic mammary cancer.' *Am. J. Surg.* **99**, 544.

— — Harrold, C. C., West, C. D., Li, M. C., MacLean, J. P. and Lipsett, M. B. (1955). 'Hypophysectomy in the treatment of advanced cancer.' *Trans. Ass. Am. Phys.* **68**, 101.

— Whitmore, W. F., West, C. D., Farrow, J. H. and Randall, H. T. (1953). (Clinical and metabolic studies of bilateral adrenalectomy for advanced cancer in man.' *Surgery* **34**, 543.

Perrault, M., LeBeau, J., Klotz, B., Sicard, J. and Clavel, B. (1952). 'L'hypophysectomie totale dans le traitement du cancer du sein. Premier cas français—Avenir de la méthode.' *Thérapie* **7**, 290.

Plunkett, E. R. (1957). 'Effect of cobalt 60 radiation on pituitary functions in humans.' *Canad. Cancer Conf.* **2**, 294.

Popjak, G. (1940). 'The pathway of pituitary colloid through the hypothalamus.' *J. Path. Bact.* **51**, 83.

Ray, B. S. (1957). 'Surgical hypophysectomy in patients with cancer.' In *Hypophysectomy*, p. 33, Ed. by O. H. Pearson. Springfield, Ill.; Thomas.

Riskaer, N., Munthe, C. W. and Hommelgaard, J. (1961). 'Transsphenoidal hypophysectomy in metastatic cancer of the breast.' *Archs Otol.* **74**, 483.

Rothenberg, S., Jaffe, H. L., Putnam, P. J. and Shimkin, B. (1955). 'Hypophysectomy with radio-active chromic phosphate in treatment of cancer.' *Archs. Neurol. Psychiat.* **73**, 193.

Schaeffer, J. P. (1924). 'Some points in regional anatomy of optic pathways with special reference to tumors of hypophysis cerebri and resulting ocular changes.' *Anat. Rec.* **28**, 243.

Scott, W. W. and Walker, A. E. (1952). Quoted in 'Man lives minus pituitary.' *Science News Letters* **61**, 98.

Sheehan, H. L. and Summers, V. K. (1949). 'The syndrome of hypopituitarism.' *Q. Jl Med.* **18**, 319.

Shimkin, M. B., Boldrey, E. B., Kelly, K. H., Bierman, H. R., Ortega, P. and Naffziger, H. C. (1952). 'Effects of surgical hypophysectomy in a man with malignant melanoma.' *J. clin. Endocr.* **12**, 439.

Stewart, H. J. and Forrest, A. P. M. (1969). 'Early pituitary implantation with yttrium 90 for advanced breast cancer.' *Lancet* **2**, 816.

Talairach, J. and Tournoux, P. (1955). 'Technique stéréotoxique de la chirurgie hypophysaire par voie nasale.' *Neurochir.* **1**, 127.

— — (1958). 'Technique de la pose d'un pellet d'or radio-actif dans l'hypophyse et suites opératoires.' In *Problemes Actuels d'Endocrinologie et de Nutrition*, p. 1. Paris; Expansion Scientific François.

Taylor, S. G. (1962). 'Endocrine ablation in disseminated mammary carcinoma.' *Surgery Gynec. Obstet,* **115**, 443.

Tobias, C. A. (1958). 'Pituitary irradiation with energy proton beams: a preliminary report.' *Cancer Res.* **18**, 121.

Vasquez-Lopez, E. (1953). 'The structure of the rabbit neurohypophysis.' *J. Endocr.* **9**, 30.

Walpole, A. L. and Paterson, E. (1949). 'Synthetic oestrogens in mammary cancer.' *Lancet* **2**, 783.

Wense, G. (1969). 'Ergebnisse der Radiohypophysectomie beim metastsierenden— Mamma carcinom unter Berücksichtigung des Geschlechts-chromatin.' *Langenbeck's Arch. Klin. Chir.* **323**, 339.

Whitaker, B. L. (1961). 'Plasma glucoronidase as an index of hormone dependency of breast tumours.' *Br. J. Cancer* **15**, 868.

Wilson, C. B., Winternitz, W. W., Berton, V. and Sizemore, G. (1966). 'Stereotoxic cryosurgery of pituitary gland in carcinoma of breast and other disorders.' *J. Am. med. Ass.* **198**, 587.

Wilslocki, G. B. (1937). 'The meningeal relations of the hypophysis cerebri. II. An embryological study of the meninges and blood vessels of the human hypophysis.' *Am. J. Anat.* **61**, 95.

— and King, L. S. (1936). 'The permeability of the hypophysis and hypothalamus to vital dyes with a study of the hypophyseal vascular supply.' *Am. J. Anat.* **58**, 412.

Xuereb, G. P., Prichard, M. M. and Daniel, P. M. (1954). 'The hypophysial portal system of vessels in man.' *Q. U. expl Physiol.* **39**, 199.

Yuhl, E. I. et al (1955). 'Clinical results of radio yttrium hypophysectomy.' *Surg. Forum* **6**, 489.

Zercas, N. I. (1969). 'Stereotaxic radiofrequency surgery of the normal and the abnormal pituitary gland.' *New Eng. J. Med.* **280**, 429.

# 15

# Tumour Response and the Completeness of Pituitary Ablation

## K. Fotherby and Frances James

## INTRODUCTION

Beatson (1896) first demonstrated that ovariectomy in women could be used to produce a remission of breast cancer, although the rationale behind this method of treatment did not become apparent until later. After it had been shown that in pre-menopausal women the ovary produced a variety of steroids, it was suggested that the absence of circulating oestrogens was responsible for the improvement in the condition of some of these patients. The suggestion that oestrogens may be secreted by the adrenal cortex, or may arise from precursors secreted by this gland, gave rise to the possibility that the failure of some patients to respond to ovariectomy may have been due to oestrogens of adrenocortical origin. Accordingly adrenalectomy was tried as a therapeutic procedure.

The possibility that the incidence of response to combined ovariectomy and adrenalectomy was less than might be expected on account of persistent secretion from remnants of adrenocortical tissue, led to the suggestion that removing the anterior pituitary (the source of the trophic hormones controlling the adrenal cortex and ovary) might be a more effective way of reducing the secretion of steroidal compounds. In addition it was thought that hypophysectomy might also have an extra advantage in eliminating the secretion of prolactin which could possibly be involved in the carcinogenic process. The development of the techniques of hypophysectomy during the mid 1950s provided the surgeons with a method of testing this hypothesis.

312

A number of techniques have been described for the elimination of the hypophysis. The major reports are of surgical methods including trans-ethmoidal, trans-sphenoidal or trans-frontal approaches, the implantation into the sella turcica of radiation sources (mainly yttrium-90), a combination of these techniques or the use of external irradiation, ultrasonic or cryogenic procedures. The various techniques available, together with their advantages and disadvantages and the incidence of side-effects, have been reviewed by Schurr (1966), Lore (1966) and Norrell et al. (1970). On the whole the incidence of response to hypophysectomy in patients with advanced breast cancer has been little different from that observed after ovariectomy and adrenalectomy. As in the case of the latter two techniques, where it is extremely difficult to determine whether all sources of steroid production have been eliminated, it is also difficult to determine the completeness or otherwise of hypophysectomy.

In spite of the obvious importance of such studies, very few attempts have been made to assess whether completeness of hypophysectomy is related to the response of the disease to the operation. This is undoubtedly due to the difficulties involved in assessing the completeness of hypophysectomy. The latter can be assessed either by a microscopic examination of the sella turcica after the death of the patient, or some attempt must be made during life to determine the extent to which functional pituitary tissue remains. The usefulness of these two approaches is compared later.

The functional activity of any remaining pituitary tissue could be determined either directly by estimation of any of the trophic hormones secreted by the pituitary, or indirectly by measuring changes which result from the action of these trophic hormones on their target organs, e.g. radio-iodine uptake by the thyroid or cortisol secretion from the adrenal. The latter may lack sensitivity whilst, with regard to the former, there are practical difficulties involved in such estimations which have not yet been overcome and which are discussed in more detail below.

## BIOCHEMICAL ESTIMATION OF PITUITARY HORMONES

The anterior pituitary is known to secrete six hormones—growth hormone (GH), thyroid stimulating hormone (TSH), adrenocorticotrophic hormone (ACTH), follicle stimulating hormone (FSH), luteinizing hormone (LH) and prolactin. Methods available for the estimation of these hormones or the effects they produce on their end organs and which are relevant on the grounds of sensitivity, are considered below. Most of the trophic hormones can now be estimated in plasma by radioimmunoassay procedures which probably provide the most sensitive method of assay presently available. They are considered briefly below and for more details of these procedures the book by Kirkham and Hunter (1971) should be consulted. In general the values to be reported in

313

this section for the levels of the various hormones in plasma are only a guide and in some cases the values obtained would depend upon the standard used in the estimations and the particular type of assay used.

The secretory activity of the anterior pituitary is controlled by regulatory substances produced in the hypothalamus, which pass to the pituitary via the portal venous system. These regulatory substances, the releasing factors, appear to be fairly small peptides and a separate releasing factor is responsible for stimulating the release of each pituitary hormone. In the case of GH, LH, FSH, TSH and ACTH, secretion of the releasing factor by the hypothalamus, or administration of the synthetic releasing factor, stimulates the release of the trophic hormone. However, in the case of prolactin, the reverse is true and the regulatory factor acts in an inhibitory manner and hence has become known as the prolactin inhibitory factor. For more details regarding these releasing factors the article by Schally and Kastin (1970) should be consulted.

## Growth hormone

The estimation of growth hormone in plasma and the usefulness of such assays has been reviewed by Greenwood (1967). The secretion of growth hormone is discontinuous so that the plasma concentration may change rapidly, the plasma half-life of the hormone being between 20 and 40 minutes. Values reported for growth hormone in plasma range from undetectable levels to about 5 µg/ml and a single HGH assay is of limited value. The values obtained for the level of growth hormone in plasma depend upon the physiological situation at the time the sample is taken.

Because of the low levels found in normal subjects, the functional capacity of the pituitary to secrete growth hormone can only be determined by using stimulation tests. Growth hormone secretion can be stimulated in a number of ways: by exercise, by fasting, by a decrease in the blood sugar level such as that following administration of insulin, by arginine infusion, by surgery or after administration of vasopressin, epinephrine, histamine and pyrogens. Women tend to have higher growth hormone levels than men, and growth hormone levels in males can be increased by administration of oestrogens. The ability of plasma growth hormone levels to increase after performance of a stimulation test, and particularly the insulin hypoglycaemia test, is a sensitive index of the function of the hypothalamic–pituitary axis (Mitchell et al., 1970; Jacobs and Nabarro, 1969). However, in patients with advanced breast cancer who may be severely ill, such tests must be carried out with caution.

## Corticotrophin

For details regarding the radioimmunoassay of ACTH in plasma the article by Berson and Yalow (1968) should be consulted. The normal range reported is from 0 to 100 pg/ml and the plasma half-life of ACTH is about 30 minutes.

As in the case of GH, levels of ACTH in plasma vary markedly during the day, the highest levels being found between 8 a.m. and 10 a.m. and the lowest values in the evening. The width of the normal range makes the interpretation of a single estimation of little value and it is necessary to use stimulation tests. Administration of vasopressin to normal subjects leads to a doubling of the plasma concentration, and insulin hypoglycaemia produces about a four fold increase. Plasma levels of ACTH can also be increased by administration of Metyrapone, an inhibitor of cortisol synthesis in the adrenal, or the administration of pyrogen.

Donald (1971) found that the fasting levels of ACTH in patients with hypopituitarism were not clearly differentiated from normal values, and the insensitivity of the method as a whole makes it quite unsuitable for use in hypophysectomized patients. Even stimulation tests do not bring the values in hypophysectomized patients anywhere near measurable levels. Since ACTH acts on the adrenal to increase the secretion of cortisol, an alternative indirect method of judging the ACTH level would be to measure plasma cortisol levels and their changes in response to stimuli, but it is unlikely that this method would be sensitive enough to detect minor changes at low plasma cortisol levels.

## Thyrotrophic hormone

Methods available for the radioimmunoassay of thyroid stimulating hormone and the clinical applications of the estimations have been reviewed by Hall (1972). The concentration of TSH in blood of normal subjects was found to be less than 3 μunits/ml and the mean value only about twice the lowest detectable amount. Due to these low values and the lack of sensitivity of the method, there is great difficult in distinguishing normal from sub-normal levels, and several euthyroid individuals have been found to have undetectable levels of serum TSH; consequently estimation of TSH levels in hypophysectomized subjects are of little value.

No alteration in the level of TSH in plasma was produced by changing the blood glucose concentration, exercise, fasting, surgery or administration of lysine vasopressin. Administration of oestrogen produces a variable response. Administration of thyrotrophin releasing factor, which is a tripeptide, produces a rapid increase in TSH concentrations in serum with a peak between 20 and 30 minutes after intravenous injection. However, the peak is only two to four times the basal value so that the test does not appear to be adequate for use in hypophysectomized patients.

Other measurements of thyroid function, such as $^{131}I$ uptake, protein bound iodine levels or tri-iodothyronine levels in serum may give an indirect indication of TSH levels in plasma. Joplin (1965) measured the 48-hour thyroid uptake of $^{131}I$ in patients with breast cancer before and after

315

implantation of yttrium-90 and found that tests carried out after the thirteenth post-operative day were a good index of the permanent thyroid function. Fourteen of fifteen patients with a mean post-implantation level of less than 21 per cent developed clinical myxoedema suggesting that effective elimination of thyrotrophin secretion had been obtained.

## Gonadotrophins

The gonadotrophins, FSH and LH, are both glycoproteins with molecular weights of between 30,000 and 40,000. The values found for the concentration of FSH and LH in serum by various investigators in normal human subjects have been summarized by Saxena et al. (1969). In men, and in women during the menstrual cycle except for the mid-cycle peak, the ratio of LH to FSH in serum is about 1, whereas in women at the mid-cycle peak it is about 2. Post-menopausal women are characterized by a relatively larger amount of FSH and the ratio obtained is about 0·5. The actual levels of the hormones in plasma show a large increase after the menopause and in post-menopausal subjects the concentration of FSH ranges from 42 to 250 miu/ml and that of LH from 40 to 90 miu/ml. Administration of the luteinizing hormone releasing factor, which is a decapeptide, stimulates the secretion of LH and also causes a smaller and a later rise in FSH.

Gonadotrophins are also known to be excreted in large amounts in the urine of ovariectomized or post-menopausal women. Although their estimation by bioassay procedures is relatively imprecise they can also be estimated in urine by radioimmunoassay procedures (Stevens, 1969). Estimation of gonado-trophins in plasma or urine, particularly from ovariectomized or post-menopausal women should therefore provide a sensitive means of assessing pituitary function.

## Prolactin

It has now been well established that prolactin, as distinct from growth hormone, does exist in humans, although in the past there has been much controversy over the matter. Growth hormone appears to have some intrinsic prolactin activity; the two hormones are not fully distinguished in bioassays and they are also difficult to separate, particularly since the amount of growth hormone in the pituitary greatly exceeds that of prolactin. Prolactin and growth hormone have similar molecular weights of about 21,500 but can be distinguished by electrophoretic techniques. Some of the properties of human prolactin have been reviewed by Sherwood (1971), Gala (1971) and by Friesen (1972). Prolactin appears to be produced in the erythrosinophyllic cells of the pituitary in contrast to growth hormone which appears to be produced in other acidophil cells. Hwang, Guyda and Friesen (1971) have described a radioimmunoassay for human prolactin in which human growth hormone and the placental lactogen do not show any significant cross reaction.

Although the normal range of values for adults is reported to be between 0 and 30 ng/ml, only 30 per cent of females have concentration above 15 ng/ml, and the sensitivity of the assay is not therefore suitable for the determination of prolactin in hypophysectomized women. As indicated above, the hypothalamus appears to produce a factor which inhibits the pituitary production of prolactin, and interference with the secretion of prolactin-inhibiting factor leads to a secretion of prolactin. The control of prolactin is further complicated by the suggestion that a prolactin-stimulating factor may also exist.

Thus it can be seen that few of the trophic hormones of the anterior pituitary can be determined with a sensitivity suitable for estimation of the residual activity of the pituitary after hypophysectomy.

## BIOCHEMICAL ASSESSMENT OF COMPLETENESS OF PITUITARY ABLATION

Attempts to assess residual pituitary function after hypophysectomy have been few. Li et al. (1955) found that in 28 of 35 patients with breast cancer who had undergone surgical hypophysectomy which was considered to be complete, the [131]I uptake at 48 hours was below the normal range. This finding was substantiated at a Symposium to discuss this topic. Fraser and Joplin (1959), Forrest, Sim and Stewart (1959) and Baron (1959) all concluded that the most useful index of completeness of hypophysectomy available at that time was the [131]I uptake by the thyroid. Fraser and Joplin found that patients could be divided clinically into two groups. Of those who were corticosteroid-dependent and where hypophysectomy was presumed adequate, in 16 out of 19 of these patients, the 48 hour radioiodine uptake was less than 25 per cent. In 5 of 9 patients who were cortisone-independent and where there was presumably some functional tissue remaining, the uptake was normal, i.e. 25–40 per cent. Forrest et al. tried to correlate the degree of ablation with the amount of gonadotrophins in urine but of 4 patients treated by implantation of radon seeds, no gonadotrophins were detected in the urine despite incomplete anatomical destruction of the gland in 3 of the subjects. However, at the time of the above studies the range of assays available was limited.

No properly designed study using modern methods of estimating gonadotrophins have been carried out in breast cancer patients. Saxena et al. (1969) present a few results obtained in hypophysectomized subjects. In 7 subjects submitted to surgical hypophysectomy, both LH and FSH concentrations varied from 0 to about 8 miu/ml. In patients implanted with yttrium-90, the values were rather higher, from 0 to 42 miu/ml in the case of LH and up to 78 miu/ml in the case of FSH (mean values for LH and FSH

317

were 15 and 17 respectively). No clinical details are given of these patients but the figures would suggest that, both in those subjected to surgical hypophysectomy and those implanted with yttrium, some degree of pituitary function still remained. With regard to the estimation of gonadotrophins it should be noted that the values obtained by biological assay and radioimmunoassay do not always agree.

Histological examination of the sella of 16 of 19 women subjected to surgical hypophysectomy (Luft and Olivecrona, 1959) showed that complete removal of the pituitary was obtained in only a few cases; in the others, however, only small amounts of pituitary tissue remained. At least 9 of the patients retained some thyroid function, as judged by $^{131}$I uptake. Peck and Olson (1963) carried out a detailed investigation of 44 patients with breast cancer subjected to a trans-frontal hypophysectomy, section of the pituitary stalk and application of Zenker's fluid to the empty sella. Their relatively crude biochemical measurements (urinary gonadotrophins and 17-oxosteroids, PBI and $^{131}$I uptake) suggested that hypophysectomy was complete in 38 cases and no hypophyseal tissue was detected on microscopic examination of random sections of the sella.

McCullagh et al. (1965) studied 29 patients with carcinoma of the breast treated by implanation of yttrium-90 into the pituitary. No response to Metyrapone administration was observed in 21 subjects whereas the remaining 8 did respond. In 3 of the patients who showed no response to Metyrapone the PBI remained within the normal range. In the Metyrapone responsive group, 7 of the 8 patients maintained normal thyroid function tests, suggesting a retention of pituitary function to a variable extent, and none of the 8 patients had objective remissions although 3 had some subjective relief. Of the 21 patients who had no response to Metyrapone and in whom hypopituitarism presumably had been produced, 19 had subjective evidence of remission and 10 of these 19 had objective remissions. Measurement of urinary gonadotrophins showed no correlation with the other biochemical measurements. Autopsy was possible in 13 patients; in 7 patients, 95–100 per cent of the pituitary had been destroyed, in 4 patients, 85–94 per cent and in 2 patients 75–84 per cent.

In more recent studies, Stewart et al. (1971) compared changes in plasma growth hormone levels during insulin hypoglycaemia in 30 women who had received implants of yttrium-90 in the pituitary for advanced breast cancer with those of a control series of 28 women with breast cancer with intact pituitaries. In the latter group a normal response was found, growth hormone levels increasing from 7·5 ng/ml to a mean maximum of about 35 ng/ml. Of the 30 patients with breast cancer who were implanted, 13 failed to show a rise in the plasma levels of growth hormone and this was also associated with a low fasting level (less than 4 ng/ml); 11 patients failed to show a rise to insulin hypoglycaemia but had fasting levels above 4 ng/ml. A further 6 patients showed a marked rise (greater than 4 ng/ml) but in only 1 subject did the increase exceed 20 ng/ml.

The various tests for thyroid function which were carried out correlated only moderately well with the plasma growth hormone responses. Low values for the PBI were only found when the growth hormone response was absent but normal or high levels of PBI were found in some patients with an absent growth hormone response. The range of values obtained in the three groups for the $^{131}$I uptake test was wide. The mean value in the group with a positive growth hormone response was significantly higher than that of the other two groups. In 6 of these patients the sella turcica was examined histologically *post mortem*. In 2 patients who had shown a positive growth hormone response, only 60 per cent of the gland had been destroyed. In the remaining 4 patients 80 per cent or more of the gland was destroyed, 2 of these patients showing no response and 2 an intermediate response to insulin hypoglycaemia.

These results, showing a variation in the response of growth hormone secretion to implantation of yttrium-90, are in agreement with the results of Wright et al. (1969) who studied patients with diabetic retinopathy who had been treated in this way. Of 36 patients studied, 2 had growth hormone levels greater than 20 ng/ml, in 9 patients it was between 5 and 20 ng/ml, and in 6 between 1 and 5 ng/ml.

Teuscher et al. (1970) obtained similarly variable results in 12 patients with diabetic retinopathy and concluded that it was difficult to obtain complete endocrine ablation. Hypophysectomy was carried out by a trans-sphenoidal approach, the emptied sella was inspected with an operating microscope and Zenker's solution was also applied. Although hypophysectomy was judged to be complete at the time of the operation, variations were obtained in post-operative hormonal activity. In only 6 of the patients was there an immediate and continuing decrease in growth hormone secretion and in a further four the immediate decrease was followed by a secondary rise. The Metyrapone test was positive in 3 patients post-operatively, indicating an ability to secrete ACTH. In some of the patients there was decreased thyroid function as evidenced by a low serum PBI and decreased $^{131}$I uptake.

Parisset et al. (1971) reviewed 110 patients with diabetic retinopathy treated with yttrium-90 implants and classified the degree of pituitary ablation achieved at three months as complete, intermediate or slight. Those classified as complete required thyroid and steroid maintenance, their insulin requirement fell by 50 per cent and impotence or amenorrhoea developed provided that the patients were normal in these respects before implantation. Growth hormone estimations were carried out in some of these subjects and all showed values of less than 2 ng/ml. Those classified as slight showed no steroid or thyroid dependence, had no alteration in sexual function and the fall in insulin requirement was less than 50 per cent. Growth hormone levels in these patients varied between 4·2 and 32 ng/ml. Those patients falling between these two groups were classified as intermediate and showed varying degrees of pituitary deficiency. Two patients in this group had low growth hormone values of less than 2 ng/ml while the remaining 10 had values of 3–18 ng/ml.

An interesting finding was made by Reed and Pizey (1967) who suggested that the appearance of diabetes insipidus, presumably due to stalk damage, was related to the completeness of hypophysectomy. Of their 95 patients, 63 developed diabetes and in 38 this condition lasted at least three months. Only 7 of 29 patients who did not develop diabetes showed tumour response to hypophysectomy and only 4 survived longer than six months, whereas 36 of the 63 who developed diabetes responded to treatment and 29 survived at least six months. Of all the patients who lived more than six months, 88 per cent had diabetes insipidus; thus the development of this condition appeared to correlate with an improved response rate in the patients.

## HISTOLOGICAL ASSESSMENT OF COMPLETENESS OF PITUITARY ABLATION

Edelstyn, Gleadhill and Lyons (1969) considered that hypophysectomy as a clinical procedure had not achieved the status which it should have done in the treatment of breast cancer, partly because of the indiscriminate selection of patients but also because of the incomplete removal of the hypophysis, the remnants of the gland remaining not being detected until autopsy. However, it would appear that the number of patients undergoing pituitary ablation where the sella turcica has been examined *post mortem* by serial sectioning is very few. Pearson and Ray (1960) studied a series of 45 autopsies on patients treated by trans-frontal hypophysectomy. No pituitary tissue was detected in 21 of these subjects and, in a further 10, only small clumps of cells were seen, but in 13 between 1 and 10 per cent of the glands still remained intact and in 1 almost the whole gland had escaped ablation.

In reviewing techniques used by previous investigators Edelstyn, Gleadhill and Lyons (1964) also came to the conclusion that total removal of the pituitary by either the trans-cranial or the trans-ethmoidal route was difficult and in their own series they followed surgical hypophysectomy by the implantation into the fossa of yttrium-90 suspended in wax. They claimed that patients who received this combined treatment had an increased incidence and duration of objective remission compared with those who had only a surgical hypophysectomy. Atkins et al. (1957) carried out histological examination of the pituitary fossa in six patients who had been hypophysectomized by the trans-frontal route and estimated that 1–10 per cent of the tissue was still present; five of these six patients failed to respond to treatment although Falconer (1963) found that if up to 10 per cent of the total volume was left behind, patients could still obtain a remission.

The amount of pituitary tissue which must remain for the gland to function relatively normally is uncertain. Sheehan (1961) carried out an extensive analysis of the pituitary at autopsy in patients who had had hypopituitarism as a result of post-partum necrosis. He found that after a large necrosis remnants of the anterior lobe could be found in three places but particularly in the pars tuberalis; 10–20 per cent of the anterior lobe may remain here and this appears to be sufficient to keep the patients in relatively good health. Fraser and Joplin (1961) also concluded that about 90 per cent of the gland had to be destroyed before Simmonds' disease became evident. Sheehan found that in some cases where almost total destruction was considered to have occurred, 1–2 per cent of the original tissue may remain. He also found that, despite destruction of most of the anterior lobe, some patients retained function of the target organs and that there was considerable variability in this, the loss of function not following any regular pattern. The nasopharyngeal pituitary, which was examined in only two cases, had the same size and shape as in normal patients and did not show any signs of hypertrophy.

This is of interest in view of the suggestion of Muller (1958) that hypertrophy of the pharyngeal hypophysis might occur and could explain the failure of some of the patients to respond to hypophysectomy. This tissue is known to contain both chromophobe and chromophil cells. The findings of Notter (1959) agree with those of Sheehan in that the pharyngeal hypophysis was detected in four of eleven patients but it was concluded not to have any functional significance. No evidence for hypertrophy of the pharyngeal pituitary was found by van Buren and Bergenstal (1960). One patient who survived seven months showed no chromophil cells in the pharyngeal pituitary which contained only chromophobe cells. The volume of pharyngeal tissue seemed insignificant in view of the fact that about 1 cu. mm of pituitary tissue remained in the sella turcica. No mitotic activity was detected in the retained fragments of the pituitary tissue, suggesting that little regeneration took place. After section of the pituitary stalk and removal of varying portions of the pituitary, an initial state of severe hypopituitarism developed that was not proportional to the amount of pituitary gland removed.

The status of the pharyngeal hypophysis has been reviewed by McGrath (1968, 1969). She concludes that in many hypophysectomies, the pharyngeal hypophysis would remain intact and could be an active source of pituitary hormones post-operatively, despite the fact that it has a volume of about only one thousandth of that of the sella hypophysis. She also presented evidence to suggest that extracts prepared from the pharyngeal hypophysis may show both growth hormone and prolactin activity.

## CONCLUSION

It will be obvious from the preceding discussion that the assessment of the completeness of procedures for ablating anterior pituitary tissue is difficult.

Accurate assessment whilst the patient is still living depends upon whether present techniques are sensitive enough to measure either the small amounts of pituitary hormones which may be secreted from residual tissue or the bio-chemical changes that these hormones may produce. As has been shown, the sensitivity of the methods available is just about adequate to measure normal levels but inadequate to measure the very low levels found after removal of most of the pituitary. The more complete the hypophysectomy, the more difficult becomes the detection of small amounts of hormones being produced. More work therefore needs to be devoted to the measurement of the trophic hormones by more sensitive methods.

The stimulation of trophic hormone secretion by use of synthetic hypothalamic releasing factors is of limited application in assessing the completeness of hypophysectomy since, in general, the increase produced by the administration of the releasing factors is only of the order of 100–200 per cent. In the future, synthesis of antagonists to the releasing factors may prove to be a simple way of achieving the equivalent of a hypophysectomy. It is also possible that some of the target organs also maintain some function despite lack of the trophic hormones from the pituitary; aldosterone secretion, for example, which is controlled mainly by a mechanism not involving the pituitary, is maintained despite the lack of ACTH.

It is clear that if biochemical measurements are to be used to assess the completeness of pituitary ablation, they should be carried out over extended periods of time with follow-up of the patients for as long as possible. Biochemical measurements should also be correlated with the state of the sella turcica and any other pituitary remnants which are detected *post mortem* (Norrell et al., 1970). As noted by Peck and Olson (1963) it is difficult to relate completeness of hypophysectomy to the incidence of regression but it could be related to the length of remission. It is possible that the pituitary remnants may have a phase of regeneration so that the pituitary could function better later rather than immediately post-operatively. Alternatively it is possible that the pituitary remnants may atrophy after a period of months and lose any function which they may have had earlier. Assessment of pituitary function soon after operation may be of importance since signs of remission often occur in this early phase, but there seems to be no information regarding pituitary function at the time that any remission obtained disappears.

It is clear also, however, that even post-mortem examination by histological means leaves a number of questions unanswered. One point that needs to be taken into consideration is that detection of one or a group of trophic hormones may not indicate the production of all. This may mean, if the residual tissue is capable of functioning, that there is little correlation between the total amount of tissue surviving and the failure of the patients to respond to the operation. This aspect deserves closer consideration than it has received hitherto. It might be expected that any pituitary remnants which do remain would be working at maximal capacity.

More work needs to be done to establish how much pituitary tissue needs to be destroyed to produce a clinical response in breast cancer and to find out how much trophic hormone is needed to stimulate the end organs. An anatomically complete hypophysectomy may not be necessary to produce a functional hypophysectomy. Good clinical responses have been obtained in patients where up to 20 per cent of pituitary tissue remained.

When patients with breast cancer do respond to hypophysectomy it is not known whether the response is due to the lack of any one particular hormone or whether it results from a general effect on metabolism as a result of a lack of most of the pituitary hormones. Pearson and Ray (1959) gave small doses of oestrogens to five patients with breast cancer hypophysectomized several weeks previously. None of the patients showed evidence of reactivation of the tumour during the 30–60 day period of treatment, suggesting that oestrogens did not stimulate growth of the mammary cancer in the absence of the pituitary. Ikkos, Luft and Olivecrona (1961) obtained a remission in four patients who were hypophysectomized after a previous ovariectomy and adrenalectomy. Such results suggest that pituitary factors, other than those concerned with the control of sex hormone production, influence the growth of hormone-dependent breast cancer in humans.

## REFERENCES

Atkins, H. J. B., Falconer, M. A., Hayward, J. L. and MacLean, K. S. (1957). 'Adrenalectomy and hypophysectomy for advanced cancer of the breast.' *Lancet* **272**, 489.
Baron, D. N. (1959). 'Investigation of anterior pituitary function after surgical hypophysectomy.' *Proc. R. Soc. Med.* **53**, 88.
Beatson, G. T. (1896). 'On the treatment of inoperable cases of carcinoma of the breast.' *Lancet* **2**, 104.
Berson, S. A. and Yalow, R. S. (1968). 'Radioimmunoassay of ACTH in plasma.' *J. clin. Invest.* **47**, 2725.
van Buren, J. M. and Bergenstal, D. M. (1960). 'An evaluation of graded hypophysectomy in man. A quantitative functional and anatomical study.' *Cancer* **13**, 155.
Doar, J. W., Wynn, V. and Webb, P. J. (1970). 'Comparison of tests of hypothalamo-pituitary-adrenocortical function in pituitary disease.' *J. Endocr.* **48**, 47.
Donald, R. A. (1971). 'Plasma immunoreactive corticotrophin and cortisol response to insulin hypoglycemia in normal subjects and patients with pituitary disease.' *J. clin. Endocr.* **32**, 225.
Edelstyn, G. A., Gleadhill, C. A. and Lyons, A. R. (1964). 'Attempted total hypophysectomy in advanced breast cancer. Report on a new method using both surgery and radiation.' *Br. J. Surg.* **51**, 32.
— — — (1969). 'A rational approach to hypophysectomy.' *Br. J. Surg.* **56**, 64.

Falconer, M. A. (1963). 'Hypophysectomy—neurosurgical aspect.' *Proc. R. Soc. Med.* **56**, 390.

Forrest, A. P. M., Brown, D. A. P., Morris, S. R. and Illingworth, C. F. W. (1956). 'Pituitary radon implant for advanced cancer.' *Lancet* **1**, 399.

— Sim, A. W. and Stewart, H. J. (1959). 'Pituitary function tests after radioactive implantation of the pituitary.' *Proc. R. Soc. Med.* **53**, 84.

Fraser, R. and Joplin, G. F. (1959). 'Discussion on the assessment of endocrine function after hypophysectomy or pituitary destruction.' *Proc. R. Soc. Med.* **53**, 81.

— — (1961). In *Modern Trends in Endocrinology—2*, p. 69, Ed. by H. Gardiner-Hill. London; Butterworths.

Friesen, H., Belanger, C., Guyda, H. and Hwang, P. (1972). 'The synthesis and secretion of placenta lactogen and pituitary prolactin.' In *Lactogenic Hormones,* Ed. by G. E. W. Wolstenholme and J. Knight, pp. 83–110. Edinburgh; Churchill Livingstone.

Gala, R. R. (1971). 'Prolactin production by the human anterior pituitary cultured *in vitro*.' *J. Endocr.* **50**, 637.

Greenwood, F. C. (1967). 'Growth hormone.' In *Hormones in Blood*, Vol. 1, pp. 195–231, Ed. by C. H. Gray and A. L. Bacharach. London; Academic Press.

Hall, R. (1971). 'The immunoassay of thyroid-stimulation hormone and its clinical applications.' *Clin. Endocr.* **1**, 115.

Hwang, P., Guyda, H. and Friesen, H. (1971). 'A radioimmunoassay for human prolactin.' *Proc. natn Acad. Sci.* **68**, 1902.

Ikkos, D., Luft, R. and Olivecrona, H. (1961). 'Hypophysectomy in the treatment of malignant tumours in man.' *Mem. Soc. Endocr.* **10**, 95.

Jacobs, H. S. and Nabarro, J. D. N. (1969). 'Tests of hypothalamic-pituitary-adrenal function in man.' *Q. Jl Med.* **38**, 475.

Joplin, G. F. (1965). 'Therapeutic pituitary ablation by needle implantation.' *Ph.D. Thesis,* University of London.

Kirkham, K. E. and Hunter, W. M. (Eds.) (1971). *Radioimmunoassay Methods.* Edinburgh; Livingstone.

Li, M. C., Rall, J. E., Maclean, J. P., Lipsett, M. B., Ray, B. S. and Pearson, O. H. (1955). 'Thyroid function following hypophysectomy in man.' *J. clin. Endocr.* **15**, 1228.

Lore, J. M. (1966). 'Transseptal transsphenoidal hypophysectomy.' *Am. J. Surg.* **112**, 577.

Luft, R. and Olivercrona, H. (1959). 'Hormone treatment of carcinoma of the breast—hypophysectomy.' In *Cancer*, Vol. 6, pp. 265–273, Ed. by R. W. Raven. London; Butterworths.

McCullagh, E. P., Feldstein, M. A., Tweed, D. C. and Dohn, D. F. (1965). 'A study of pituitary function after intrasellar implantation of $^{90}$Yttrium.' *J. clin. Endocr.* **25**, 832.

McGrath, P. (1968). 'Prolactin activity and human growth hormone in pharyngeal hypophyses from embalmed cadavers.' *J. Endocr.* **42**, 205.

— (1969). 'The extra-sella post-hypophysectomy remnant.' *Br. J. Surg.* **56**, 64.

Mitchell, M. L., Byrne, M. J., Sanchez, Y. and Sawin, C. T. (1970). 'Detection of growth-hormone deficiency. The glucagon stimulation test.' *New Engl. J. Med.* **282**, 539.

Muller, W. (1958). 'On the pharyngeal hypophysis.' In *Endocrine Aspects of Breast Cancer*, pp. 106–110, Ed. by A. R. Currie. Edinburgh; Livingstone.

Norrell, H., Alves, A. M., Winternitz, W. W. and Maddy, J. (1970). 'A clinicopathologic analysis of cryohypophysectomy in patients with advanced cancer.' *Cancer* **25**, 1060.

Notter, G. (1959). 'A technique for destruction of the hypophysis using $Y^{90}$-spheres.' *Acta radiol. (Stockh.)* Suppl. 184.

Parisset, A., Kohner, E. M., Cheng, H. and Fraser, T. R. (1971). 'Diabetic retinopathy. New vessels arising from the optic disc. II. Response to pituitary ablation by $Y^{90}$ implant.' *Diabetes* **20**, 824.

Pearson, O. H. and Ray, B. S. (1959). 'Results of hypophysectomy in the treatment of metastatic mammary cancer.' *Cancer* **12**, 85.

— — (1960). 'Hypophysectomy in the treatment of metastatic mammary cancer.' *Am. J. Surg.* **99**, 544.

Peck, F. C. and Olson, K. B. (1963). 'The treatment of advanced breast cancer by hypophysectomy.' *N. Y. St. J. Med.* **63**, 2191.

Reed, P. I. and Pizey, N. C. (1967). 'Trans-sphenoidal hypophysectomy in the treatment of advanced breast cancer.' *Br. J. Surg.* **54**, 369.

Saxena, B. B., Leyendecker, G., Chen, W., Gandy, H. M. and Peterson, R. E. (1969). 'Radioimmunoassay of follicle-stimulating and luteinizing hormones by chromato-electrophoresis.' *Acta endocr. (Kbh).* Suppl. **142**, 185.

Schally, A. V. and Kastin, A. J. (1970). 'The role of sex steroids, hypothalamic LH-releasing hormone and FSH-releasing hormone in the regulation of gonadotrophin secretion from the anterior pituitary gland.' In *Advances in Steroid Biochemistry and Pharmacology*, Vol. 2, pp. 41–69, Ed. by M. H. Briggs. London; Academic Press.

Schurr, P. H. (1966). 'Techniques and effects of hypophysectomy, pituitary stalk section and pituitary transplantation in man.' In *The Pituitary Gland*, Vol. 2, pp. 22–48, Ed. by G. W. Harris and B. T. Donovan. London; Butterworths.

Sheehan, H. L. (1961). 'Atypical hypopituitarism.' *Proc. R. Soc. Med.* **54**, 43.

Shenkin, A., Nuki, G., Lindsay, R. M., Whaley, K., Downie, W. W. and Dick, W. C. (1970). 'The lysine-vasopressin test: an evaluation of two methods of administration in non-corticosteroid treated and corticosteroid-treated patients with rheumatoid arthritis.' *J. Endocr.* **47**, 1.

Sherwood, L. M. (1971). 'Human prolactin.' *New Engl. J. Med.* **284**, 774.

Stevens, V. C. (1969). 'Discrepancies and similarities of urinary FSH and LH patterns as evaluated by different assay methods.' *Acta endocr.* Suppl. **142**, 338.

Stewart H. J., Benson, E. A., Roberts, M. M., Forrest, A. P. M. and Greenwood, F. C. (1971). 'Pituitary function after yttrium implants as measured by plasma growth hormone levels.' *J. Endocr.* **50**, 41.

Teuscher, A., Escher, F., Konig, H. and Zahnd, G. (1970). 'Long-term effects of transsphenoidal hypophysectomy on growth hormone, renal function and eyeground in patients with diabetic retinopathy.' *Diabetes* **19**, 502.

Wright, A. D., Kohner, E. M., Oakely, N. W., Hartog, M., Joplin, G. F. and Fraser, T. R. (1969). 'Serum growth hormone levels and the response of diabetic retinopathy to pituitary ablation.' *Br. med. J.* **2**, 346.

# 16

# The Role of Brain Catecholamines in Treatment

## Basil A. Stoll

### INTRODUCTION

Ablation of either the ovaries, adrenals or pituitary gland, or therapy with large doses of androgen, will cause tumour regression in about one-third of pre-menopausal women with advanced breast cancer. The mechanism of tumour regression is uncertain, and most attempts to explain it in the past were based on the observation that each of the methods mentioned can interfere with the availability of oestrogen, which was assumed necessary for maintaining the growth of hormone-dependent mammary cancer. Neverthe-less, numerous investigators who were trying to establish such a relationship, found no association between clinical response of the tumour to oophor-ectomy, adrenalectomy or hypophysectomy on the one hand, and the continued excretion of small amounts of oestrogen on the other (see Chapter 12).

Because of this uncertainty as to the role of oestrogen in the human tumour, information has been sought from experimental mammary tumour systems, particularly in rodents. Both in the spontaneous virus-dependent tumour in the mouse, and in the carcinogen-induced tumour in the rat, it has been found that prolactin is the hormone principally responsible for stimulating and maintaining the growth of these tumours (see Chapters 2 and 12). The dimethylbenzanthracene (DMBA)-induced rat mammary tumour, first introduced by Huggins, Briziarelli and Sutton (1959), is the most widely investigated of these experimental tumours, and it has been shown that, similarly to the human tumour, a proportion of the tumours regress after either oophorectomy, adrenalectomy, hypophysectomy or androgen administration.

Whereas prolactin administration will reactivate this experimental tumour after hypophysectomy, oestradiol administration will not. This and related experimental observations (see Chapter 2) have raised doubts as to whether ovarian hormones are at all necessary for the growth of the tumour as long as prolactin levels are high enough (Pearson, 1972). However, an alternative view is that ovarian hormones are required to sensitize the tumour to the effect of prolactin (Dao, 1972). It is most important when reviewing and drawing conclusions from such experimental evidence, not to confuse the role of prolactin and oestrogen in the hormonal *genesis* of the tumour with their possible importance in the *maintenance* of human mammary cancer.

The oestrogen dependence theory was given new support when it was shown that some breast cancers can concentrate oestradiol from the blood (see Chapter 12). It was then suggested that the level of circulating and excreted oestrogen does not necessarily indicate the hormone interaction at the target tissue, and therefore that excreted hormone levels may not be relevant to the problem. This suggestion is supported by a recent report where it is claimed that the presence of high affinity oestradiol receptor protein in the tumour can be very closely correlated with the likelihood of tumour regression following endocrine therapy (Jensen et al., 1972). However, a later report suggests that the *in vivo* uptake of oestradiol by the tumour cannot predict its response to endocrine ablation, oestrogen or androgen therapy (Braunsberg et al., 1973).

Oestrogen dependence cannot, of course, explain the clinical observation of regression of breast cancer in about one-third of post-menopausal patients after high dosage oestrogen therapy—the so-called oestrogen 'responsiveness'. Furthermore, a similar response has been reported in 4 out of 23 pre-menopausal patients after treatment with *very high* oestrogen dosage—up to 1 g diethyl-stilboestrol daily (Kennedy, 1962). To explain these cases of oestrogen responsiveness, it is usually suggested that there is a varied cell population in human mammary cancer, different clones being either oestrogen-dependent or oestrogen-responsive, prolactin-dependent or prolactin-responsive, androgen-dependent or androgen-responsive, while some are completely unresponsive to all hormonal change (Furth, 1972).

## HYPOPHYSEAL FACTORS INFLUENCING BREAST CANCER MAINTENANCE

Apart from experimental evidence there is clinical evidence also that, in addition to oestradiol, one or more pituitary trophic hormones play a part in maintaining the growth of hormone-dependent mammary cancer. It has been observed that, whereas oestrogen administration can reactivate breast cancer after control by oophorectomy, it does not do so after hypophysectomy (Pearson and Ray, 1959), presumably because of the absence of a pituitary factor which is essential for tumour stimulation. The importance of a pituitary factor *other than* gonadotrophin and ACTH has recently been emphasized by the results of a controlled clinical trial, which showed trans-frontal hypophysectomy superior to adrenalectomy and oophorectomy in the palliation of advanced breast cancer (Hayward et al., 1970). Hypophysectomy was significantly, though not overwhelmingly, superior both in the proportion of patients responding, and in the duration of tumour response (see Table 16.1).

TABLE 16.1

Randomized Comparison of Bilateral Adrenalectomy and Trans-frontal Hypophysectomy in Breast Cancer (Hayward et al., 1970)

|  | Bilateral adrenalectomy | Trans-frontal hypophysectomy |
|---|---|---|
| Total cases | 77 | 70 |
| Response rate | 23% | 36% |
| Mean remission | 26·3 months | 37·1 months |
| Mean survival of responders | 31·6 months | 40·8 months |

Nevertheless, it is possible that either gonadotrophin, ACTH, prolactin or growth hormone may play a role in maintaining the growth of human mammary cancer. Gonadotrophin excretion levels always rise sharply after oophorectomy, and it may be important that an association has been noted between a higher gonadotrophin excretion and a greater likelihood of breast cancer regression after therapeutic oophorectomy in pre-menopausal women (Scowen and Hadfield, 1955; Pommatau et al., 1963). This finding was based upon a bioassay method, and now that sensitive radioimmunoassay methods have been established for FSH and LH, it is possible that estimation of their separate levels after therapeutic oophorectomy in breast cancer may provide information on a possible relationship to tumour growth (see Chapter 6).

The finding mentioned above suggested that gonadotrophin might play a part in the control of breast cancer activity, and led me to attempt a trial of gonadotrophin therapy in advanced breast cancer, although Segaloff et al. (1954) had previously reported absence of response to FSH derived from species other than the human. In 14 patients with advanced breast cancer, a trial of human chorionic gonadotrophin (the only widely available form of human gonadotrophin), yielded no objective evidence of tumour response (Stoll, 1964). Nevertheless, to decide this question confidently requires a trial of either human pituitary or human menopausal gonadotrophin, and to date this has not been possible because of inadequate supplies of these preparations.

A role has been postulated for ACTH in maintaining the growth of hormone responsive breast cancer, and the suggestion appears to be supported by the palliative results achieved by the operation of bilateral adrenalectomy with or without oophorectomy. ACTH is thought to be the pituitary trophic hormone which stimulates the secretion of oestrogens from the adrenal cortex, particularly after the menopause and particularly in patients with advanced disease (see Chapter 5). Suppression of ACTH release is thought by some to explain the benefit observed from corticosteroid treatment in advanced breast cancer; although in my opinion, such benefit is more likely to be due to non-specific and anti-oedema effects of corticosteroids (Stoll, 1963).

Finally, the prolactin–growth hormone complex has been suspected for many years to play a role in maintaining the growth of hormone-dependent mammary cancer in the human (Hadfield, 1956; Pearson, 1957; Stoll, 1958). Very recently, human prolactin has been separated from growth hormone and is now capable of measurement by biological assay and radioimmunoassay (see Chapter 9). Although absolute values recorded by each method on the same sample may differ, most assays provide a substantially similar range in different physiological states. Several groups are currently investigating the changes in serum prolactin levels in relation to clinical response to endocrine therapy in patients with breast cancer.

It should be pointed out that growth hormone also may be important in maintaining the growth of breast cancer. It has been noted that human growth hormone is chemically more closely related to human placental lactogen than it is to the growth hormones of other species (Geschwind, 1972). Even in its pure form, human growth hormone possesses intrinsic mammotrophic activity, and will affect the animal bioassay systems used for assay of human prolactin. It may be important too that the release of both growth hormone and prolactin is stimulated by oestrogen administration, and it is thought possible that they act synergistically in promoting the growth of mammary carcinoma (Meites, 1972).

## DOPAMINE AND HYPOTHALAMIC REGULATION

Recent research has established that the release of anterior pituitary trophic hormones can be controlled by noradrenergic neurones whose cell bodies lie in the arcuate nucleus, and whose neurohormones stimulate controlling centres in the median eminence of the hypothalamus (see Chapters 7 and 8). Activity of these centres is thought to involve the synthesis and release of catecholamines in the hypothalamus. The hypothalamic catecholamines then act as neuro-transmitters to release specfic releasing factors for individual trophic hormones from the adjacent anterior pituitary tissue. Individual releasing factors exist for growth hormone, ACTH and thyrotrophin, and it has been suggested that LH and FSH share the same releasing factor, called LHRF (Schally, Arimura and Bowers, 1968). All these releasing factors have been identified as fairly simple polypeptides and some have been synthesized. In the case of prolactin, however, the hypothalamic regulating factor seems to act in an inhibitory manner, and is known as prolactin inhibiting factor (PIF), its true nature being uncertain.

The possibility of a selective pharmacological 'hypophysectomy' has been investigated for many years (Stoll, 1956) and hope of achieving it was stimulated recently, when it was shown that catecholamines are involved in the release of anterior pituitary hormones. By using agents which influence the transmission, dissipation, synthesis or receptor site action of catecholamines such as dopamine, the possibility was also presented of either stimulating or inhibiting the release of specific pituitary trophic hormones.

Because of the different regulating mechanism for prolactin, it is possible to achieve differential effects upon hormonal release by such a method. It is possible by pharmacological methods to inhibit prolactin release, and at the same time stimulate gonadotrophin, growth hormone and ACTH release, or vice versa, according to whether dopamine is increased or decreased. If the roles of these individual pituitary trophic hormones in breast cancer were firmly established, therapy of this type would clearly be preferable to hypophyseal ablation by surgery or radiation. These latter methods are not only undiscriminating in their ablation of *all* trophic hormone secretory tissue, but they also involve life-long replacement therapy by cortisone and thyroxine.

The hypothalamic controlling centres contain specific target receptors whose activity can be modulated by several mechanisms. The best known is the long feedback mechanism triggered mainly by steroid hormones secreted by the peripheral target organs, but there is also a short feedback mechanism involving inhibition of the controlling centres by the pituitary hormones themselves. Finally, the hypothalamic centres are affected by impulses from the cerebral cortex and limbic systems. The orbital region of the prefrontal cortex of the rabbit has been shown to be involved in the release of prolactin (Tindal and Knaggs, 1972). A possible implication may be that emotional or psychological factors may influence the development and progress of mammary cancer in the human by acting through such cerebral pathways (see Chapter 19).

As mentioned above, neural activity in the region of the hypothalamus is thought to involve the synthesis and release of catecholamines, and it has been confirmed that the regional administration of dopamine in experimental animals can affect the release of anterior pituitary hormones. Hypothalamic infusion of dopamine has been shown to depress the serum level of prolactin in rats, either by facilitating the release of PIF (Kamberi, Mical and Porter, 1971), or by a direct effect on the anterior pituitary tissue (Birge et al., 1971). It also raises the serum level of LH (Schneider and McCann, 1969) presumably by stimulation of LHRF secretion from the hypothalamus.

Dopamine activity in the hypothalamus can be stimulated or depressed pharmacologically. Dopamine activity in the brain of rats can be increased by administration of levodopa, a dopamine precursor (Carlsson, 1959). On the other hand, dopamine activity in the brain can be depressed by neuroleptic agents such as reserpine (Carlsson et al., 1958), phenothiazines such as chlorpromazine (Sulman, 1959), psychotropic stimulants such as dextro-amphetamine and imipramine, anti-histamines such as meclizine, and anti-hypertensive agents such as α-methyl dopa. Thus, for example, chlorpromazine administration will cause a rise in prolactin release and fall in growth hormone release, and levodopa will do just the opposite (see Chapter 18).

Certain ergot alkaloids such as ergocornine and ergocryptine can also depress prolactin secretion, partly by acting on the hypothalamus (Wuttke, Cassell and Meites, 1971), and partly by a direct effect on anterior pituitary tissue (Lu, Koch and Meites, 1971; Malven and Hoge, 1971). On the other hand, the administration of thyrotrophin releasing hormone (TRH) causes a rapid increase in serum prolactin level. It is uncertain whether this is mediated by the TSH–thyroid axis or by a direct action on the prolactin secreting tissue of the anterior pituitary gland (L'Hermite et al., 1972). There is also doubt as to whether TRH is the physiological PRF or whether it acts by inhibiting the effect of PIF on the anterior pituitary tissue (see Chapter 8).

## EFFECT OF DOPAMINE ON PROLACTIN RELEASE

The evidence in Chapter 2 suggests that prolactin is a major influence in stimulating mitotic activity in the DMBA-induced rat mammary tumour. If this experimental observation can be extended to the human (an extrapolation which is discussed later in this chapter), it is logical to attempt to inhibit prolactin release from the anterior pituitary gland in aiming at the hormonal control of advanced breast cancer. It has been noted above that prolactin levels in the blood can be depressed by increasing dopamine levels in the hypothalamus of the rat, and there is considerable evidence that the neuroendocrine regulation of prolactin secretion in the human is similar to that in the rodent (Sherwood, 1971; Friesen, 1971).

Theoretically, dopamine transmission in the hypothalamus can be increased or dopamine receptors stimulated by the following methods:

(1) Administration of levodopa (Carlsson and Hillard, 1962), a precursor which is rapidly converted to dopamine in the brain by the action of dopa decarboxylase. It is of particular interest that the administration of levodopa to rats with DMBA-induced hormone responsive mammary carcinoma has been shown to cause significant growth inhibition, both in the size and number of the tumours (Meites et al., 1972). It has been suggested that levodopa breakdown in the peripheral blood can be delayed by the concurrent administration of a dopa decarboxylase inhibitor which cannot cross the

blood–brain barrier (Pletscher and Bartholini, 1971; Vesell et al., 1971). This could theoretically lead to an even higher concentration of levodopa in the brain.

(2) Inhibiting dopamine deamination by administration of a monoamine oxidase inhibitor such as iproniazid (Lu and Meites, 1971) or pargyline (Donoso et al., 1971). Again it is of interest that both these agents have been shown to inhibit the growth of DMBA-induced hormone responsive murine mammary carcinoma (Nagasawa and Meites, 1970; Meites et al., 1972). Given in combination with levodopa, agents of this group have been used experimentally to potentiate the effect of levodopa in counteracting dopamine depletion in the brain due to reserpine administration (Hornykiewicz, 1966). In clinical practice, however, MAO inhibitors cannot be administered concurrently with levodopa.

(3) Prolonging dopamine action by inhibiting the re-uptake of dopamine by nerve endings. Anti-cholinergic agents such as benztropine, benzhexol and orphenadrine, which have been proved useful in the treatment of Parkinsonism, are said to inhibit catecholamine receptor uptake (Coyle and Snyder, 1969; Farnebo, Fuxe and Hamberger, 1970). They may therefore be able to prolong dopamine action when given in combination with levodopa.

(4) Stimulation of dopamine receptors in the brain by agents such as apomorphine (Anden et al., 1967; Lal et al., 1972). The side effects from effective doses of this agent preclude its clinical usage in the therapy of breast cancer.

It was decided that for a clinical trial in breast cancer the simplest and safest of these methods was the administration of levodopa, which has had extensive clinical trial in the treatment of Parkinsonism. It is a 3 : 4-hydroxy-phenylalanine isomer which is able to pass the blood–brain barrier and is thought to undergo transformation to dopamine in the brain (Hornykiewicz, 1966). The oral administration of levodopa to rats has been shown to lower the serum level of prolactin (Donoso et al., 1971), and similarly the oral administration of levodopa to normal women at a dose of 0·25 to 0·5 g has been shown to depress prolactin levels (Hwang, Guyda and Friesen, 1971; Malarkey, Jacobs and Daughaday, 1971). It may be important that administration of such a dose of levodopa also causes a *rise* in the serum level of growth hormone (Eddy et al., 1971; Kansal, Talbert and Buse, 1971; Sherman, 1971) and in the level of FSH (Dickey, Marks and Stevens, 1971).

The serum level of prolactin found both in normal and in cancer-bearing non-pregnant women is usually below the threshold of detection for the bioassay method, but is usually within the range of a good immunoassay method. The administration of levodopa to normal women does not always yield a *sustained* depression of prolactin levels (see later), but given to patients with non-puerperal galactorrhoea associated with high serum prolactin levels, it usually causes a marked fall, although rarely to normal levels (Malarkey,

Jacobs and Daughaday, 1971; Kleinberg, Noel and Frantz, 1971; Turkington, 1972; Hwang, Guyda and Friesen, 1971).

The effect of levodopa on pituitary hormone release in young people is not clear. In the case of pre-pubertal children with short stature, a single dose of 0·25 to 0·5 g levodopa caused a similar rise in serum growth hormone level to that seen in adults, although there was no effect on the TSH, FSH, LH or cortisol levels (Hayek and Crawford, 1972). On the other hand, it has been reported that in normal young adults, levodopa administration fails to change the serum level of either growth hormone or TSH (Burton et al., 1971).

It has been noted above that a single dose of 0·25 to 0·5 g levodopa will lower serum prolactin levels in normal human subjects. The degree and duration of the fall in prolactin level need to be defined. According to most of the observations, the minimal level of prolactin is not reached until at least an hour after the administration of 0·5 g levodopa, and although some degree of depression is maintained for four to six hours, the minimum level is maintained for only about two hours. According to the above reports also, increase of levodopa dosage to 1·0 or 1·5 g does not appreciably increase the magnitude of the fall in the prolactin level.

There seems no advantage, therefore, in exceeding an individual dose of 0·5 g and, in addition, by not exceeding a daily total dosage of 2 g levodopa, the side effects of the agent are kept down to a minimum (Godwin-Austen, Frears and Bergmann, 1971).

Because of the delay before reponse, and the limited duration of response to each individual dose, a dosage of 0·5 g levodopa four times daily will lead to fluctuation in the serum prolactin level. In addition there is said to be a natural diurnal rhythm in the serum prolactin level in mammals, the highest level being in the evening and night (Koch, Chow and Meites, 1971; L'Hermite, 1972). Fluctuations in the serum level are also related to stress so that, for example, exercise causes a rise in the serum prolactin level, and a minor procedure such as proctoscopy can double the serum prolactin level (Noel et al., 1972).

It is not surprising, therefore, that after several days' administration of 0·5 g levodopa at four-hourly intervals to a pre-menopausal woman, the serum prolactin level was reported to be lowered only to the extent of about 50 per cent (Minton and Dickey, 1972). Another report notes that, although individual doses of 0·5 g levodopa may cause a fall of 50–97 per cent in the serum prolactin level within 90 minutes, the administration of 0·5 g four times daily could not achieve a sustained suppression of the level because of the presence of surges (Malarkey, Jacobs and Daughaday, 1971). Finally, Pearson (1972) has reported that levodopa administration in ten women for up to two months caused no constant change in the mean serum prolactin level.

To aim at a continuously low level, it would therefore appear desirable to prolong the effect of each dose pharmacologically, and one way of prolonging the concentration of levodopa in the brain is to inhibit dopamine re-uptake in the nerve endings. The synaptic activity of both dopamine and noradrenaline in the brain is thought to be terminated by the membrane uptake system. Cholinergic drugs like benztropine, diphenhydramine, benzhexol and orphenadrine are able to inhibit catecholamine receptor uptake both in the corpus striatum and in the hypothalamus (Coyle and Snyder, 1969; Farnebo, Fuxe and Hamberger, 1970). Their combination with levodopa has been claimed to prolong the effect of each individual dose of levodopa in the treatment of Parkinsonism (Hughes et al., 1971).

The most potent inhibitor of dopamine re-uptake across the neuronal membrane is said to be benztropine (Cogentin) (Farnebo, Fuxe and Hamberger, 1970; Coyle and Snyder, 1969). It is a synthetic compound formed by combining the tropine and benzhydryl portions of the atropine and benadryl molecules respectively, and therefore possesses both anti-cholinergic and anti-histaminic properties. It is slowly excreted and a single dose of 1–2 mg at night is claimed to maintain blood concentration for up to 24 hours. This dosage was therefore used in combination with levodopa in the clinical trial reported. Its major side-effects are a dry mouth and a soporific tendency.

## CLINICAL TRIAL OF LEVODOPA

As mentioned above, levodopa administration has been shown to depress the serum level of prolactin both in the human and in experimental animals. It has been given to rats with DMBA-induced mammary carcinoma and its trial was found to cause significant growth inhibition both in the size and in the numbers of tumours (Meites et al., 1972). Concurrently, I reported on a trial of levodopa administration in a group of 12 post-menopausal patients with soft-tissue manifestation of advanced recurrent breast cancer (Stoll, 1972). All the selected cases showed actively progressing soft-tissue tumour, which was beyond the control of surgery or radiotherapy. It is my considered opinion that exploratory clinical trials of new agents should be on patients with superficial soft tissue lesions which can be measured and photographed serially. All metastatic lesions in the patient must show regression for significant response to endocrine therapy to be recorded, and in my clinical experience, existing parameters of the growth of bone and visceral metastases (involving, as they do, interpretations of radiography and scintigraphy) do not lend themselves to accurate assessment of objective response to endocrine therapy (Stoll, 1969).

The initial dosage of levodopa was 0·25 g orally at four-hour intervals and was increased by twice-weekly increments to a maintenance dose of 0·5 g four times daily. This was well tolerated except for occasional episodes of postural hypotension and intermittent nausea in some patients. These symptoms were much more severe when attempts were made to raise the dose level above 2 g daily. Symptoms of tremor and involuntary movements, which are occasionally noted in the treatment of Parkinsonian patients with levodopa, were not encountered at the dose level prescribed.

Anti-emetics were avoided, especially those of the phenothiazine series, because of their tendency to antagonize catecholamine action upon the hypothalamus, and those containing pyridoxin hydrochloride because it tends to antagonize the effect of levodopa (Evered, 1971). No other local or systemic treatment was permitted, but in 5 out of the 12 patients, Cogentin 1–2 mg at night was added in the hope of prolonging the concentration of dopamine in the brain, as has been discussed above.

After two months' therapy with levodopa alone or with added Cogentin, there was no evidence of even the earliest tumour regression in any of the cases. Therefore, in the 7 patients receiving levodopa alone, oestrogen therapy was added in the form of Premarin, 1·25 mg four times daily. This mixture of conjugated oestrogens was selected because it is usually well tolerated with only rare complaints of nausea. At the end of three months of combined therapy, i.e. five months after commencement of levodopa therapy, 3 out of the 7 patients showed a minimum of 50 per cent decrease in volume of measurable tumour. The first objective evidence of tumour regression in these cases was noted after six weeks of combined treatment, although the relief of skin itching over the nodules was noted after only two or three weeks' treatment.

Combination therapy was continued in these 3 patients, but the mean duration of tumour regression was only eight months. In none of the cases was tumour regression complete. Nevertheless, it is important to note that *none of these 3 patients had responded to at least three months of oestrogen therapy given prior to the institution of levodopa therapy*. In all cases, the treatment-free intervening period was more than two months and the disease was progressing when the combination therapy was instituted.

Before discussing possible deductions from these observations, it may be useful to review subsequently reported trials of levodopa treatment in advanced breast cancer. Friesen (1972) reports objective evidence of regression in nodular infiltration in 1 out of 6 patients, and Pearson (1972) objective response in 2 out of 7 patients on similar dosage of levodopa to that noted above. One of these latter cases had nodular infiltration of the skin and the other bone metastases, and only partial suppression of the prolactin level was noted in these patients. Finally, Dickey and Minton (1972) report dramatic relief of pain from similar dosage of levodopa in 2 out of 6 patients with bone metastases. In one of the patients who was pre-menopausal, the prolactin level was reduced by approximately 50 per cent as a result of therapy.

If one adds the above four small series together, one finds that objective response from up to 2 g levodopa daily is claimed in only 3 out of 31 cases of breast cancer. Can this be ascribed to the *moderate* suppression of prolactin level which has been observed in such cases, especially in view of the observation that minute levels of prolactin are sufficient to maintain tumour growth in DMBA-induced mammary carcinoma in rats?

The use of Cogentin in an attempt to prolong the duration of action of the levodopa appeared to offer no clinical advantage in the few patients treated. It is possible that trials of levodopa in combination with dopa decarboxylase inhibitors, as suggested earlier in the section, might lead to a higher concentration of levodopa in the brain and hence to a greater or more prolonged depression of the prolactin level. However, my preliminary observations suggest that a combination of levodopa with oestrogen increases the likelihood of regression of breast cancer in post-menopausal women and its possible mechanism will now be discussed.

## ROLE OF PROLACTIN AND OESTROGEN IN BREAST CANCER

Another clinical attempt at prolactin inhibition in the treatment of breast cancer has recently been reported using 2-Br-α-ergocryptine (European Breast Cancer Group, 1972). It has been noted that certain ergot alkaloids (including 2-Br-α-ergocryptine), which markedly depress the secretion and release of prolactin from the anterior pituitary in the rat, also inhibit the growth of DMBA-induced mammary carcinoma (Heuson, Waelbroeck and Legros, 1970).

In the clinical trial reported, however, there was no evidence of tumour regression in any of the 19 post-menopausal patients receiving up to 15 mg of 2-Br-α-ergocryptine daily for six weeks (see Chapter 17). Although serial prolactin levels were not measured in these trial patients, it has been shown that such treatment will cause a marked fall in the serum prolactin level in women with non-puerperal galactorrhoea. The trial in breast cancer has been criticized both because of its short duration, and also the absence of controls. Nevertheless, it appears that, as in the case of levodopa, either the suppression of prolactin was not adequate or prolonged enough to affect tumour growth to any extent, or alternatively, some factor other than prolactin stimulates breast cancer growth in post-menopausal women.

The role of prolactin in the stimulation of human mammary cancer has been questioned recently because of reports that basal prolactin levels are low in the serum of middle aged and post-menopausal women with or without breast cancer (Turkington, 1972; Hwang, Friesen and Guyda, 1972). In spite of these reports, L'Hermite (1972) has shown a very wide range of prolactin level in older women, with occasionally very high levels above the age of 70, although levels around the time of the menopause tend to be low. Moreover, Pearson (1972) has shown the mean basal level of serum prolactin in 24 patients with breast cancer to be significantly higher than normal, and, using the outdated pigeon crop assay, Berle and Voigt (1972) have shown assayable levels of prolactin of 15 of 37 patients with breast cancer, compared with 4 of 55 comparable control patients. It should also be pointed out that the prolactin levels noted in the breast cancer patients referred to above, were probably basal levels, and as noted earlier, circadian fluctuations are usual and stress can cause surges to appear in the level.

The disappointing tumour response to levodopa or 2-Br-α-ergocryptine administration may result from their inability to reduce serum prolactin to a sufficiently low level. In DMBA-induced rat mammary carcinoma, even minute levels of serum prolactin may be associated with evidence of uninhibited tumour growth. It is also possible that in the stimulation of breast cancer, the level of prolactin receptors in the target may be more important than the serum prolactin level. It has been shown that stimulation of lactation in mammary tissue may be associated with a very wide range of serum prolactin levels (Friesen, 1972), and this wide range of target sensitivity may apply to malignant mammary tissue also.

However, two other recent observations have led to doubt as to whether the growth of human mammary cancer is always stimulated by prolactin. It has assumed for many years that high dosage of oestrogen caused a fall in the serum prolactin level, and that this was the mechanism whereby oestrogen therapy caused regression of breast cancer (Kim, 1965). However, a recent report suggests that the effect of high dose oestrogen therapy in women (ethinyl oestradiol 3 mg daily), is to cause a very marked and immediate *rise* in the serum prolactin level (L'Hermite and Heuson, 1973; Kwa, 1972). Another recent finding is that in five of eight patients who showed regression of breast cancer after pituitary stalk section, the serum prolactin level *rose* and remained elevated during the period of remission (Turkington, Underwood and van Wyk, 1971). This is particularly difficult to explain in view of the fact that ablation of the pituitary gland by surgery or radiation is followed by regression of breast cancer in about one-third of cases. Serum prolactin levels in such cases fall to very low levels although they may return to normal after three to six months (Friesen, 1972).

It has also been noted (Kennedy, 1962) that the same tumour may respond first to high dosage of oestrogen, and later when resistance develops, it may respond to oophorectomy. It has been noted by the author that a tumour may respond first to oestrogen therapy and then to hypophysectomy (Stoll, 1969). The explanation which has been put forward for apparently paradoxical responses by breast cancer (both to high dose oestrogen therapy and to oophorectomy, both to pituitary stalk section and to hypophysectomy) is that mammary carcinoma includes a variety of mutant cell types differing in specific hormonal sensitivity. It is suggested that some are prolactin-dependent and others prolactin-responsive; some are oestrogen-dependent and others oestrogen-responsive; some are androgen-dependent and some androgen-responsive; some independent of any hormonal control (Furth, 1972). It is suggested also that different clones may co-exist in the same individual so that the more rapidly growing clones will tend to outgrow one which is restrained and thus the type of hormonal responsiveness changes.

It is possible, however, to interpret these 'paradoxical' responses without recourse to this somewhat anarchistic explanation. It is suggested in Chapter 3 that there are two ways by which mammary cancer can be made to undergo regression—one associated with withdrawal of prolactin and oestrogen (as occurs following endocrine ablation) and the other with their increase to a high level. This hypothesis is based on the assumption that *low* levels of prolactin and oestrogen lead to mitotic stimulation and extensive cell proliferation in mammary tissue, part of the role of oestrogen being to sensitize the mammary epithelium to the stimulating effect of prolactin (Nagasawa and Yanai, 1971). On the other hand, *high* levels of prolactin and oestrogen can cause functional stimulation of mammary tissue, with minimal cell proliferation but marked alveolar differentiation and secretory changes leading to the synthesis of milk protein.

If the breast cancer has retained its capacity for stimulation by these hormones, withdrawal of both prolactin and oestrogen will decrease mitotic activity. On the other hand, increase of the hormonal concentration at the target to a high level may lead to secretory stimulation and subsequently also to decrease of mitotic activity. The morphological characteristics of this carcinostatic effect are discussed in detail in Chapter 3 but it is important to note here that functional stimulation need not go as far as a morphologically secretory appearance in order to be associated with tumour regression. As has been pointed out (Hilf, Michel and Bell, 1967), 'when the biochemical impetus is directed towards secretion, growth of the neoplasm is significantly reduced, implying that energy is being channelled into protein synthesis for purposes other than cell multiplication'. These theoretical considerations are not merely conjectural but have been applied, as a working hypothesis, to the oestrogen therapy of breast cancer (see Chapter 3).

## PREDICTION OF HORMONAL SENSITIVITY

In view of the uncertainty as to the mechanism of the different types of hormonal therapy, it would obviously be of considerable advantage to determine the specific hormonal sensitivity of each individual breast cancer before instituting therapy. The problem is being approached through three different channels. The first is to measure the concentration in the urine or serum of steroids such as oestrogen, androgen or corticosteroids, or of pituitary trophic hormones such as prolactin, growth hormone or gonado-trophin. The second is to measure the levels of individual hormone receptor sites in the tumour including those for oestradiol, progesterone or prolactin. The third is to bioassay the effect of various hormones or hormone combinations upon a biopsy specimen of the tumour maintained in organ culture.

Let us assume, for simplicity, that the mitotic activity of breast cancer depends mainly on the oestradiol–prolactin ratio at the tumour cell, then the sensitivity to therapy will depend on the following hormonal and tumoral factors:

## Hormonal factors

(1) The concentration of prolactin and oestradiol in the serum, taking into account that the former may show gross fluctuations through each 24 hours.

(2) The receptor site levels for prolactin and oestradiol in the tumour, taking into account that estimations may vary grossly because of clonal heterogeneity at different sites of the tumour (Braunsberg et al., 1973).

(3) The modifying effect of prolactin on oestradiol utilization in the cell—either by increasing the affinity of the target cell or by affecting the level of enzymes concerned with the transport or conversion of the steroid.

(4) The modifying effect of oestradiol on the utilization of prolactin by the cell (Meites, Cassell and Clark, 1971).

(5) The possibility of a biphasic temporal response if (3) and (4) are not synchronous. Thus, in a patient receiving oestrogen therapy, there may be a time difference between the local effect of oestrogen on the tumour cell and its indirect effects on prolactin secretion, release or utilization.

## Tumoral factors

(1) The heterogeneity of the cell population at each tumour site and the genetically determined sensitivity of each clone to the two hormones.

(2) The overall rate of growth and the degree of differentiation in the tumour. This may determine the predominance of a carcinostatic or a carcinocidal effect (see Chapter 3).

(3) The stage of tumour growth—this will determine the stage in progression to autonomy (Furth, 1972), and its relation to immune response mechanisms (Keast, 1970).

(4) The size and site of the lesions and the effect of previous treatment upon each lesion—mainly in relation to vascular factors.

Because of the complexity of the above hormonal and tumoral factors, it would seem highly unlikely on a theoretical basis, that measurement either of hormone levels in the blood or of receptor site levels in the tumour (or even of both), will lead to an absolute correlation with the responsiveness of the tumour to endocrine manipulation. The moderate degree of success achieved by a discriminant such as that of Bulbrook, in predicting a greater or lesser likelihood of response to endocrine ablation, probably reflects a genetically determined association of a specific hormonal environment with a tumour of specific growth characteristics.

Estimation of the level of both oestradiol and prolactin receptors may provide more significant information if it can be assumed that receptor binding determines hormonal dependence or responsiveness. The technique is certainly simpler and possibly more reliable than that of organ culture. However, the high degree of correlation claimed by Jensen et al. (1972) between clinical response and oestradiol receptor level in the tumour is somewhat remarkable in view of the report by Braunsberg et al. (1973) that the *in vivo* uptake of oestradiol by the tumour does not predict its response to endocrine ablation, oestrogen or androgen therapy.

Because of the difficulty in elucidating the relative roles of each hormone separately in maintaining the growth of breast cancer *in vivo*, it has been suggested that an *in vitro* system such as organ culture might be better able to define the roles of each hormone singly or in combination. Furth (1972) and Dao (1972) have examined the effect of prolactin in stimulating DNA synthesis in experimental mammary carcinoma in organ cultures containing tritiated thymidine. On the other hand, Chayen, Altmann and Bitensky (1970) and Salih et al. (1972) have examined the effect of oestradiol in enhancing pentose shunt activity in organ cultures of human mammary cancer. Although the technique does not measure nucleotide incorporation, it permits reading within 24 hours, and has the added advantage that histochemical localization makes the method independent of the well known cellular heterogeneity of breast cancer specimens. The latter authors have shown by this method that 32 per cent of 50 specimens showed enhancement with sheep prolactin and of these about one-third responded to oestradiol also. Such a method (utilizing *human* prolactin), may be useful in predicting responsiveness to hypophysectomy but only of the clone which has been sampled, and only if taken in conjunction with the post-operative reduction in serum prolactin and oestradiol levels achieved in each patient.

However, it seems unlikely that such a method can provide an individualized bioassay capable of predicting sensitivity to other methods of endocrine therapy such as oophorectomy, adrenalectomy, androgen, oestrogen or progestin therapy. Response in organ culture cannot take into account changes in the endocrine environment of the tumour *in vivo*, resulting from the influence of steroid metabolites, homeostatic mechanisms, indirect effects of administered hormones or interactions with endogenous hormones.

## EFFECT OF LEVODOPA ON BREAST CANCER ACTIVITY

Facilitation of the carcinostatic effect (see Chapter 3) may explain the regression of breast cancer noted above in the three patients receiving levodopa and oestrogen after failing to respond to treatment by oestrogen alone previously. Regression of a tumour by the carcinostatic mechanism after high dosage oestrogen therapy involves stimulation of its functional activity, and this requires the presence of an adequate level of prolactin as well as oestrogen. High dosage of oestrogen stimulates prolactin release in post-menopausal women (L'Hermite and Heuson, 1973), but the added levodopa in our patients may have been necessary to sensitize a failing hypothalamic feedback mechanism (Stoll, 1972).

As discussed in Chapter 10, there is considerable evidence that the hypothalamic threshold to feedback mechanisms tends to rise as the menopause is approached, and further with advancing age. This can be corrected by levodopa administration, but to explain our cases of tumour regression following its combination with high dosage of oestrogen, one would have to assume that the effect of oestrogen in stimulating prolactin release would be great enough to overcome the tendency for levodopa to diminish prolactin release by increasing dopamine and thus PIF levels.

The fall in hypothalamic sensitivity with advancing age may be due to dopamine depletion, similar to that noted in the nigrostriatal system in the case of idiopathic Parkinsonism. It has been shown that the hypothalamic threshold in the oestrogen–gonadotrophin feedback tends to rise as the menopause is approached (Neumann et al., 1970; Adamopoulos, Lorraine and Dove, 1971). This also occurs after oophorectomy (Davidson, 1969) and with advancing age (Dilman, 1971). It has been suggested that monoamine oxidase levels in the hypothalamus are increased after the menopause (Kobayashi, Kobayashi and Kato, 1964; Tryding, Tufvesson and Nilsson, 1972), and with advancing age (Robinson et al., 1972) and that this may lead to an accelerated breakdown of dopamine (see Chapter 19).

Levodopa therapy in breast cancer may thus act by correcting decreased sensitivity of the hypothalamic feedback mechanism. However, it is interesting that while levodopa administration has been reported to yield dramatic relief of the pain associated with bone metastases of breast cancer, such pain relief is usually not followed by objective evidence of tumour regression. If it is more than a placebo effect, it is reminiscent of the pain relief following hypophyseal ablation (see Chapter 14). It is not impossible that levodopa may influence the conductivity of centripetal fibres carrying pain stimuli to the thalamic centres.

It has also been suggested by Papaioannou (1972) that levodopa may cause remission in breast cancer by stimulating the immune response. Levodopa is the metabolic precursor not only of dopamine but also of noradrenaline, and it has been suggested that the function of the lymphocyte may be influenced by its noradrenaline content which is normally high. It has been shown that alpha adrenergic stimulation increases lymphocyte transformation *in vitro*, while reserpine, an alpha blocker, reduces cellular and humoral immunity and causes atrophy of the thymus (Hadden, 1971). Levodopa may thus stimulate the immune response by virtue of its being a precursor of an alpha adrenergic energizer.

It is also pointed out by Papaioannou that levodopa administration increases the level of growth hormone in the blood, presumably by stimulating secretion of the growth hormone releasing factor (Boyd, Lebovitz and Pfeiffer, 1970). Growth hormone is said to increase development of lymphoid tissue, while the presence of antibody against this hormone will depress lymphoid development. It is suggested, therefore, that levodopa may stimulate the immune response by a dual mechanism of catecholamine and growth hormone release.

## THE MENOPAUSE AND BREAST CANCER ACTIVITY

There are numerous clinical observations suggesting that hormonal readjustment around the time of the menopause may slow the activity of breast cancer. Thus the proportion of patients presenting with breast cancer falls sharply between the ages of 50 and 55 (Clemmesen, 1948, 1965; Anderson et al., 1950). Spontaneous regression is more common in breast cancer around the time of the menopause (Smithers et al., 1952). The average recurrence-free interval is longer in patients in whom the natural menopause intervenes after mastectomy (Clemmesen, 1948; Hadfield and Holt, 1956). Survival rates are significantly higher for patients developing cancer between the ages of 41 and 50 (Richards, 1948; Delarue, 1955). Radiologically sclerotic and slow growing metastases in bone are more common in patients whose recurrence-free interval spans the menopause (Stoll, 1969).

These observations have been generally interpreted to reflect the sudden fall in circulating oestrogen level which occurs at the time of the menopause. It is also possible that they reflect a fall in serum prolactin level associated with the rise in gonadotrophin secretion which occurs at the menopause. A reciprocal relationship between prolactin and gonadotrophin secretion is found in patients with non-puerperal galactorrhoea (Besser and Edwards, 1972). A reciprocal relationship has been shown in the rat between pituitary secretion of gonadotrophin and prolactin (Ben-David, Danon and Sulman, 1971).

The mechanism may be a crowding out of the acidophil prolactin secreting cells by the proliferation of the basophil gonadotrophin secreting cells (Cozen and Nelson, 1961; Perlow, 1964). It is the rise of gonadotrophin secretion and not the fall in oestrogen secretion which causes the serum prolactin level to fall in the rat after oophorectomy (Ben-David, Danon and Sulman, 1971) (see Chapter 6). The mechanism may involve an effect on the hypothalamic feedback controlling prolactin secretion but it is not clear whether it is the FSH or the LH moiety which is the major antagonist to prolactin in this respect.

As mentioned earlier in this chapter, observations by Scowen and Hadfield (1955) and Pommatau et al. (1963) suggested that a higher mean level of gonadotrophin excretion after oophorectomy predicts a greater likelihood of tumour regression in breast cancer patients. There are clinical observations which point to the same conclusion. The incidence of severe menopausal flushing is thought to run parallel to that of high serum levels of gonadotrohin, because of the observation that the frequency of flushes is reduced by stilboestrol administration, parallel to its reduction of gonadotrophin excretion levels (Smith and Albert, 1955). The persistence of severe flushes following prophylactic oophorectomy at the time of mastectomy, is regarded as a good prognostic sign because it is usually found to be associated with the absence of clinical evidence of tumour recurrence (Stoll, 1969). The appearance of tumour recurrence in such women often coincides with recent decrease in the intensity and frequency of flushes.

## CONCLUSION

Recent research emphasizes the need for pituitary trophic hormones in addition to oestrogen in stimulating the growth of both experimental and human mammary cancer.

Recent observations that various agents could influence the levels of dopamine in the brain have suggested the possibility of a selective pharmacological 'hypophysectomy'. Its application to the treatment of advanced breast cancer must await the outcome of current trials of agents with selective inhibitory effects upon pituitary trophic hormone secretion and release.

Idiopathic or induced depletion of dopamine in the hypothalamus may decrease the sensitivity of the hypothalamic centres to feedback mechanism, and it is possible that levodopa priming may improve the limited benefit which has been achieved in the past from endocrine therapy in late breast cancer. A group of 12 post-menopausal patients with recurrent soft-tissue manifestations of breast cancer were given 2 g levodopa daily (with or without added Cogentin) for a period of two months with no significant effect on the tumour growth. However, continuation of levodopa with the addition of oestrogen therapy led to objective evidence of regression in 3 out of 7 cases, none of whom had responded previously to at least three months of oestrogen therapy alone. To account for this, it is suggested that the administration of levodopa may correct the decreased sensitivity of the hypothalamic feedback mechanism.

Based on morphological evidence in regressing mammary carcinoma, the hypothesis is suggested that tumour regression can be achieved either by withdrawal of prolactin and oestrogen, as in endocrine ablative surgery, or by raising them to a high level, as in oestrogen therapy. The latter can cause stimulation of maturation and differentiation in the tumour leading to a decrease in mitotic activity. As the release of prolactin from the anterior pituitary gland depends on feedback mechanisms, the integrity of the hypothalamic mechanisms is important in the endocrine therapy of breast cancer.

## REFERENCES

Adamopoulos, D. A., Lorraine, J. A. and Dove, C. A. (1971). 'Endocrinological studies in women approaching the menopause.' *J. Obstet. Gynaec. Br. Cwlth.* **78**, 62.

Anden, N. E., Rubenson, A., Fuxe, K. and Hökfelt, T. (1967). 'Evidence for dopamine receptor stimulation by apomorphine.' *J. Pharm. Pharmac.* **19**, 627.

Anderson, E., Reed, S. C., Huseby, R. A. and Oliver, C. P. (1950). 'Possible relationship between menopause and age at onset breast cancer.' *Cancer (Phil.)* **3**, 410.

Ben-David, M., Danon, A. and Sulman, F. G. (1971). 'Evidence of antagonism between prolactin and gonadotrophin secretion. Effect of metallibure on perphenazine induced prolactin secretion in ovariectomised rats.' *J. Endocr.* **51**, 719.

Berle, P. and Voigt, K. D. (1972). 'Plasma prolactin levels in women with breast cancer.' *Acta endocr.* Suppl. **159**, 38.

Besser, G. M. and Edwards, C. R. W. (1972). 'Galactorrhoea.' *Br. med. J.* **2**, 280.

Birge, V. A., Jacobs, L. S., Hammer, C. T. and Daughaday, W. H. (1971). 'Catecholamine inhibition of prolactin secretion by isolated rat adenohypophysis.' *Endocrinology* **86**, 120.

Boyd, A. E., Lebovitz, H. E. and Pfeiffer, J. B. (1970). 'Stimulation of human growth hormone secretion by L-Dopa.' *New Engl. J. Med.* **283**, 1425.

Braunsberg, H., James, V. H. T., Irvine, W. T., James, F., Jamieson, C. W., Sellwood, R. A., Carter, A. E. and Hulbert, M. (1973). 'Prognostic significance of oestrogen uptake by human breast cancer tissue.' *Lancet* **1**, 163.

Burton, J. L., Libman, L. J., Hall, T. and Schuster, S. (1971). 'Levodopa in acne vulgaris.' *Lancet* **2**, 370.

Carlsson, A. (1959). 'The occurrence, distribution and physiological role of catecholamines in the nervous tissue.' *Pharmac. Rev.* **11**, 490.

— and Hillard, N. A. (1962). 'Formation of phenolic acids in brain after the administration of 3,4,dihydroxyphenylalanine.' *Acta phys. Scand.* **55**, 95.

— Lindquist, M., Magnusson, T. and Waldron, B. (1958). 'On the presence of 3-hydroxytyramine in the brain.' *Science* **107**, 471.

Chayen, P., Altmann, F. P. and Bitensky, L. (1970). 'Response of human breast cancer to steroid hormones in vitro.' *Lancet* **1**, 869.

Clemmesen, J. (1948). 'Carcinoma of the breast: Results from statistical research.' *Br. J. Radiol.* **21**, 583.

— (1965). 'Statistical studies in the aetiology of malignant neoplasms. 1. Review of results.' *Acta path. microbiol. scand.* Suppl. **174**, 254.

Coyle, J. T. and Snyder, S. H. (1969). 'Antiparkinsonian drugs. Inhibition of dopamine uptake in the corpus striatum as a possible mechanism of action.' *Science* 889.

Cozen, D. A. and Nelson, M. M. (1961). 'Effect of ovariectomy on the follicle stimulating and interstitial cell stimulating content of the anterior pituitary of the rat.' *Endocrinology* **68**, 767.

Dao, T. L. (1972). In *Prolactin and Carcinogenesis* (4th Tenovus Workshop), p. 189, Ed. by A. R. Boyns and K. Griffiths. Cardiff; Alpha Omega Alpha.

Davidson, J. M. (1969). In *Frontiers in Endocrinology*, p. 343, Ed. by W. F. Ganong and L. Martini. Oxford University Press.

Delarue, N. C. (1955). 'Fundamental concepts determining a philosophy of treatment in mammary carcinoma.' *Canad. med. Ass. J.* **73**, 597.

Dickey, R. P. and Minton, J. P. (1972). 'Levodopa relief of bone pain from breast cancer.' *New Engl. J. Med.* **286**, 843.

— Marks, B. and Stevens, V. C. (1971). 'Effect of levodopa on human and rat FSH and LH.' *Endocr. Soc. USA Meet.* 281.

Dilman, V. M. (1971). 'Age associated elevation of hypothalamic threshold to feedback control and its role in development, ageing and disease.' *Lancet* **1**, 1211.

Donoso, A. O., Bishop, W., Fawcett, C. P., Krulich, L. and McCann, S. M. (1971). 'Effect of drugs that modify brain monoamine concentration on plasma gonadotrophin and prolactin levels in the rat.' *Endocrinology* **89**, 774.

Eddy, R. L., Lloyd Jones, A., Chakmakjian, Z. H. and Silverthorne, M. C. (1971). 'Effect of levodopa on human hypophyseal hormone release.' *Endocr. Soc. USA Meet.* 336.

European Breast Cancer Group (1972). 'Clinical trial of 2-Br-a-ergocryptine (C B154) in advanced breast cancer.' *Europ. J. Cancer* **8**, 155.

Evered, D. F. (1971). 'L-Dopa as a vitamin B6 antagonist.' *Lancet* **1**, 94.

Farnebo, L. O., Fuxe, K., and Hamberger, B. (1970). 'Effect of some anti-Parkinsonian drugs on catecholamine neurones.' *J. Pharm. Pharmac.* **22**, 733.

Friesen, H. G. (1971). 'Human placental lactogen and human pituitary lactogen.' *Clin. Obstet. Gynec.* **14**, 669.

— (1972). In *Prolactin and Carcinogenesis* (4th Tenovus Workshop), p. 64, Ed. by A. R. Boyns and K. Griffiths. Cardiff; Alpha Omega Alpha.

Furth, J. (1972). In *Prolactin and Carcinogenesis* (4th Tenovus Workshop), p. 137, Ed. by A. R. Boyns and K. Griffiths. Cardiff; Alpha Omega Alpha.

Geschwind, I. I. (1972). In *Prolactin and Carcinogenesis* (4th Tenovus Workshop), p. 1, Ed. by A. R. Boyns and K. Griffiths. Cardiff; Alpha Omega Alpha.

Godwin-Austen, R. B., Frears, C. C. and Bergmann, S. (1971). 'Incidence of side effects from levodopa during the introduction of treatment.' *Br. med. J.* **1**, 267.

Hadden, J. W. (1971). 'Sympathetic modulation of immune response.' *New Engl. J. Med.* **285**, 178.

Hadfield, G. (1956). 'Recent research in physiology of breast applied to mammary cancer.' *Br. med. J.* **1**, 1507.

— and Holt, J. A. G. (1956). 'The physiological castration syndrome in breast cancer.' *Br. med. J.* **2**, 972.

Hayek, A. and Crawford, J. D. (1972). 'L-Dopa and pituitary hormone secretion.' *J. clin. Endocr.* **34**, 764.

Hayward, J. L., Atkins, H. J. B., Falconer, M. A., Maclean, K. S., Salmon, C. F. W., Schurr, P. H. and Sheheen, C. H. (1970). 'Clinical trials comparing hypophysectomy with adrenalectomy, and with transethmoidal hypophysectomy.'

In *Breast Cancer* (2nd Tenovus Workshop), p. 50, Ed. by C. A. F. Joslin and E. N. Gleave. Cardiff; Alpha Omega Alpha.

Heuson, J. C., Waelbroeck, C. and Legros, N. (1970). 'Growth inhibition of rat mammary carcinoma and endocrine changes produced by 2 Br α ergocryptine.' *Europ. J. Cancer* **6**, 353.

Hilf, R., Michel, I. and Bell, C. (1967). 'Biochemical responses of normal and neoplastic mammary tissue to hormonal treatment.' *Recent Progr Hormone Res.* **23**, 229.

Hornykiewicz, O. (1966). 'Dopamine and brain function.' *Pharmac. Rev.* **18**, 925.

Huggins, C., Briziarelli, G. and Sutton, H. Jnr. (1959). 'Rapid induction of mammary carcinoma in the rat and the influence of hormones on the tumours.' *J. expl Med.* **109**, 25.

Hughes, R. C., Polgar, J. C., Weightman, D. and Walton, J. N. (1971). 'Levodopa in Parkinsonism. The effects of withdrawal of anticholinergic drugs.' *Br. med. J.* **2**, 487.

Hwang, P., Friesen, H. G. and Guyda, H. J. (1972). See Chapter 9.

— Guyda, H. J. and Friesen, H. (1971). 'A radioimmunoassay for human prolactin.' *Proc. natn Acad. Sci.* **68**, 1902.

Jensen, E. V., Block, G. E., Smith, S., Kyser, K. and Desombre, E. R. (1972). In *Oestrogen Target Tissue and Neoplasia,* Ed. by T. L. Dao. University of Chicago Press.

Kamberi, J. A., Mical, R. F. and Porter, J. C. (1971). 'Effect of anterior pituitary perfusion and intraventricular injection of catecholamines on prolactin release.' *Endocrinology* **88**, 1012.

Kansal, P. C., Talbert, O. R. and Buse, M. G. (1971). 'Effect of levodopa on serum thyroxine and growth hormone.' *Proc. Endocr Soc. USA Meet.* 337.

Keast, D. (1970). 'Immunosurveillance and cancer.' *Lancet* **2**, 710.

Kennedy, B, J. (1962). 'Massive oestrogen administration in premenopausal women with metastatic breast cancer.' *Cancer (Phil.)* **15**, 641.

Kim, U. (1965). 'Pituitary function and hormonal therapy of experimental breast cancer.' *Cancer Res.* **25**, 1146.

Kleinberg, D. L. and Frantz, A. G. (1971). 'Human prolactin measurement in plasma by in vitro bioassay.' *J. clin. Invest.* **50**, 1557.

Kobayashi, T., Kobayashi, P. and Kato, R. (1964). 'Effect of sex steroids on the choline acetylase activity in the hypothalamus of female rats.' *Endocr. Jap.* **11**, 9.

Koch, Y., Chow, Y. F. and Meites, J. (1971). 'Direct inhibition by ergocornine of pituitary prolactin release.' *Endocrinology* **89**, 229.

Kleinberg, D. L., Noel, G. L. and Frantz, A. G. (1971). 'Chlorpromazine stimulation and levodopa suppression of plasma prolactin in man.' *J. clin. Endocr.* **33**, 873.

Kwa, H. G. (1972). In *Prolactin and Carcinogenesis* (4th Tenovus Workshop), Ed. by A. R. Boyns and K. Griffiths. Cardiff; Alpha Omega Alpha.

Lal, S., de la Vega, C. E., Sourkes, T. L. and Friesen, H. G. (1972). 'Effect of apomorphine on human growth hormone secretion.' *Lancet* **2**, 661.

L'Hermite, M. (1972). In *Prolactin and Carcinogenesis* (4th Tenovus Workshop), p. 81, Ed. by A. R. Boyns and K. Griffiths. Cardiff; Alpha Omega Alpha.

— and Heuson, J. C. (1973). 'Stimulation of basal serum prolactin levels by oral ethinyl oestradiol.' In Press.

L'Hermite, M., VanHaelst, L., Copinschi, G., Leclerq, R., Golstein, J., Bruno, O. D. and Robyn, C. (1972). 'Prolactin release after injection of TRH in man.' *Lancet* 1, 763.

Lu, H., Koch, Y. and Meites, J. (1971). 'Direct inhibition by ergocornine of pituitary prolactin release.' *Endocrinology* **89**, 229.

— and Meites, J. (1971). 'Inhibition by L-dopa and MAO inhibitors of pituitary prolactin release. Stimulation of methyldopa and d-amphetamine.' *Proc. Soc. expl Biol. Med.* **137**, 480.

Malarkey, W. B., Jacobs, L. S. and Daughaday, W. (1971). 'Levodopa suppression of prolactin in non-puerperal galactorrhoea.' *New Engl. J. Med.* **285**, 1160.

Malven, P. V. and Hoge, W. R. (1971). 'Effect of ergocornine on prolactin secretion by hypophyseal homografts.' *Endocrinology* **88**, 445.

Meites, J. (1972). In *Prolactin and Carcinogenesis* (4th Tenovus Workshop), p. 54, Ed. by A. R. Boyns and K. Griffiths. Cardiff; Alpha Omega Alpha.

— Cassell, E. and Clark, J. (1971). 'Estrogen inhibition of mammary tumor growth in rats. Counteraction by prolactin.' *Proc. Soc. expl Biol. Med.* **137**, 1225.

— Lu, K. H., Wuttke, W., Welsch, C. W., Nagasawa, H. and Quadri, S. K. (1972). 'Recent studies on function and control of prolactin secretion in rats.' *Recent Progr Hormone Res.* **28**, 471.

Minton, J. P. and Dickey, R. P. (1972). 'Prolactin, FSH and LH in breast cancer. Effect of levodopa and oophorectomy.' *Lancet* 1, 1069.

Nagasawa, H. and Meites, J. (1970). 'Suppression by ergocornine and iproniazid of carcinogen induced mammary tumours in rats. Effect on serum and pituitary prolactin.' *Proc. Soc. expl Biol Med.* **135**, 469.

— and Yanai, R. (1971). 'Increased mammary gland response to pituitary mammotropic hormone by oestrogen in rats.' *Endocr. Jap.* **17**, 53.

Neumann, F., Wallrabe, R. von B., Elger, W., Steinbeck, H., Hanh, J. B. and Kramer, M. (1970). 'Aspects of androgen dependent events as studied by anti-androgens.' *Recent Progr Hormone Res.* **26**, 337.

Noel, G. L., Suh, H. K., Stone, G. and Frantz, H. G. (1972). 'Prolactin response to surgery and other forms of stress in men and women.' *Clin. Res.* **20**, 435.

Papaioannou, A. N. (1972). 'Prolactin, levodopa and immune response in breast cancer.' *Lancet* 2, 226.

Pearson, O. H. (1957). 'Observations on the role of androgens and estrogens in body balance.' *Archs intern Med.* **100**, 724.

— (1972). In *Prolactin and Carcinogenesis* (4th Tenovus Workshop), p. 154, Ed. by A. R. Boyns and K. Griffiths. Cardiff; Alpha Omega Alpha.

— and Ray, B. S. (1959). 'Results of hypophysectomy in the treatment of metastatic mammary carcinoma.' *Cancer (Phil.)* **12**, 85.

Perlow, A. F. (1964). 'Effect of ovariectomy on pituitary and serum gonadotrophins in the mouse.' *Endocrinology* **74**, 102.

Pletscher, A. and Bartholini, C. (1971). 'Selective rise in brain dopamine by inhibition of extracerebral levodopa decarboxylation.' *Clin. Pharmac. Ther.* **12**, 334.

Pommatau, E., Poulain, S., Dargent, M. and Mayer, M. (1963). 'FSH levels in postmenopausal or castrated women with advanced mammary cancer. Effect of adrenalectomy.' *Cancer Chemother. Abst.* 1280.

Richards, G. E. (1948). 'Mammary cancer—the place of surgery and of radiotherapy in its management.' *Br. J. Radiol.* **21**, 109.

Robinson, D. S., Nies, A., Davis, J. N., Bunney, W. E., Davis, J. M., Colbirn, R. W., Bourne, H. R., Shaw, D. M. and Coppen, H. J. (1972). 'Ageing, monoamines and monoamine oxidase levels.' *Lancet* **1**, 290.

Salih, H., Flax, H., Brander, W. and Hobbs, J. R. (1972). 'Prolactin dependence in human breast cancers.' *Lancet* **2**, 1103.

Schally, A. V., Arimura, A. and Bowers, C. U. (1968). 'Hypothalamic neurohormones regulating anterior pituitary function.' *Recent Progr Hormone Res.* **24**, 497.

Schneider, H. P. and McCann, S. M. (1969). 'Possible role of dopamine as transmitter to promote discharge of LH releasing factor.' *Endocrinology* **85**, 121.

Scowen, E. F. and Hadfield, G. (1955). 'Mammotrophic activity of extracts of human urine.' *Cancer (Phil.)* **8**, 890.

Segaloff, A., Gordon, D., Carabasi, R. A., Horvat, B. N., Schlosser, J. V. and Murison, P. J. (1954). 'Hormonal therapy in cancer of the breast.' *Cancer (Phil.)* **7**, 758.

Sherman, L. (1971). Personal communication.

Sherwood, L. M. (1971). 'Human prolactin.' *New Engl. J. Med.* **284**, 774.

Smith, R. A. and Albert, A. (1955). 'Effect of estrogen on urinary gonadotrophin.' *Proc. Mayo Clin.* **30**, 617.

Smithers, D. W., Rigby Jones, P., Galton, D. A. G. and Payne, P. N. (1952). 'Cancer of the breast—a review.' *Br. J. Radiol.* Suppl. **4**, 1.

Stoll, B. A. (1956). 'P-hydroxypropiophenone for advanced breast cancer.' *Med. J. Aust.* **2**, 181.

— (1958). In *Modern Trends in Endocrinology—1*, p. 212, Ed. by H. Gardiner-Hill. London; Butterworths.

— (1963). 'Corticosteroids in the therapy of advanced mammary cancer.' *Br. med. J.* **2**, 210.

— (1964). 'Hormones and breast cancer.' *Br. med. J.* **2**, 755.

— (1969). In *Hormonal Management in Breast Cancer*. London; Pitman.

— (1972). 'Breast cancer and brain catecholamines. A hypothesis.' *Lancet* **1**, 431.

Sulman, F. G. (1959). 'The mechanism of the push and pull principle. 2. Endocrine effects of hypothalamic depressants and the phenothiazine group.' *Archs Inst. Pharmacodyn. Ther.* **118**, 298.

Tindal, J. S. and Knaggs, G. S. (1972). 'Pathways in the forebrain of the rabbit concerned with the release of prolactin.' *J. Endocr.* **52**, 253.

Tryding, N., Tufvesson, G. and Nilsson, S. (1972). 'Ageing, monamines and monoamine oxidase levels.' *Lancet* 489.

Turkington, R. W. (1972). In *Prolactin and Carcinogenesis* (4th Tenovus Workshop), p. 39, Ed. by A. R. Boyns and K. Griffiths. Cardiff; Alpha Omega Alpha.

— Underwood, L. E. and van Wyk, J. J. (1971). 'Elevated serum prolactin levels after pituitary stalk section in man.' *New Engl. J. Med.* **285**, 707.

Vesell, E. S., Ng, L., Passananti, G. T. and Chase, T. N. (1971). 'Inhibition of drug metabolism by levodopa in combination with a dopa decarboxylase inhibitor.' *Lancet* **2**, 370.

Wuttke, W., Cassell, E. and Meites, J. (1971). 'Effect of ergocornine on serum. prolactin and LH and on hypothalamic content of PIF and LRF.' *Endocrinology* **88**, 737.

# 17

# The Role of Prolactin Inhibition
# in Treatment

## J. C. Heuson

In view of the fact that, as yet, the role of prolactin in human breast cancer is highly speculative and still derived from indirect evidence, it is advisable to review this evidence before discussing the problem of prolactin inhibition. Therefore, this chapter will be divided into two parts: the first will be devoted to the role of prolactin in the growth of experimental and human breast cancer. The second will discuss prolactin inhibition proper, as a new therapeutic approach to breast cancer.

## ROLE OF PROLACTIN IN THE GROWTH OF MAMMARY CANCER

### Experimental tumours

The experimental mammary tumour most extensively and conclusively studied from the point of view of hormone-dependence is the DMBA-induced mammary carcinoma of the Sprague–Dawley rat (Huggins, Briziarelli and Sutton, 1959; Huggins, Grand and Brillantes, 1961). Maintenance of tumour growth in this system involves ovarian hormones: oestrogen (Huggins, Briziarelli and Sutton, 1959) and progesterone (Huggins, Briziarelli and Sutton, 1959; Takahashi and Simpson, 1970), prolactin (Nagasawa and Yanai, 1970; Pearson, 1967; Pearson et al., 1969) and insulin (Heuson and Legros, 1972; Heuson, Legros and Heimann, 1972). Oestrogens reactivate growth of the tumours from their regressed state after oophorectomy but not after hypophysectomy (Pearson, 1967). In contrast, ovine prolactin (Pearson,

1967) or bovine prolactin (Nagasawa and Yanai, 1970) reactivate tumour growth after oophorectomy + adrenalectomy (Nagasawa and Yanai, 1970) or hypophysectomy (Pearson, 1967).

Bovine growth hormone is inactive under these conditions (Nagasawa and Yanai, 1970; Pearson, 1967). It cannot be ruled out with certainty from the data given in these studies, however, that doses of growth hormone higher than those used might have had some activity. This role of prolactin in the DMBA-induced carcinogenesis is further supported by the effect of tranquillizing drugs, such as the phenothiazine derivatives, which are potent stimulators of prolactin secretion (Lu et al., 1970; Pearson et al., 1969). It was found that perphenazine strongly enhances tumour appearance and growth (Heuson et al., 1972; Pearson et al., 1969), even after oophorectomy and adrenalectomy (Pearson et al., 1969).

An important point which requires elucidation is whether the oestrogens have a direct effect on growth at the tumour tissue level, thus synergizing with peptide hormones, or whether they merely stimulate prolactin secretion and thereby tumour growth. The first hypothesis is likely in view of the fact that such synergism has been clearly demonstrated in the normal mammary tissue (Lyons, Li and Johnson, 1958; Nagasawa and Yanai, 1971) and that the tumour tissue contains oestrogen receptors, like other target organs of the oestrogens (King, Gordon and Steggles, 1969). However, oestradiol-17$\beta$, alone or in combination with prolactin, failed to stimulate DNA synthesis in organ cultures of rat mammary tumours, while prolactin exerted a marked stimulating effect; these culture experiments were carried out in the presence of insulin and cortisol (Welsch and Rivera, 1972). The relevance of these *in vitro* observations to the *in vivo* situation is unknown.

The role of prolactin in rat mammary tumour growth is further substantiated by the effects of drugs that specifically inhibit prolactin secretion. Among these drugs, ergot alkaloids have been most extensively studied. They produce various endocrine effects that have been recognized since 1951. Ergocornine suppresses deciduoma formation and implantation (Shelesnyak, 1954), terminates pseudo-pregnancy and early pregnancy (Carlsen, Zeilmaker and Shelesnyak, 1961) and inhibits lactation (Zeilmaker and Carlsen, 1962). Other ergot alkaloids, α-ergocryptine and 2-Br-α-ergocryptine (CB 154) also inhibit fertility and lactation in the rat (Flückiger and Wagner, 1968). CB 154 interferes with function and normal involution of the corpora lutea in the rat leading to their accumulation (Heuson, Waelbroeck-Van Gaver and Legros, 1970).

All these effects are consistent with the operation of a single mechanism, namely inhibition of prolactin secretion. Prevention of the ergocornine induced interruption of pregnancy by simultaneous administration of prolactin provided evidence in favour of this interpretation (Shelesnyak, 1958). Determinations of blood prolactin level by radioimmunoassay brought about a direct demonstration that ergocornine (Nagasawa and Meites, 1970), CB 154 (Heuson et al., 1972) and other ergot alkaloids (Shaar and Clemens, 1972) markedly inhibit prolactin secretion. The mechanism of this inhibition has been investigated. It was found that ergocornine increases the PIF content of the hypothalamus, which suggests that the drug acts in part via the hypothalamus (Wuttke, Cassell and Meites, 1971). Ergocornine, however, also inhibits prolactin secretion by direct action on the pituitary cells. This was demonstrated in organ culture experiments which showed that the level of prolactin in the medium is depressed by the addition of ergocornine or CB 154 during culture (Pasteels and Ectors, 1970; Pasteels et al., 1971).

Electron microscopic studies of organ cultures of rat pituitaries suggest that the inhibitory effect of ergocornine is due to suppression of exocytosis of the prolactin granules, without gross interference with the synthesis of prolactin and granule formation (Ectors, Danguy and Pasteels, 1972). Direct inhibition by ergocornine of pituitary prolactin release also occurs *in vivo*, as demonstrated conclusively in experiments involving hypophyseal homografts (Lu, Koch and Meites, 1971; Malven and Hoge, 1971; Shaar and Clemens, 1972).

In view of their selective inhibition of prolactin secretion, ergot alkaloids were studied in the DMBA-induced rat mammary tumour. CB 154 significantly inhibits tumour growth in tumour-bearing rats (Heuson, Waelbroeck-Van Gaver and Legros, 1970); it depresses tumour formation when drug administration is started shortly after DMBA (Heuson et al., 1972; Stähelin, Burckhardt-Vischer and Flückiger, 1971). Ergocornine and ergocryptine also inhibit initiation (Clemens and Shaar, 1972) and growth (Cassell, Meites and Welsch, 1971; Clemens and Shaar, 1972; Nagasawa and Meites, 1970) of the DMBA-induced tumours. Finally, it has been recently shown that ergocornine and CB 154 induce a marked regression of spontaneous mammary tumours developing in old female rats (Quadri and Meites, 1971).

Derivatives of cyclic imides have also been investigated in the DMBA-induced rat mammary tumour system. One such derivative, 1-(morpholinomethyl)-4-phtalimido-piperidindione-2,6 (CG 603) was found to inhibit tumour growth noticeably (Mückter, Frankus and Moré, 1969, 1970). Recent studies have shown that CG 603 effectively inhibits prolactin secretion in the rat (Gelato, Quadri and Meites, 1972; van der Guchten, 1971), by a mechanism as yet unsolved. It is possible that prolactin inhibition accounts for part or all of the anti-tumour activity of CG 603, although the drug produces a prolonged arrest of the oestrous cycle (Mückter, Frankus and Moré, 1969, 1970), indicating that it acts less selectively on prolactin than the ergot alkaloids, and probably interferes with the secretion of gonadotrophins.

Discussion of the effect of oestrogen antagonists on rat mammary tumour and prolactin secretion may be pertinent to this problem. As stated above, the question as to whether oestrogens at physiological doses have a direct stimulatory effect on tumour growth or an indirect effect via prolactin secretion is unsettled. Whatever the answer to this question may be, it has been shown that the oestrogen antagonist nafoxidine (U 11,110A Upjohn, Kalamazoo, Mich.) inhibits induction and growth of the rat mammary tumour (Heuson et al., 1972; Terenius, 1971). A possible mechanism of this effect is at the level of the tumour tissue itself by interference with oestrogen action. It was found, however, that nafoxidine decreased about six fold the stimulating effect of oestradiol-17β on prolactin secretion in oophorectomized rats (Heuson et al., 1972). Inhibition of prolactin secretion by nafoxidine may therefore conceivably account for part or all of the anti-tumour effect of this drug.

These pharmacological studies, especially those relating to the ergot alkaloids, which appear to act as selective inhibitors of prolactin secretion in the rat, support the concept that prolactin plays a major part in the initiation and growth of the rat mammary tumour. Because of the similarities between the rat tumour and the human breast cancer, these studies may form the basis for new approaches to the endocrine treatment of the human disease.

Before ending this paragraph, it should be stressed that stimulation of experimental mammary tumour growth by prolactin is not a universal phenomenon. Thus, it was shown that the R3230AC tumour, a transplantable, hormone-sensitive mammary carcinoma of the Fisher rat, instead of being stimulated, is inhibited under various conditions involving increased prolactin secretion. Such conditions are administration of ovine prolactin, simultaneously with oestrogens (Hilf, Michel and Bell, 1967), grafting of MtTF4 mammotrophic tumour (Hilf, Bell and Michel, 1967), which secretes large amounts of prolactin as well as other hormones, and administration of fluphenazine hydrochloride (Hilf et al., 1971). The R3230AC tumour is hormone-sensitive as lactation, accompanied by an elevation of various enzyme activities, is initiated by administration of oestrogens and prolactin (Hilf, Michel and Bell, 1967). These observations indicate that hormone sensitivity should not always be equated to hormone dependence, as far as tumour growth is concerned, and that differentiation of the tumour tissue induced by hormones may sometimes lead to tumour regression.

This brief review of the role of prolactin in experimental mammary tumours has been dealing only with rat tumours. Discussion of the mouse mammary tumours has been deliberately omitted because, with few exceptions (Foulds, 1967), these tumours, once established, are autonomous. It should be said, however, that prolactin is believed to play a major part in the development of the spontaneous (Bern and Nandi, 1961) as well as hormonally-induced (Boot, 1970) mammary tumours in mice. Here again, pharmacological interference with prolactin secretion, using ergocornine and 2-Br-α-ergocryptine (CB 154) resulted in the suppression of mammary hyperplastic alveolar nodule formation (Yanai and Nagasawa, 1970) and mammary tumour appearance (Yanai and Nagasawa, 1971) in mice.

## Human mammary cancer

Surgical hypophysectomy is probably the most effective endocrine treatment of advanced breast cancer. It appeared equal in value to adrenalectomy in a retrospective study where the results from 12 North American clinics were pooled by the Joint Committee of the AMA (1961). However, a prospective randomized study, comparing hypophysectomy and adrenalectomy, of which interim reports already reveal slight but significant difference (Atkins et al., 1960), has recently been completed. It shows a definite advantage of hypophysectomy over adrenalectomy in terms of duration of remission and survival (Hayward, 1972).

These observations point to an important role of one or several pituitary hormones in the maintenance of breast cancer tissue growth. Yet it does not answer the question as to whether the role of these hormones is a direct one at the tumour tissue level or an indirect one, mediated by other endocrine glands, or both. Several investigators have attempted to answer this question.

Pearson and Ray (1959) studied the effect of hormone administration on tumour growth in patients with osseous metastases after hypophysectomy. The effect was estimated by change in pain pattern and by measurement of urinary calcium excretion and calcium balance. By these criteria, administration of 'physiological' doses of oestrogen (approximately 0·15 mg of ethinyloestradiol daily) to five patients who eventually obtained objective remissions from the hypophysectomy, failed to reactivate tumour growth. These findings are in contrast with previous studies (Pearson et al., 1954), showing that oestrogens reactivate tumour growth in cases of remissions following *oophorectomy* in pre-menopausal women. This difference of response to oestrogen administration after oophorectomy and hypophysectomy suggests that stimulation of tumour growth by the oestrogens requires the concomitant action of some hormonal factor from, or mediated by, the pituitary.

In the same study, human growth hormone (HGH, Raben's preparation), 5–15 mg daily for periods of 4–12 days, was administered to five other patients after hypophysectomy. In two of them, HGH exacerbated bone pains which had subsided after hypophysectomy, increased the calcium urinary excretion and aggravated the negative calcium balance. However, these two patients did not obtain clear-cut objective remissions of their disease from hypophysectomy. In the three other patients, HGH administration, in combination with oestrogens in two, failed to stimulate metastatic disease. These three patients obtained an objective remission from their hypophysectomy. The author's conclusion, from these preliminary observations, is that growth hormone may be an important endocrine factor in mammary cancer.

However, investigations by Lipsett and Bergenstal (1960) along the same line provided strong evidence against this interpretation. They studied the effect of HGH (various preparations from Li, Raben and Brink, 5–10 mg daily for periods of 4–96 days) on urinary calcium in 11 patients with breast cancer metastatic to bones and in 14 subjects *without cancer*. In the latter subjects, urinary calcium increased by an average of 64 mg daily (range 0–164 mg per 24 hours) under HGH administration. Among the 11 breast cancer patients, 10 had been subjected to hypophysectomy or pituitary stalk section, and 1 to oophorectomy; 6 of them were in remission. In these 6 patients, in contrast to the non cancer patients, HGH produced no elevation in urinary calcium excretion, except a very slight one in 2 patients. However, HGH administered to the 5 patients who were *not* in remission resulted in significant increases in calcium excretion averaging 93 mg daily, a response that was in the control range.

In the same study, 2 patients with 'oestrogen-dependent' tumours were in relapse and hypercalcaemic after a remission induced by oophorectomy. In both, hypophysectomy was followed by restoration of normal calcium urinary values and objective signs of remission. Those patients were then treated for consecutive periods of 5–6 days with HGH (2·5 mg b.i.d.) and ethinyloestradiol (0·05 mg daily), either singly or in combination. In neither case was there any significant effect of the treatment on urinary calcium excretion values. Finally, 5 patients in remission received an ovine prolactin preparation (15 i.u./mg, 50–100 mg/24 hours for periods of 6–12 days). None of them experienced hypercalcaemia or increase in pain. It is not stated whether these patients in remission had been subjected to hypophysectomy or to stalk section. This missing information could have been of paramount importance for interpretation of the data, as will be apparent below in the discussion on pituitary stalk section.

These studies by Pearson and Ray (1959) and by Lipsett and Bergenstal (1960) agree in suggesting that oestrogens alone, unlike in pre-menopausal patients after oophorectomy (Lipsett and Bergenstal, 1960; Pearson et al., 1954), are unable to reactivate tumour growth in hypophysectomized patients and that HGH is not the pituitary hormone with which they can synergize to promote breast cancer growth. Pearson and Ray's initial contention of an important role of HGH was seemingly a misinterpretation of preliminary data not involving control patients. Thus, the data by Lipsett and Bergenstal showed that the changes in calcium balance induced by HGH in *non-responders* to hypophysectomy were similar to those observed in the *non-cancer* controls.

With respect to the failure to reactivate tumour growth with ovine prolactin as reported by Lipsett and Bergenstal, this observation does not rule out the possibility that human prolactin is involved in the process. First, ovine prolactin has not been conclusively shown to be mammotrophic in the human species. Moreover, the dosage may be critical and may not have been large enough; thus, in adreno-ovariectomized rats bearing DMBA-induced mammary tumours, administration of ovine prolactin reactivates tumour growth in doses of 2·5 mg but not 1·25 mg, given twice daily (Nagasawa and Yanai, 1970). In addition, it is not stated in Lipsett and Bergenstal's paper, whether prolactin was administered after hypophysectomy or after hypophyseal stalk section. Finally, combination of oestrogens and prolactin was not tested in these experiments.

Preliminary results presented by McCalister and Welbourn (1962) are relevant to the foregoing remarks. They injected ovine prolactin (500 i.u. daily for three days) in ten patients *before* hypophysectomy for advanced mammary cancer with osseous metastases and in nine control subjects without evidence of metabolic or bone disease. They found that prolactin produced a slight but significant elevation of the urinary calcium excretion in the control subjects. A significantly greater elevation occurred in the six patients who subsequently responded favourably to hypophysectomy, while no elevation occurred in the four patients who failed to respond. In this series, prolactin was administered to patients who had not been subjected to major ablative procedures and therefore were not deprived of their endogenous sources of oestrogen. The positive effect of prolactin reported in this study may then be tentatively explained by a synergistic action of the endogenous oestrogens.

Particularly relevant to the problem of prolactin and human breast cancer are the results of pituitary stalk section in the treatment of this disease. This operation was performed by cutting the pituitary stalk immediately above the sella turcica and inserting a diaphragm made up of a tantalum plate (Antony et al., 1969; Dugger, van Wyk and Newsome, 1958) or of a polyethylene disc (Ehni and Eckles, 1959). The purpose of placing a diaphragm was to avoid or retard revascularization from the hypothalamus. This procedure induced a fair rate of objective remissions, ranging from 33 to 54 per cent. Yet, its therapeutic value cannot be accurately assessed in these small series of cases because of lack of control groups subjected to a treatment of known efficacy, such as hypophysectomy. Nevertheless, the important fact is that it apparently did produce tumour regression.

The endocrine mechanism of this effect has been investigated. The procedure produces partial infarction of the anterior lobe but does not cause its disappearance. The surviving cells amount to about one-quarter of the preoperative volume of the anterior lobe, and are indistinguishable histologically from those of a normal pituitary (Ehni and Eckles, 1959). Pituitary stalk section resulted in a decreased output of TSH and gonadotrophin, although to a lesser extent than after hypophysectomy (Ehni and Eckles, 1959). Plasma

355

levels of growth hormone, in the fasting state as well as in response to insulin hypoglycaemia, progressively fell to undetectable values (Antony et al., 1969). Urinary excretion of 17-ketosteroids and of 17-hydroxycorticosteroids dropped to the low levels observed in hypopituitarism; response to ACTH was frequently diminished or absent, suggesting that varying degrees of adrenal atrophy had occurred; the response to hypoglycaemia or pyrogen, however, was usually as great as that obtained by ACTH (van Wyk et al., 1960).

The remarkable finding, however, in regard to the subject under discussion, is the observation that lactation occurred post-operatively, in several patients, precisely in those who derived benefit from the procedure (Ehni and Eckles, 1959). It suggested that the pituitary remnant was secreting large amounts of a lactogenic hormone. This interpretation was confirmed by measurement of serum prolactin levels after pituitary stalk section in patients with breast cancer (Turkington, Underwood and van Wyk, 1971). Serum prolactin was measured by the rate of induction of the specific milk protein $^{32}$P-casein in organ cultures of C3H/HeJ mouse mammary gland. It was found that, of the 11 patients subjected to stalk section for metastatic breast carcinoma, 8 showed objective remission of their disease for periods ranging from seven months to twelve years; 5 of the 8 had noticeably elevated prolactin levels during the period of remission. Lack of elevation could possibly be explained in 2 of the 3 others by a long period of storage of the serum at $-20°C$, but not in the third. Among the 3 patients who showed no objective remission, 2 had elevated prolactin levels.

These endocrine studies do not give a definite explanation of the mechanism by which pituitary stalk section induces regression of breast cancer. The most likely one is that it acts as a result of the decreased secretion of pituitary hormones (growth hormone, gonadotrophins) or of adrenal hormones. Ovarian secretions are not involved because in most of the cases of remission described by Antony et al. (1969) the patients had previously been subjected to oophorectomy. A role of growth hormone is unlikely for reasons already discussed. A role of the gonadotrophins is also unlikely, because they have not been found to play a direct part in normal or tumorous mammary tissue growth in any experimental system. It is therefore likely that pituitary stalk section induces tumour regression by a decrease in secretion of the adrenal hormones. It has been shown that large amounts of oestradiol are produced in post-menopausal women under ACTH stimulation and that the ovaries do not appreciably contribute to this production (Barlow, Emerson and Saxena, 1969). A decrease in ACTH secretion after stalk section could thus conceivably result in a suppression of oestrogen production from the adrenals and thereby induce tumour regression.

Another conclusion that one can derive from the results of pituitary stalk section is that a very marked stimulation of prolactin secretion does not preclude the occurrence of tumour regression induced by deprivation of another hormone. Prolactin alone, even in very high concentrations, is unable to sustain growth of the tumour tissue. Some other hormone, possibly oestrogen, has to act simultaneously. Although these observations cast some doubt upon the possible role of prolactin in human breast cancer, pituitary stalk section offers a unique opportunity of clarifying the situation. If one assumes that prolactin–oestradiol is the combination that sustains growth of hormone-dependent breast cancer, then administration of physiological doses of oestradiol after pituitary stalk section should reactivate tumour growth, which it failed to do after hypophysectomy, as discussed above.

Treatment of advanced breast cancer by 'pharmacological' doses of oestrogens offers another example of an effective means of achieving breast cancer regression despite stimulation of prolactin secretion. The fact that large doses of oestrogens do indeed stimulate prolactin secretion in patients is demonstrated by the results of preliminary measurements shown in Table 17.1.

Another explanation that could conceivably account for the remissions obtained by pituitary stalk section or by oestrogen administration is that the resulting increase in prolactin secretion causes by itself tumour regression in some cases. These cases need not be the same as those responding to ablative procedures. It is generally accepted that response or failure to respond to hormone administration is not a good indicator of the probability of a favourable response to ablative procedures. It is also known that oestrogen administration can produce remissions at the time of a relapse after a favourable response to adrenalectomy (Devitt, 1966; Keating, Yone Moto and Byron, 1968) but that it never occurs after hypophysectomy (Lipsett and Bergenstal, 1960; Pearson and Ray, 1959). This is consistent with the hypothesis that prolactin would be the mediator of oestrogen-induced remissions. Oestrogen–prolactin combination can indeed produce mammary tumour regression: this has been demonstrated in an experimental tumour of the rat, tumour R3230AC, as referred to above (Hilf, Bell and Michel, 1967; Hilf et al., 1971). This possibility in human breast cancer is admittedly highly speculative. It cannot be dismissed, however, and is amenable to experimentation.

## PROLACTIN INHIBITION IN THE TREATMENT OF ADVANCED BREAST CANCER

Until the recent introduction of specific bioassays and radioimmunoassays (see Chapter 9), nothing was known about human prolactin and regulation of its secretion. Since then only very little and incomplete data have been published on physiological and pharmacological inhibition of prolactin secretion. Therefore, the writing of this paragraph is somewhat premature and the data presented will be inconclusive. It is likely that much more will be

## TABLE 17.1

Stimulation of Basal Serum Prolactin (HPr)* Levels by Oral Ethinyloestradiol, 1 mg Three Times Daily, in Post-menopausal Women (mU/ml)

| Subject | Baseline | | | After ethinyloestradiol (EO) | | | Statistical significance |
|---|---|---|---|---|---|---|---|
| | Mean ±SE | Period before EO (days) | No. of determinations | Mean ±SE | Period after EO (days) | No. of determinations | |
| G.E. | 573 ±55 | 20 | 9 | 946 ±138 | 8 | 6 | $p < 0.025$ |
| DK.C. | 427 ±26 | 10 | 6 | 1,067 ±123 | 11 | 5 | $p < 0.01$ |
| DS.M. | 90 ±3 | 6 | 5 | 210 ±25 | 9 | 7 | $p < 0.01$ |

After M. L'Hermite and J. C. Heuson, to be published.
* HPr was measured in serum samples collected in the morning by a radioimmunoassay (Midgley and L'Hermite, to be published) extended from the method described by Davis et al., *Biol. Repr.* (1971), **4**, 145.

known at the time when this book is published. Yet it may be worth reviewing the pioneer work that has already been carried out in this field.

The use of inhibitors of prolactin secretion in advanced breast cancer is based on the assumption that prolactin is one of the hormones involved in the maintenance of breast cancer growth. This assumption has been discussed in the preceding paragraph. It is based only on indirect evidence and therefore should be considered as a working hypothesis. At this stage, the use of specific inhibitors may thus serve the double purpose of adding information to the basic problem of the role of prolactin in breast cancer, and offering a new therapeutic approach.

Since the first clinical trials (European Breast Cancer Group, 1972a, b) with potential inhibitors of prolactin secretion were undertaken long before the first information on their actual efficacy as inhibitors in the human was known, the discussion will be presented, for the sake of clarity, in the reverse of the chronological order of the studies.

Among the ergot alkaloids, only 2-Br-α-ergocryptine (CB 154) has been investigated in humans. It was administered to three patients for treatment of non-puerperal galactorrhoea (Lutterbeck et al., 1971). A more or less complete suppression of milk secretion was obtained with doses ranging from 3 to 9 mg daily. Complete cessation of galactorrhoea was achieved by Copinschi et al. (1973) in a male patient suffering from a prolactin-producing pituitary tumour, with CB 154 at doses of 3 to 5 mg daily. In this patient radioimmunoassay determinations showed a progressive decline of the serum prolactin concentration from extremely high levels to nearly normal values. The only data available to us on the effect of CB 154 in normal female subjects were kindly provided by del Pozo and Friesen and are shown in Table 17.2. Prolactin determinations were carried out by the radioimmunoassay method described by Hwang, Guyda and Friesen (1971). These data show that CB 154 given as a single oral dose of 4 mg produced a marked and prolonged decrease in the serum prolactin levels.

TABLE 17.2

Inhibition of Basal Serum Prolactin (HPr) Levels with a Single 4 mg Oral Dose of CB 154 in 4 Normal Women (Normal Range < 30 ng/ml)

| Subject | Baseline | | — | Post-CB 154 | | | |
|---------|----------|------|-----|-------------|-----|-----|-----|
| HSi | 21 | 30·5 | —— 5·2 | 4 | 4 | 4·6 | 6·5 |
| BCl | 30·5 | 23 | —— 6·8 | 4·3 | 9·6 | 8·8 | 9·1 |
| MMa | 34 | 22 | —— 4·4 | 3·8 | 4·1 | 5·0 | 5·7 |
| ILi | 11 | 11·3 | —— 3·6 | 3·0 | 3·2 | 3·4 | 8·0 |
| Time (hours) | − 2 | − 1 | —— 2·5 | 5 | 8 | 12 | 24 |

E. del Pozo and H. Friesen, to be published.

L-dopa is another compound which was recently found to inhibit prolactin secretion in the rat (Donoso et al., 1971) and in man. Malarkey, Jacobs and Daughaday (1971) studied the effect of L-dopa in five patients suffering from non-puerperal galactorrhoea and in five normal pre-menopausal female subjects. Among the galactorrhoeic patients, elevations of serum prolactin measured by radioimmunoassay were found in three patients with pituitary tumours and in one of two patients with functional pituitary disorders. In all five patients oral administration of 0·5 g of L-dopa produced a noticeable fall (70–97 per cent) in serum prolactin within 90 minutes. Administration of 0·5 g four times daily for three days did not achieve a sustained suppression of serum prolactin levels; it was still possible to demonstrate the inhibitory effect of single doses, although dramatic rebound elevations above the base levels were a prominent feature in some cases. One patient received L-dopa in increasing doses up to 3·0 g per day for six weeks. Although single doses still depressed serum prolactin by 48 per cent, the base level remained unchanged and the galactorrhoea persisted. L-dopa produced some decrease in serum prolactin levels in the normal subjects, although evaluation of the effect was obscured by the sensitivity of the assay.

Kleinberg, Noel and Frantz (1971) studied the effect of L-dopa on plasma prolactin, as measured by a bioassay. Ingestion of 0·5 g of L-dopa produced a marked fall in plasma prolactin within one to two hours in four patients shown to have consistently elevated prolactin levels from various causes. The same authors also showed that 0·5 g of L-dopa totally suppressed the elevation of plasma prolactin induced by a single injection of 12·5 to 25 mg of chlorpromazine. Minton and Dickey (1972) measured serum prolactin by radioimmunoassay in a pre-menopausal woman suffering from breast cancer. They found that prolactin fell by 50 per cent after four days on L-dopa given orally at doses of 250 mg every four hours for two days and 500 mg every four hours for the next two days. The same 50 per cent fall occurred within 20 hours after oophorectomy was performed.

The potential therapeutic activity of inhibitors of prolactin secretion in breast cancer has been investigated by the European (EORTC) Breast Cancer Group. An EORTC type I clinical trial of CB 154 (2-Br-α- ergocryptine) was conducted in patients with advanced breast cancer (EBCG, 1972a), according to the protocol of the Group (GECA, 1967). Nineteen post-menopausal patients received increasing oral doses of CB 154 up to 5 mg three times daily for six weeks. None of them showed signs of objective tumour regression. The calculated 95 per cent confidence interval for the rate of CB 154-induced remissions in the population of patients in this study is from 0 to 18 per cent. The probability that CB 154, which was given here at maximum tolerated doses, induces remission is therefore quite small. One may object that the EORTC type I studies, such as this, do not include a control group receiving a treatment of known efficacy, and that therefore one cannot rule out the fact that the patients studied belonged to a highly biased population of poor-risk patients, unlikely to benefit from any treatment. The objection is valid although it can be partly overcome by 'historical' controls.

The European Breast Cancer Group, whose composition has not changed since this study, has recently carried out a type I clinical trial with nafoxidine (U 11, 100 A), an oestrogen antagonist, which induced 8 remissions out of 24 patients (33 per cent) (EBCG, 1972c). Another trial currently in progress conducted by this group compares nafoxidine and ethinyloestradiol on a randomized basis. The number of remissions as yet are 19 out of 50 patients with nafoxidine (38 per cent), and 11 out of 46 patients with ethinyloestradiol (24 per cent) (EBCG, 1972d). These 'historical' controls give a high degree of confidence that the patient population of the Group is not usually grossly biased. Another objection is that the patients were treated for a rather short period of only six weeks which was selected because a majority of patients receiving large doses of CB 154 experienced discomfort from digestive intolerance (nausea, vomiting). In conclusion, there is a high probability that CB 154 is virtually inactive as a treatment for advanced breast cancer, although a controlled trial may appear necessary to reach a definitive conclusion.

The European Breast Cancer Group has completed another clinical trial with a potential inhibitor of prolactin secretion, the cyclic imide 1-(morpholinomethyl)-4-phtalimido-piperidindione-2,6 (CG 603) (EBCG, 1972b). This compound was selected because it was shown to inhibit growth of the DMBA-induced mammary tumour (Mückter, Frankus and Moré, 1969, 1970) and to inhibit prolactin secretion (Gelato, Quadri and Meites, 1972; van der Guchten, 1971) in the rat. Experiments are in progress to study the effect of CG 603 and its derivatives on prolactin secretion in patients (L'Hermite and Heuson, 1973); 23 post-menopausal patients received CG 603 at a dose of 2·0 g daily over a period of six weeks. There was only 1 objective remission (4·3 per cent, 95 per cent confidence interval: 0·1–22·0 per cent). Again, it appears that this compound has little, if any, significant activity in breast cancer. This conclusion is subject to the same limitations as in the CB 154 trial.

Scattered preliminary reports on the use of L-dopa in advanced breast cancer begin to appear in the literature. Stoll (1972) treated seven patients who were over two years post-menopausal with L-dopa at daily oral doses of 0·25, then 0·5 g, four times daily for a period of two months. There was no objective response. However, while still on L-dopa, the patients received, in addition, 1·25 mg of Premarin four times daily for three months. Three patients showed objective regression of their cancer, although they had failed to respond to a three-month treatment with oestrogens, given before L-dopa. These results are of interest, but they are difficult to interpret in terms of prolactin secretion.

Murray, Mozaffarian and Pearson (1972) reported at the Fourth Tenovus Workshop on Prolactin and Carcinogenesis held in Cardiff on March 16–17,

1972, that, out of seven patients with advanced breast cancer who received 0·5 g of L-dopa three times daily, two showed objective regression of their cancer. Dickey and Minton (1972) reported two cases of pre-menopausal women suffering from painful bone metastases from breast cancer, requiring large doses of analgesics. They were treated with 0·25 g, then 0·5 g of L-dopa every four hours with almost immediate complete relief of the bone pains with either the low or the high dosage. Recurrence of bone pain, after a three-week period of treatment, followed its cessation also within a few hours. Re-institution of therapy again resulted in relief of pain.

It would therefore appear from these preliminary reports, that L-dopa has some therapeutic efficacy in breast cancer. The proportion of objective remission of two out of seven, reported by Pearson, is encouraging, although bearing on too small a number of patients to have any statistical meaning. The observation by Dickey and Minton on the rapidity of relief and recurrence of bone pain on commencement and cessation of therapy is puzzling, because if sedation were the result of regression of cancer deposits after a three-week period of treatment, one would not expect the pain to recur almost immediately after cessation of therapy.

These unusual observations, put together with the somewhat paradoxical finding that L-dopa seems to have therapeutic activity in breast cancer while CB 154 does not, although the latter would appear, from the admittedly sparse data available, to be at least as active as the former in inhibiting prolactin secretion, raises the question of the mechanism of action of L-dopa. Effects other than, but possibly concurrent with, prolactin inhibition should be carefully sought.

## CONCLUSION

The DMBA-induced mammary carcinoma of the rat often serves as an experimental model for the human breast cancer. Its growth depends upon various hormones, among which prolactin plays a major role. Whether oestrogens synergize with prolactin to promote growth at the tumour tissue level, or simply stimulate prolactin which in turn enhances tumour growth, has not yet been decided. Tumour growth may be influenced by pharmacological interference with prolactin secretion: stimulation of prolactin secretion by phenothiazine derivatives enhances tumour growth, whereas inhibition of it by ergot alkaloids, cyclic imide derivatives, and possibly oestrogen antagonists depress tumour growth. These observations, besides their fundamental interest, may form the basis of new therapeutic approaches to the treatment of breast cancer.

Some transplantable tumours of the rat behave in the opposite way to the DMBA-induced ones: they regress as a result of increased prolactin stimulation.

Hormone-dependent breast cancer seems to depend upon some hormonal factor from, or mediated by, the pituitary. Unlike in oophorectomized patients, oestrogens fail to reactivate breast cancer after hypophysectomy. Human growth hormone administered in amounts large enough to produce definite anabolic effects is unable to reactivate tumour growth in hypophysectomized patients, whether given with or without oestrogens. Ovine prolactin has no clear-cut effect under similar circumstances. However, critical appraisal of the information available fails to rule out a role of prolactin in breast cancer.

Pituitary stalk section dramatically raises the serum prolactin level, although it induces objective regression of breast cancer. It is conceivable that oestrogen deprivation after stalk section is responsible for the anti-tumour effect of the latter. Minimum levels of both hormones acting together would then be required to sustain breast cancer growth, irrespective of the extent to which individual hormones are stimulated. Administration of 'pharmacological' doses of oestrogens also enhances prolactin secretion. The possibility that high concentrations of prolactin would alone cause tumour regression under such circumstances cannot be entirely dismissed and is amenable to clinical experimentation. The responsiveness of some human breast cancers would then be reminiscent of that of the transplantable rat mammary tumours.

2-Br-α-ergocryptine (CB 154) is an effective inhibitor of prolactin secretion in patients with pathological elevations of serum prolactin, as well as in normal subjects. L-dopa is also effective, although seemingly to a lesser degree. Indeed the available data are too sparse to allow accurate comparison.

An EORTC type I clinical trial of CB 154 at maximum tolerated doses in advanced breast cancer failed to produce any objective tumour regression. This failure suggests that CB 154 is virtually non-active in breast cancer, possibly because depression of prolactin secretion is not deep enough. Critical appraisal of the CB 154 clinical trial indicates that it leaves some doubt as to the complete inefficacy of the drug. Another EORTC clinical trial studied a cyclic imide derivative, CG 603, which inhibits prolactin secretion and mammary tumour growth in the rat. This compound also showed little, if any, activity in advanced breast cancer.

Scattered preliminary reports on the use of L-dopa in advanced breast cancer begin to appear in the literature. Two cases of objective regression have been reported. Relief of bone pains due to metastatic breast cancer has been described; pain sedation occurs within hours of initiation of therapy and vanishes within hours of its cessation. Evaluation of these results raises some questions as to the mechanism of action of L-dopa. A careful search for effects other than, but possibly concurrent with, prolactin inhibition should be pursued.

363

## ACKNOWLEDGMENTS

Part of the author's work described in this paper was supported by a Grant from the Fonds Cancérologique de la Caisse Générale d'Epargne et de Retraite.

The author's department is affiliated to the European Organization for Research on Treatment of Cancer (EORTC) and to the Association Euratom–University of Brussels–University of Pisa.

## REFERENCES

Antony, G. J., van Wyk, J. J., French, F. S., Weaver, R. P., Dugger, G. S., Timmons, R. L. and Newsome, J. F. (1969). 'Influence of pituitary stalk section on growth hormone, insulin and TSH secretion in women with metastatic breast cancer.' *J. clin. Endocr.* **29**, 1238.

Atkins, H. J. B., Falconer, M. A., Hayward, J. L., MacLean, K. S., Schurr, P. H. and Armitage, P. (1960). 'Adrenalectomy and hypophysectomy for advanced cancer of the breast.' *Lancet* **1**, 1148.

Barlow, J. J., Emerson, K. Jnr. and Saxena, B. N. (1969). 'Estradiol production after ovariectomy for carcinoma of the breast.' *New Engl. J. Med.* **280**, 633.

Bern, H. A. and Nandi, S. (1961). 'Recent studies of the hormonal influence in mouse mammary tumorigenesis.' *Progr. expl Tumor Res.* **2**, 90.

Boot, L. M. (1970). 'Prolactin and mammary gland carcinogenesis. The problem of human prolactin.' *Int. J. Cancer* **5**, 167.

Carlson, R. A., Zeilmaker, G. H. and Shelesnyak, J. (1961). 'Termination of early (pre-nidation) pregnancy in the mouse by single injection of ergocormine methanesulphonate.' *J. Reprod. Fert.* **2**, 369.

Cassell, E. E., Meites, J. and Welsch, C. W. (1971). 'Effects of ergocornine and tumors in rats.' *Cancer Res.* **31**, 1051.

Clemens, J. A. and Shaar, C. J. (1972). 'Inhibition by ergocornine of initiation and growth of 7,12-dimethylbenzanthracene-induced mammary tumors in rats: effect of tumor size.' *Proc. Soc. expl Biol. Med.* **139**, 659.

Copinschi, G., L'Hermite, M., Pasteels, J. L. and Robyn, C. (1973). '2-Br-α-ergocryptine (CB 154) inhibition of prolactin secretion and galactorrhoea in a case of pituitary tumor.' Paper presented at the Second International Seminar on Reproductive Physiology and Sexual Endocrinology, Brussels, 1972. Basel; Karger.

Devitt, J. E. (1966). 'Successful estrogen therapy for postadrenalectomy relapses of breast cancer.' *Canad. med. Ass. J.* **94**, 929.

Dickey, R. P. and Minton, J. P. (1972). 'Levodopa relief of bone pain from breast cancer.' *New Engl. J. Med.* **286**, 843.

Donoso, A. O., Bishop, W., McCann, S. M. et al. (1971). 'Effects of alterations in brain monoamine concentrations on plasma prolactin.' Paper presented at the Fifty-third Annual Meeting of the Endocrine Society. San Francisco, June 24–26, 1971.

Dugger, G. S., van Wyk, J. J. and Newsome, J. F. (1958). 'Transection of the hypophyseal stalk in the management of metastatic carcinoma.' *Am. Surg.* **24**, 603.

Ectors, F., Danguy, A. and Pasteels, J. L. (1972). 'Ultrastructure of organ cultures of rat hypophyses exposed to ergocornine.' *J. Endocr.* **52**, 211.

Ehni, G. and Eckles, N. E. (1959). 'Interruption of the pituitary stalk in the patient with mammary cancer.' *J. Neurosurg.* **16**, 628.

European Breast Cancer Group (1972a). 'Clinical trial of 2-Br-α-ergocryptine (CB 154) in advanced breast cancer.' *Europ. J. Cancer* **8**, 387.

— (1972b). 'Clinical trial of the cyclic imide 1-(morpholinomethyl)-4-phtalimido-piperidindione-2, 6 (CG 603) in advanced breast cancer.' *Europ. J. Cancer* **8**, 157.

— (1972c). 'Clinical trial of nafoxidine, an oestrogen antagonist, in advanced breast cancer.' *Europ. J. Cancer* **8**, 387.

— — (1972d). Unpublished.

Flückiger, E. and Wagner, H. R. (1968). '2-Br-α-ergokryptin: Beeinflussung von Fertilität und Laktation bei der Ratte.' *Experientia* **24**, 1130.

Foulds, L. (1967). 'Biology of hormone-dependent tumours.' In *Hormone in Genese und Therapie des Mammacarcinoms*, p. 3. Berlin; Akademie Verlag.

GECA (1967). 'Protocole pour les essais cliniques de traitement des cancers mammaires humains en phase avancée.' *Europ. J. Cancer* **2**, 201.

Gelato, M., Quadri, S. K. and Meites, J. (1972). 'Inhibition of prolactin release by a thalidomide-related compound (CG 603).' *Proc. Soc. expl. Biol. Med.* **140**, 167.

Hayward, J. L. (1972). 'Endocrine therapy of advanced breast cancer.' Paper presented at the Breast Cancer Task Force Treatment Subcommittee, National Cancer Institute, Bethesda, January 31, 1972.

Heuson, J. C., Waelbroeck-Van Gaver, C. and Legros, N. (1970). 'Growth inhibition of rat mammary carcinoma and endocrine changes produced by 2-Br-α-ergocryptine, a suppressor of lactation and nidation.' *Europ. J. Cancer* **6**, 353.

— and Legros, N. (1972). 'Influence of insulin deprivation on growth of the 7,12-dimethylbenz(a)anthracene-induced mammary carcinoma in rats subjected to alloxan diabetes and food restriction.' *Cancer Res.* **32**, 226.

— — and Heimann, R. (1972). 'Influence of insulin administration on growth of the 7,12-dimethylbenz(a)-anthracene-induced mammary carcinoma in intact, oophorectomized, and hypophysectomized rats.' *Cancer Res.* **32**, 233.

— Waelbroeck, C., Legros, N., Gallez, G., Robyn, C. and L'Hermite, M. (1972). 'Inhibition of DMBA-induced mammary carcinogenesis in the rat by 2-Br-α-ergocryptine (CB 154), an inhibitor of prolactin, secretion, and by nafoxidine (U 11,100 A), an estrogen antagonist.' Paper presented at the Second International Seminar on Reproductive Physiology and Sexual Endocrinology, Brussels, 1972. *Gynec. Invest.* **2**, 130.

Hilf, R., Michel, I. and Bell, C. (1967). 'Biochemical responses of normal and neoplastic mammary tissue to hormonal treatment.' *Recent Progr. Hormone Res.* **23**, 229.

— Bell, C. and Michel, I. (1967). 'Influence of the mammotrophic tumor MtTF4 on the growth and biochemistry of the R3230AC mammary carcinoma and mammary glands.' *Cancer Res.* **27**, 482.

— — Goldenberg, H. and Michel I. (1971). 'Effect of fluphenazine HC1 on

R3230AC mammary carcinoma and mammary glands of the rat.' *Cancer res.* **31**, 1111.

Huggins, C., Briziarelli, G. and Sutton, H. Jnr. (1959). 'Rapid induction of mammary carcinoma in the rat and the influence of hormones on the tumors.' *J. expl Med.* **109**, 25.

— Grand, L. C. and Brillantes, F. P. (1961). 'Mammary cancer induced by a single feeding of polynuclear hydrocarbons, and its suppression.' *Nature, Lond.* **189**, 204.

Hwang, P., Guyda, H. and Friesen, H. (1971). 'A radioimmuno-assay for human prolactin.' *Proc. natn Acad., Sci.* **68**, 1902.

Joint Committee on Endocrine Ablative Procedures in Disseminated Mammary Carcinoma (1961). *J. Am. med. Ass.* **175**, 137.

Keating, J. L., Yone Moto, R. H. and Byron, R. L. (1968). 'Cytotoxic drug and hormone therapy after adrenalectomy for advanced breast cancer.' *Surgery Gynec. Obstet.* **127**, 538.

King, R. J. B., Gordon, J. and Steggles, A. W. (1969). 'The properties of a nuclear acidic protein fraction that binds [6, 7-$^3$H] oestradiol–17β.' *Biochem. J.* **114**, 649.

Kleinberg, D. L., Noel, G. L. and Frantz, A. G. (1971). 'Chlorpromazine stimulation and L-dopa suppression of plasma prolactin in man.' *J. clin. Endocr.* **33**, 873.

L'Hermite, M. and Heuson, J. C. (1973). To be published.

Lipsett, M. B. and Bergenstal, D. M. (1960). 'Lack of effect of human growth hormone and ovine prolactin on cancer in man.' *Cancer Res.* **20**, 1172.

Lu, K. H., Amenomori, Y., Chen, C. L. and Meites, J. (1970). 'Effects of central acting drugs on serum and pituitary prolactin levels in rats.' *Endocrinology* **87**, 667.

— Koch, Y. and Meites, J. (1971). 'Direct inhibition by ergocornine of pituitary prolactin release.' *Endocrinology* **89**, 229.

Lutterbeck, P. M., Pryor, J. S., Varga, L. and Wenner, R. (1971). 'Treatment of non-puerperal galactorrhoea with an ergot alkaloid.' *Br. med. J.* **3**, 228.

Lyons, W. R., Li, C. H. and Johnson, R. E. (1958). 'The hormonal control of mammary growth and lactation.' *Recent Progr. Hormone Res.* **14**, 219.

McCalister, A. and Welbourn, R. B. (1962). 'Stimulation of mammary cancer by prolactin and the clinical reponses to hypophysectomy.' *Br. Med. J.* **1**, 1669.

Malarkey, W. B., Jacobs, L. S. and Daughaday, W. H. (1971). 'Levodopa suppression of prolactin in nonpuerperal galactorrhea.' *New Engl. J. Med.* **285**, 1160.

Malven, P. V. and Hoge, W. R. (1971). 'Effect of ergocornine on prolactin secretion by hypophyseal homografts.' *Endocrinology* **88**, 445.

Minton, J. P. and Dickey, R. P. (1972). 'Prolactin, F.S.H. and L.H. in breast cancer: effect of levodopa and oophorectomy.' *Lancet* **1**, 1069.

Mückter, H., Frankus, E. and Moré, E. (1969). 'Experimental therapeutic investigations with 1-(morpholinomethyl)-4-phtalimido-piperidindione-2,6 on dimethylbenzanthracene-induced tumors of Sprague-Dawley rats.' *Cancer Res.* **29**, 1212.

— — — (1970). 'Experimental investigations with 1-(morpholinomethyl)-4-phtalimidopiperidindione-2,6 and drostanolone proprionate in dimethyl-benzanthracene-induced tumors of Sprague-Dawley rats.' *Cancer Res.* **30**, 430.

Murray, R. M. L., Mozaffarian, G. and Pearson, O. H. (1972). 'Prolactin levels with L-dopa treatment in metastatic breast carcinoma.' In *Prolactin and Carcinogenesis*

(4th Tenovus Workshop), p. 158, Ed. by A. R. Boyns and K. Griffiths. Cardiff; Alpha Omega Alpha.

Nagasawa, H. and Meites, J. (1970). 'Suppression by ergocormine and iproniazid of carcinogen-induced mammary tumors in rats; effects on serum and pituitary prolactin levels.' *Proc. Soc. expl Biol. Med.* **135**, 469.

— and Yanai, R. (1970). 'Effects of prolactin or growth hormone on growth of carcinogen-induced mammary tumors of adreno-ovariectomized rats.' *Int. J. Cancer* **6**, 488.

— — (1971). 'Increased mammary gland response to pituitary mammotropic hormones by estrogen in rats.' *Endocrinol. Jap.* **18**, 53.

Pasteels, J. L. and Ectors, F. (1970). 'Mode d'action de l'ergocormine sur la sécrétion de prolactine.' *Arch. Int. Pharmac. Thérapie*, **186**, 195.

— Danguy, A., Frérotte, M. and Ectors, F. (1971). 'Inhibition de la sécrétion de prolactine par l'ergocornine et la 2-Br-α-ergocryptine: action directe sur l'hypophyse en culture.' *Ann. Endocr.* **32**, 188.

Pearson, O. H. (1967). 'Biological problems regarding hormonal surgery.' In *Major Endocrine Surgery for the Treatment of Cancer of the Breast in Advanced Stages*, p. 215, Ed. by M. Dargent and C. Romieu. Lyon; SIMEP.

— and Ray, B. S. (1959). 'Results of hypophysectomy in the treatment of metastatic mammary carcinoma.' *Cancer* **12**, 85.

— West, C. D., Hollander, V. P. and Treves, N. E. (1954). 'Evaluation of endocrine therapy for advanced breast cancer.' *J. Am. med. Ass.* **154**, 234.

— Llerena, O., Llerana, L., Molina, A. and Butler, T. (1969). 'Prolactin-dependent rat mammary cancer: a model for man?' *Trans. Ass. Am. Phycns* **82**, 225.

Quadri, S. K. and Meites, J. (1971). 'Regression of spontaneous mammary tumors in rats by ergot drugs.' *Proc. Soc. expl Biol. med.* **138**, 999.

Shaar, C. J. and Clemens, J. A. (1972). 'Inhibition of lactation and prolactin secretion in rats by ergot alkaloids.' *Endocrinology* **90**, 285.

Shelesnyak, M. C. (1954). 'Ergotoxine inhibition of deciduoma formation and its reversal by progesterone.' *Am. J. Physiol.* **179**, 301.

— (1958). 'Maintenance of gestation of ergotoxine-treatred pregnant rats by exogenous prolactin:' *Acta endocr.* **27**, 99.

Stähelin, H., Burckhardt-Vischer, B. and Flückiger, E. (1971). 'Rat mammary cancer inhibition by a prolactin suppressor, 2-bromo-α-ergokryptine (CB 154).' *Experientia* **27**, 915.

Stoll, B. A. (1972). 'Brain catecholamines and breast cancer: a hypothesis.' *Lancet* **1**, 431.

Takahashi, T. and Simpson, W. L. (1970). 'Hormone responsiveness of the transplanted tumors obtained from DMBA-induced mammary tumors.' *Tohoku J. expl. Med.* **101**, 93.

Terenius, L. (1971). 'Anti-oestrogens and breast cancer.' *Europ. J. Cancer* **7**, 57.

Turkington, R. W., Underwood, L. E. and van Wyk, J. J. (1971). 'Elevated serum prolactin levels after pituitary-stalk section in man.,' *New Engl. J. Med.* **285**, 707.

Van der Guchten, A. A. (1971). 'The effect of 1-(morpholinomethyl)-4-phtalimido-piperidindione-2,6 and drostanolone on the plasma prolactin concentration of oestrone-treated orchidectomized R-Amsterdam rats.' *Europ. J. Cancer* **7**, 581.

367

van Wyk, J. J., Dugger, G. S., Newsome, J. F. and Thomas, P. Z. (1960). 'The effect of pituitary stalk section on the adrenal function of women with cancer of the breast.' *J. clin. Endocr.* **20**, 157.

Welsch, C. W. and Rivera, E. M. (1972). 'Differential effects of estrogen and prolactin on DNA synthesis in organ cultures of DMBA-induced rat mammary carcinoma.' *Proc. Soc. expl Biol. Med.* **139**, 623.

Wuttke, W., Cassell, E. and Meites, J. (1971). 'Effects of ergocornine on serum prolactin and LH, and on hypothalamic content of PIF and LRF.' *Endocrinology* **88**, 737.

Yanai, R. and Nagasawa, H. (1970). 'Suppression of mammary hyperplastic nodule formation and pituitary prolactin secretion in mice induced by ergocornine or 2-bromo-α-ergocryptine.' *J. natn Cancer Inst.* **45**, 1105.

— — (1971). 'Inhibition by ergocornine and 2-Br-α-ergocryptin of spontaneous mammary tumor appearance.' *Experientia* **27**, 934.

Zeilmaker, G. H. and Carlsen, R. A. (1962). 'Experimental studies on the effect of ergocornine methanesulphonate on the luteotrophic function of the rat pituitary gland.' *Acta endocr.* **41**, 321.

# 18

# The Effects of Drugs on Human Hypophysiotrophic Functions

## Lawrence Sherman and Howard D. Kolodny

We have access to all the information of the biosphere, arriving as elementary units in the stream of solar photons. When we have learned how they are rearranged against randomness, to make, say, springtails, quantum mechanics and the late quartets, we may have a clearer notion how to proceed.

Lewis Thomas, 1971

## INTRODUCTION

Advances in understanding neuroendocrine control mechanisms have been spectacular. Alteration of human anterior pituitary function by drugs apparently acting on hypophysiotrophic areas of the hypothalamus has been accomplished in the last decade, and pharmacological control of these areas may be close at hand.

Several of the many clinical conditions associated with abnormal hypothalamic control of the anterior pituitary are already under pharmacological attack. These include non-puerperal galactorrhoea of various origins, and acromegaly and gigantism. Non-hormonal agents that affect hypothalamic function are also being studied for their effects on hormone-dependent tumours, including breast carcinoma.

There is considerable evidence that brain catecholamines play an important role in anterior pituitary function, and that drugs affecting their metabolism affect secretion of anterior pituitary hormones (Chapters 7 and 8; Anton-Tay and Wurtman, 1971; Sherman and Kolodny, 1971). In this chapter we concentrate on agents that affect brain catecholamines and alter anterior pituitary function in man, stressing the hormones most consistently affected by these agents—growth hormone, prolactin, and gonadotrophins. Because these hormones (particularly prolactin) have been suspected of inciting or supporting development of breast carcinoma, discussion of agents altering their secretion is singularly appropriate to this volume.

## EFFECTS ON GROWTH HORMONE

The hypothalamus, by secreting a neurohormone called growth hormone releasing factor (GRF), controls growth hormone release from the anterior pituitary. GRF is one of several hormones synthesized in hypothalamic neurons, secreted in the region of the median eminence into the hypothalamic hypophysio-portal system, and transported to the anterior lobe by passage

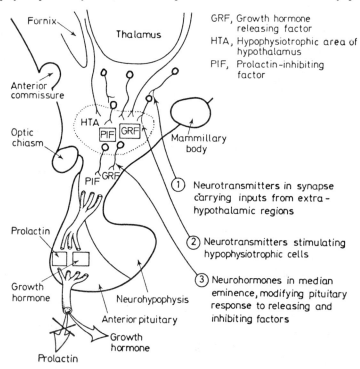

GRF, Growth hormone releasing factor
HTA, Hypophysiotrophic area of hypothalamus
PIF, Prolactin-inhibiting factor

① Neurotransmitters in synapse carrying inputs from extra-hypothalamic regions

② Neurotransmitters stimulating hypophysiotrophic cells

③ Neurohormones in median eminence, modifying pituitary response to releasing and inhibiting factors

*Figure 18.1. Diagram of mid-sagittal section of hypothalamus and pituitary in man, showing some suggested mechanisms controlling secretion of growth hormone and prolactin. Possible sites and modes of action of brain catecholamines are numbered. The recently isolated hypothalamic hormone, growth hormone-release inhibiting factor (GIF), is not shown. Also not shown is thyroid releasing hormone (TRH), which in addition to its action on the thyrotrophic cells of the anterior pituitary, acts as a prolactin releasing factor.*

down the pituitary stalk *(Figure 18.1)*. These hypophysiotrophic hormones are presumably responsible for maintaining normal structure and function of the anterior pituitary. Synthesis and release of most anterior pituitary hormones, including growth hormone, occur primarily in response to stimulatory action of hypophysiotrophic hormones. Specific adrenergic effects on growth hormone secretion have been noted, suggesting direct participation of adrenergic mechanisms in hypothalamic control of growth hormone secretion in man. It is now speculated that norepinephrine (and possibly dopamine) controls the release of GRF, and consequently growth hormone, by stimulating alpha-adrenergic receptors in the hypothalamus (Müller and Pecile, 1968; Müller et al., 1970).

## Chlorpromazine

Results of animal experiments demonstrate that the phenothiazines, widely used as tranquillizers, depress thermoregulatory, pressor and endocrine functions of the hypothalamus (Jarvik, 1970; de Wied, 1967). Among hypothalamic-controlled endocrine functions antagonized by chlorpromazine are secretion of gonadotrophins in intact mice and rats; stress-induced release of ACTH; and the normal inhibitory influence on prolactin and melanocyte-stimulating hormone (de Wied, 1967). The few animal experiments on the effect of chlorpromazine on growth hormone have generally given similar results. Chronic administration of the drug interferes with growth both in mice and rats. This growth retardation may result from inhibition of growth hormone secretion, for repeated injections of growth hormone can overcome the effect (Sulman, 1959; Cranston, 1958). Chlorpromazine alone appears not to affect pituitary growth hormone content in rats, but completely suppresses release of growth hormone after insulin-induced hypoglycaemia (Müller et al., 1967a, b); Müller and Pecile, 1968). This suppression of the growth hormone response to hypoglycaemia is not found when chlorpromazine administration is followed by intracarotid infusion of rat pituitary stalk–median-eminence extracts, believed to contain GRF (Müller et al., 1967a, b). Thus, chlorpromazine seems to suppress growth hormone by acting on the central nervous system, not the anterior pituitary.

Chlorpromazine also decreases serum growth hormone (measured by radioimmunoassay) in man. Benjamin, Casper and Kolodny (1969) found that in patients with galactorrhoea associated with chronic chlorpromazine use, the normal rise in serum growth hormone (HGH) concentration seen four to six hours after an oral glucose load was diminished *(Figure 18.2)*. A later investigation by Sherman et al. (1971) showed that one-week administration of chlorpromazine to normal subjects significantly decreased fasting HGH concentration and attenuated the usual HGH response to hypoglycaemia without inducing lactation *(Figure 18.3)*. Ability of chlorpromazine to blunt

371

the rise in serum HGH produced by hypoglycaemia was confirmed by Mims, Stein and Bethune (1972), who also found that the drug blunted the HGH response to L-dopa. The same group (Mims and Bethune, 1972) used

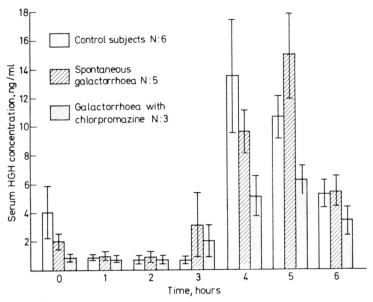

*Figure 18.2. Serum HGH during a six-hour oral glucose tolerance test in six normal women, five women with idiopathic galactorrhoea, and three women with galactorrhoea associated with chronic chlorpromazine therapy. Note suppressed HGH during fasting and at the fourth to sixth hours in this last group. Despite small number of subjects, differences between the chlorpromazine-treated group and the others were significant at the fifth hour (t=2·661, p<0·05 for comparison with control group; t=2·708, p<0·05 for comparison with group with idopathic galactorrhoea) (adapted from data of Benjamin et al., 1969)*

chlorpromazine to reduce or eliminate the normal steep increase in HGH after the onset of sleep.

By what mechanism does chlorpromazine lower blood HGH concentration? Possibilities include alteration of metabolic clearance of serum HGH; induction of a pre-pubertal state by suppression of pituitary gonadotrophins (impairment of HGH responsiveness has been noted in hypogonadal patients); non-specific pituitary suppression; and direct inhibition of hypothalamic growth hormone releasing factor (GRF). The last mechanism seems most likely.

Among drugs active on the CNS, those that interfere with availability of brain catecholamines have been demonstrated to suppress GRF release and, consequently, growth hormone secretion (Müller and Pecile, 1968). Evidence

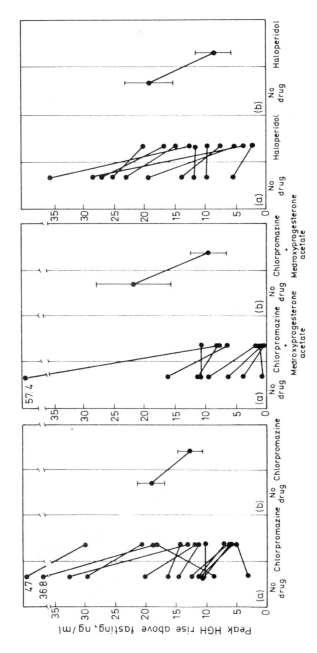

Figure 18.3. Peak serum HGH responses above fasting concentrations in three groups of control subjects. Responses were measured before and at the end of one week of oral administration of chlorpromazine (25 mg q.i.d.), chlorpromazine and medroxprogesterone acetate (10 mg q.i.d.), and haloperidol (2 mg b.i.d.). (a) individual results. (b) Means ± SEM. Decreases noted in peak HGH response above fasting levels were statistically significant for each drug regimen: t = 2·602, p < 0·025 for chlorpromazine; t = 2·572, p < 0·05 for chlorpromazine and medroxyprogesterone acetate; t = 3·890, p < 0·005 for haloperidol. Intergroup differences were not significant

for central anti-adrenergic activity of phenothiazine derivatives is well documented (de Wied, 1967; Bradley et al., 1966; O'Keefe, Sharman and Vogt, 1970; Andén, Carlsson and Haggendal, 1969). The phenothiazines antagonize excitatory actions of norepinephrine (Bradley et al., 1966), and excitatory and inhibitory actions of dopamine (York, 1972), on single neurons in the brain; and influence uptake and release of norepinephrine from brain slices (Bloom and Giarmin, 1968). Chlorpromazine appears to antagonize the action of catecholamines primarily by blocking their receptors. (It may also impair permeability of storage granules to catecholamines.)

This adrenergic receptor blockade hypothesis has been strengthened by x-ray crystallographic analysis of the molecular structures of chlorpromazine and dopamine. Using Dreiding molecular models, Horn and Snyder (1971) found that dopamine, in its solid-state conformation, is superimposable upon a portion of the known x-ray structure of chlorpromazine. *Figure 18.4* shows this similarity of conformation of the two compounds. The authors suggested that chlorpromazine, because of its ability to mimic the conformation of dopamine, may exert some of its clinical effects by interacting with dopamine-related sites and blocking the receptor sites of the catecholamine in areas of the CNS. It is noteworthy that the chlorpromazine–dopamine similarity of conformation applies also to chlorpromazine and norepinephrine, for the x-ray structure of norepinephrine is similar to that of dopamine. It is also noteworthy that molecular models indicate that the butyrophenone, haloperidol, could assume a conformation resembling portions of the phenothiazine molecule (Horn and Snyder, 1971). This would help to account for the central anti-adrenergic activity of haloperidol, and its suppressive effect on serum HGH (Kim et al., 1971).

Chronic hypersecretion of HGH in many cases of gigantism and acromegaly is non-autonomous, and in these cases appears to be under deranged hypothalamic control. Our group studied the effects of chlorpromazine on a small group of acromegalic patients. In two of four patients, a significant suppression of serum HGH was noted, with improvement of the clinical state (Kolodny et al., 1971a, b). Partial suppression of fasting serum HGH by chlorpromazine has also been reported in a child with hypothalamic tumour and gigantism (Fefferman, Costin and Kogut, 1972). Another group treated seven acromegalic patients with chlorpromazine; they found no clinical improvement in any of their patients, and significant HGH suppression in only two (Dimond et al., 1972). We have suggested that drugs able to interfere with the metabolic cycle of brain catecholamines—possibly combinations of drugs acting at different steps in the cycle—might prove effective in treating acromegalics in whom HGH hypersecretion is non-autonomous (Sherman and Kolodny, 1971). Clearly the long-term efficacy of such drug therapy in acromegaly has yet to be demonstrated.

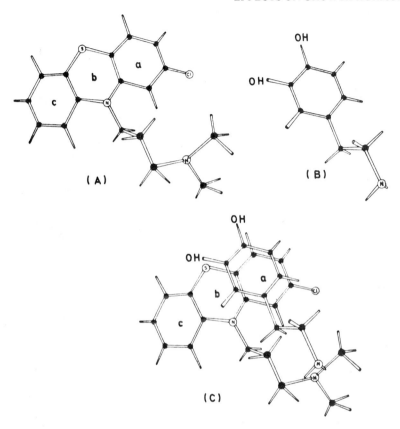

*Figure 18.4. Drawings of Dreiding molecular models of chlorpromazine and dopamine, based on their solid-state conformations established by x-ray crystallography. (A) Chlorpromazine structure. (B) Dopamine structure. (C) Illustration of dopamine superimposed on a portion of the chlorpromazine molecule*
[Reproduced from Horn and Snyder (1971) by courtesy of the Editor of *Proceedings of the National Academy of Sciences*]

## Alpha- and beta-adrenergic stimulating and blocking agents

Soon after the demonstration that hypoglycaemia produced a rapid increase in serum HGH (Roth et al., 1963), it became evident that growth hormone, like ACTH, was a 'stress' hormone. Exercise, physical trauma, psychic stress, electroshock therapy and surgery all caused an increase in serum HGH (Schalch and Reichlin, 1968)—and all were associated with increased

375

catecholamine concentrations in blood and tissue. Experiments were then performed to characterize observed effects on HGH secretion in terms of alpha and beta-adrenergic receptors. It was found that alpha-adrenergic stimulation by intravenous infusion of phenylephrine or methoxamine enhanced HGH secretion and inhibited fat mobilization, while alpha-adrenergic blockade by intravenous infusion of phentolamine inhibited HGH secretion and enhanced fat mobilization (Imura et al., 1971). Conversely, beta-adrenergic stimulation by isoproterenol inhibited, and beta-adrenergic blockade by propranolol enhanced, HGH secretion. Other studies in man (Blackard and Heidingsfelder, 1968) and in baboons (Werrbach et al., 1970) also suggested that alpha-adrenergic activity provoked release of growth hormone, while beta-adrenergic activity blocked such release.

In 1967 Irie et al. reported that a decrease in serum free fatty acid (FFA) concentration might be a potent stimulus for HGH secretion. In 1971 Cryer et al. reported the corollary finding in baboons: a rapid fall in serum growth hormone concentration associated with acute elevation of serum FFA levels induced by intravenous injection of fat and heparin. Because of these findings it is conceivable that central anti-adrenergic agents lower serum HGH levels by first stimulating fat mobilization. There was indeed evidence from the experiments with alpha- and beta-adrenergic stimulating and blocking agents (Blackard and Heidingsfelder, 1968; Imura et al., 1971) that serum HGH and FFA concentrations were inversely related. However, examination of the data reveals that in one experiment phentolamine significantly impaired serum HGH response to a standard infusion of insulin (0·1 units/kg) without increasing serum FFA concentration (Blackard and Heidingsfelder, 1968), and in the other experiment lowered the fasting HGH concentration *before* a rise in serum FFA levels occurred (Imura et al., 1971).

Although acute elevation of FFA concentrations may cause virtual cessation of growth hormone secretion (Cryer et al., 1971), present evidence indicates that central anti-adrenergic agents do not exert their attenuating effects on serum HGH by this peripheral mechanism. Our own experience is in accord with this. Our group has measured serum FFA during insulin tolerance tests in human subjects. Measurements were made before and after treatment for seven days with chlorpromazine or another central anti-adrenergic drug, haloperidol. Both drugs produced significant inhibition of the insulin-induced rise in serum HGH without affecting the FFA response to insulin (unpublished observations). Thus, a more direct effect of anti-adrenergic drugs on central catecholamine metabolism or action, resulting in inhibition of GRF release, still seems likely.

## Reserpine

Reserpine was the first of many alkaloids to be isolated and synthesized from the semi-tropical plant, *Rauwolfia serpentina*. Its sedative and hypotensive actions are well known. In animals, sedation by reserpine is associated with decreased brain levels of norepinephrine, dopamine and serotonin; CNS depression probably results from depletion of norepinephrine. Hypotension results from catecholamine depletion of peripheral structures, including the sympathetic nervous system and blood vessels. Reserpine interferes with intra-neuronal storage of catecholamines, and may decrease norepinephrine synthesis by blocking uptake of dopamine into storage granules containing dopamine-beta-oxidase, the enzyme which catalyses synthesis of norepinephrine from dopamine (Nickerson, 1970).

Müller et al. (1967a) first showed that reserpine suppressed the release of growth hormone (measured by changes in width of tibial epiphyseal cartilage) following insulin-induced hypoglycaemia in rats. They found that the blocking action of the drug did not seem to be exerted at the level of the anterior pituitary, since rats pre-treated with reserpine had normal depletion of pituitary growth hormone content after administration of rat hypothalamic extracts. It had already been shown that systemic administration of reserpine did not decrease catecholamine content in the pituitary itself (Dahlström and Fuxe, 1966).

The suppression by reserpine of the growth hormone response to hypoglycaemia seems to be due to the drug's catecholamine-depleting effect on the hypothalamus (or neurons controlling its hypophysiotrophic functions), and not its depressive effect on the CNS generally. Two lines of evidence support this contention: (1) some drugs that interfere with brain catecholamine metabolism (alpha-methyl-meta-tyrosine, alpha-methyldopa, tetrabenzine) suppress growth hormone responses to hypoglycaemia without depressing the CNS (Müller et al., 1967b; Müller and Pecile, 1968); (2) diazepam, a drug that acts on the limbic system and the reticular formation of the brain stem, and depresses the CNS, has been shown to have no effect on the growth hormone response to hypoglycaemia in man (Havard et al., 1972). The diazepam study informs us that it would be dangerous to assume that every sedative affects hypophysiotrophic functions.

The effects of reserpine on growth hormone have now been demonstrated in man by Cavagnini and Peracchi (1971). High doses of the drug (6 mg daily in two divided doses) for five days resulted in suppression of the serum HGH response to hypoglycaemia, but not arginine. The results are in accord with the idea that the central adrenergic system is essential for normal growth hormone response to hypoglycaemia, but is not involved in the response to arginine (Strauch, Modigliani and Bricaire, 1969). The results also suggest that the suppressive action of reserpine on growth hormone occurs at a central, not a peripheral, level.

## Haloperidol

Prototype of the butyrophenone group of anti-schizophrenic drugs, haloperidol is similar to chlorpromazine in being a tertiary amine compound that antagonizes the action of catecholamines in the central and peripheral nervous systems. Like chlorpromazine, it depresses the hypothalamus, as measured by an increase in lobulo-alveolar development of the mammary gland and decrease in body temperature (Mishkinsky et al., 1969). There have been few reports on the endocrine effects of haloperidol (Boris, Milmore and Trimal, 1970; Brown, 1971). Recently, our group reported significant attenuation of the serum HGH response to insulin from short-term (one week) therapy with haloperidol in ten normal subjects (Kim et al., 1971). Peak serum HGH concentration above the fasting level following rapid insulin infusion (highest concentration minus fasting concentration) was substantially reduced after the haloperidol treatment period in eight subjects. The mean peak response was $19.4 \pm 2.89$ ng/ml before, and $9.12 \pm 1.90$ ng/ml after haloperidol treatment. This difference was highly significant. Overall results of measuring the peak serum HGH were strikingly similar to those obtained with chlorpromazine *(Figure 18.3)*.

The known pharmacological effects of haloperidol suggest that the drug antagonizes excitatory actions of brain catecholamines by receptor site blockade (possibly within the hypothalamus), thus inhibiting release of GRF. Haloperidol has definite central anti-adrenergic activity. It reduces the concentration of norepinephrine and dopamine in the rat diencephalon and telencephalon (Abuzzahab, 1971), and reduces the dopamine content of the dog caudate nucleus (Himwich et al., 1970) and the mouse corpus striatum (O'Keefe, Sharman and Vogt, 1970). Its effects on hypothalamic catecholamine metabolism and on hypothalamic GRF depletion are largely unknown. A direct effect of haloperidol on the anterior pituitary or on peripheral growth hormone metabolism, resulting in lowered serum HGH, cannot be excluded.

Our group is presently studying the effects of this drug on serum HGH in acromegalic patients.

## L-Dopa (L-3,4-dyhydroxyphenylalanine)

L-dopa, precursor of the catecholamine dopamine, has been demonstrated to cross the blood–brain barrier when given peripherally (Hornykiewicz, 1970), and has been widely used to treat patients with Parkinson's disease. (The caudate nucleus, putamen, and substantia nigra of these patients are deficient in dopamine.) In the mammalian brain, catecholamines are normally concentrated in the basal ganglia, the hypothalamus, and midbrain areas exercising possible influence over hormone secretion by the anterior pituitary

(Anton-Tay and Wurtman, 1971). Experimental evidence linking brain catecholamines to growth hormone secretion (Müller et al., 1967a, b, 1970; Werrbach et al., 1970; Imura et al., 1971), and the clinical availability of L-dopa, have provided an opportunity to study the effect of this catecholamine precursor on growth hormone in man.

An increase in serum HGH following acute oral L-dopa administration was first demonstrated in patients with Parkinson's disease (Boyd, Lebovitz and Pfeiffer, 1970), and soon afterwards in normal subjects (Kansal, Talbert and Buse, 1971). In both groups a peak rise in serum HGH, unaccompanied by changes in blood glucose concentration, occurred 60–120 minutes after drug administration. In another study, the magnitude of the HGH response was dose-related for amounts of L-dopa between 250 mg and 1 g (Eddy et al., 1971). The rise in serum HGH could be attentuated, delayed or abolished by the simultaneous infusion of phentolamine (Kansal, Talbert and Buse, 1971). This suggests that L-dopa promotes HGH release through a mechanism requiring alpha-adrenergic stimulation. Although hypoglycaemia produces a rise in serum HGH by stimulating hypothalamic catecholamine activity, L-dopa reportedly fails to potentiate the serum HGH response to insulin infusion (Van Loon, 1971).

Mims, Stein and Bethune (1972), while confirming the rise in serum HGH after a single dose of L-dopa in normal subjects, found 'no such response' in patients with acromegaly. Our group found that a single oral dose (500 mg) of L-dopa caused a paradoxical decrease of greater than 50 per cent in serum HGH concentration in five of seven acromegalic patients 30–90 minutes after administration of the drug (Sherman et al., 1972). This again emphasizes the frequently non-autonomous nature of HGH hypersecretion, coupled with deranged hypothalamic control, in acromegaly; and suggests that in this disease acutely raised levels of brain catecholamines may inhibit secretion of GRF (the reverse of the normal state), and cause blood levels of HGH to be suppressed.

## EFFECTS ON PROLACTIN

Hypothalamic control of prolactin secretion, unlike that of most hormones of the anterior pituitary, is inhibitory *(Figure 18.1)*. Experimental evidence reviewed elsewhere (Chapters 1–3; Meites and Nicoll, 1966; Pasteels, 1970; McCann et al., 1972) supports the notion that prolactin release in mammals is restrained (though not completely inhibited) by the hypothalamus, and the restraint eliminated when hypothalamic control is removed. Induction of hyperprolactinaemia in patients after pituitary-stalk section demonstrates this effect in man (Turkington, Underwood and van Wyk, 1971). A remarkable finding is that plasma prolactin in man is increased by a number of stressful stimuli—including elective surgery, vigorous exercise and psychic stress (Noel et al., 1972; Friesen et al., 1972b)—that are also known to elevate serum HGH. The demonstration that hypoglycaemia, induced by rapid infusion of 0·2 units/kg of insulin in seven normal subjects, produced a five fold increase in plasma prolactin in every subject is equally remarkable (Noel et al., 1972). These results forcefully remind us that present knowledge of the role of brain catecholamines and the hypothalamus in restraining release of prolactin is incomplete.

After many years of uncertainty, it is now clear that prolactin in man exists as a hormone distinct from growth hormone (Frantz and Kleinberg, 1970; Forsyth and Myres, 1971; Hwang et al., 1971; Sherwood, 1971; Turkington, 1971a; Friesen, 1972). Although human prolactin has only recently been isolated, and its polypeptide structure only partly characterized, sensitive bioassays and heterologous and homologous radioimmunoassays have permitted its determination in normal and pathological states (Friesen, 1972; Turkington, 1972f; Forsyth and Edwards, 1972).

Blood levels of human prolactin, measured by radioimmunoassay methods, are detectable throughout life in both sexes. Physiological hyperprolactinaemia occurs in foetal life and early infancy, and in women during pregnancy and the immediate post-partum period (Forsyth and Edwards, 1972; Friesen, 1972). Elevated serum prolactin concentration has been reported in several conditions, and is sometimes, but not always, associated with abnormal lactation. These conditions include: (1) prolonged post-partum lactation (Frantz and Kleinberg, 1970; Malarkey, Jacobs and Daughaday, 1971); (2) idiopathic galactorrhoea (Forsyth et al., 1971); Turkington, 1972d); (3) pituitary and hypothalamic tumours associated with galactorrhoea (Malarkey, Jacobs and Daughaday, 1971; Friesen et al., 1972a; Turkington, 1972b); (4) about 20–30 per cent of 'non-functioning' chromophobe pituitary tumors (Friesen, 1972); (5) disseminated sarcoidosis (Turkington and MacIndoe, 1972); and (6) administration of certain drugs (Forsyth et al., 1971; Turkington, 1972e). Hyperprolactinaemia is not found, however, in patients with gynaecomastia unassociated with drug therapy (Turkington, 1972a).

Common to some of these states, it is thought, is a hypothalamic defect that prevents the normal release of the neurohormone, prolactin-inhibiting factor (PIF), and allows increased secretion of prolactin by the anterior pituitary. Turkington and MacIndoe (1972), reporting a group of patients with disseminated sarcoidosis and hyperprolactinaemia, noted one in whom autopsy revealed bilateral sarcoid granulomata in the median eminence and other hypothalamic centres, without granulomatous invasion of the anterior pituitary. These findings support the concept of hypothalamic defects that may prevent release of PIF and ultimately produce hyperprolactinaemia.

Ectopic prolactin production, independent of hypothalamic mechanisms, has also been reported by Turkington (1971b) in one patient with bronchogenic carcinoma and another with hypernephroma.

The physiological, pathological and pharmacological causes of human hyperprolactinaemia are listed in Table 18.1.

TABLE 18.1

Causes of Human Hyperprolactinaemia

(I) *Physiological*
   (A) Pregnancy (steady rise, peak just before delivery)
   (B) Post-partum
      (1) Non-nursing mothers, up to four weeks
      (2) Nursing mothers, same; suckling induces marked but transient increases during next three months
   (C) Breast stimulation in non-post-partum women
   (D) Foetal life
   (E) Early infancy
   (F) Stress: anaesthesia, surgery, exercise, acute anxiety
   (G) Hypoglycaemia


(II) *Pathological*
   (A) Hypothalamic disorders
      (1) Chiari–Frommel syndrome: pathologically prolonged post-partum lactation
      (2) Ahumada–Del Castillo syndrome: idiopathic galactorrhoea
      (3) Hypothalamic tumours: craniopharyngioma, ectopic pinealoma, metastatic tumours
      (4) Post-resection of craniopharyngioma (in children with normal or accelerated growth rates despite decreased growth hormone)
      (5) Disseminated sarcoidosis
   (B) Prolactin-secreting pituitary tumours
      (1) Forbes–Albright syndrome: pituitary tumour with galactorrhoea and (usually) amenorrhoea
      (2) Acromegaly (infrequent)
      (3) Nelson's syndrome: pituitary tumour following bilateral adrenalectomy for Cushing's syndrome
      (4) 'Non-functioning' chromophobe adenoma (20–30 per cent of cases)
   (C) Surgical transection of pituitary stalk
   (D) Primary hypothyroidism with pituitary prolactin secretion stimulated by increased secretion of thyrotrophin-releasing factor of hypothalamus
   (E) Chronic renal failure
   (F) Ectopic prolactin production by tumours
      (1) Bronchogenic carcinoma
      (2) Hypernephroma
   (G) Irritative lesions of the chest wall
      (1) Herpes zoster
      (2) Chest surgery
      (3) Trauma to intercostal nerves

*Continued*

TABLE 18.1 *(Cont.)*

(III) *Pharmacological*
    (A) Psychotropic drugs
        (1) Phenothiazines: chlorpromazine, fluphenazine, promazine, perphenazine
        (2) Tricyclic anti-depressant: amitryptyline, nortriptyline,m imipramine
        (3) Reserpine
        (4) Butyrophenones: haloperidol (Note: psychotropic drugs *without* effect on serum
            prolactin include lithium carbonate and chlordiazepoxide)
    (B) Anti-hypertensive drugs
        (1) Reserpine
        (2) Alpha-methyldopa
    (C) After discontinuance of oral contraceptives
    (D) Oestrogen therapy
    (E) Injection of thyrotrophin-releasing factor

## Chlorpromazine

It has long been known that chronic chlorpromazine therapy may be complicated by galactorrhoea. This complication occurs most often in women of child-bearing age who have never previously lactated (Apostolakis et al., 1972). Like other phenothiazines, the drug stimulates lobulo-alveolar development of the mammary gland in experimental animals (Sulman, 1970). Brain implantation with phenothiazine derivatives has shown that this mammotrophic effect occurs only with implantation in the median eminence region; no such effect has been noted with implantation outside the hypothalamus—including the pituitary gland.

It was therefore suspected that chlorpromazine administration in man resulted in increased pituitary secretion, and elevated serum levels, of prolactin. This suspicion was confirmed when sustained increases in prolactin levels were found in psychiatric patients chronically treated with chlorpromazine and other phenothiazine derivatives, including fluphenazine, promazine and perphenazine (Frantz and Kleinberg, 1970; Kleinberg and Frantz, 1971; Turkington, 1972e). Chronicity of phenothiazine therapy is not essential for sustained hyperprolactinaemia. Turkington (1972e) showed in two healthy volunteers who ingested 4 mg of perphenazine every eight hours for three days that serum prolactin levels remained elevated for ten days after cessation of the drug.

Noteworthy in the studies of patients on long-term phenothiazine treatment was the presence of elevated serum prolactin concentrations even in patients without galactorrhoea. Thus, the stimulus of hyperprolactinaemia alone is insufficient to produce inappropriate lactation. As in physiological lactation, other hormonal factors are required. A fall in oestradiol concentration precedes initiation of normal post-partum lactation; inhibition of pituitary

382

gonadotrophins, producing such a fall, may be necessary to permit lactation in patients with hyperprolactinaemia associated with ingestion of phenothiazines. The complexity of the prolactin–galactorrhoea relationship is underscored by reports of rare patients with galactorrhoea (particularly those with normal menses) whose prolactin levels were in the normal range (Kleinberg and Frantz, 1971; Forsyth and Edwards, 1972). Although hyperprolactinaemia is a frequent stimulus to galactorrhoea, it is not absolutely essential for its occurrence.

It has now been demonstrated that serum prolactin can be elevated acutely by a single intramuscular injection of chlorpromazine (Kleinberg, Noel and Frantz, 1971; Turkington, 1972c; Friesen et al., 1972a). Turkington (1972c) has taken advantage of this to develop a phenothiazine stimulation test for prolactin reserve *(Figure 18.5),* and has already demonstrated cases of isolated prolactin deficiency in women who failed to lactate in the puerperium. The acute elevation of serum prolactin produced by chlorpromazine can be prevented by L-dopa pre-treatment (Kleinberg, Noel and Frantz, 1971), a finding consistent with the opposing actions of these drugs on brain catecholamines.

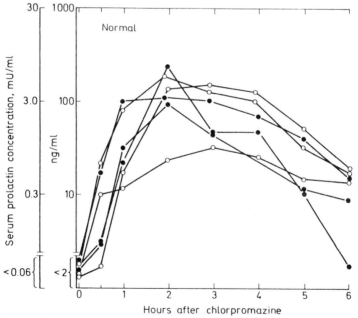

*Figure 18.5. Serum prolactin response to an intramuscular injection of chlorpromazine (50 mg) in six normal subjects. Open circles, women; closed circles, men*

[Reproduced from Turkington (1972c) by courtesy of the Editor of *Journal of Clinical Endocrinology*]

Prolactin has been implicated in mammary tumorigenesis (Mühlbock and Boot, 1959; Welsch, Clemens and Meites, 1969; Welsch, Jenkins and Meites, 1970). The observed stimulatory effect of the phenothiazines on this hormone is disturbing, in view of the use of these drugs in women with breast carcinoma—indeed, in view of their use in otherwise normal women who may be at risk. The relative infrequency of alerting symptoms (galactorrhoea, amenorrhoea) in patients with chronic hyperprolactinaemia associated with phenothiazine therapy adds a potentially sinister note to the problem of prolactin and mammary tumorigenesis.

### Reserpine

In 1970 Lu et al. showed that, in rats, a single intraperitoneal injection of reserpine produced a marked increase in serum prolactin concentration, while reducing pituitary prolactin content. Since reserpine had been shown to inhibit catecholamine activity in the hypothalamus by interfering with storage and possibly inducing depletion, and was reported to decrease hypothalamic PIF, the authors concluded that the observed stimulation of pituitary prolactin release by reserpine may have been due to interference with catecholamine—and therefore PIF—activity. At about the same time other investigators, working with *in vitro* preparations of rat pituitary after injection of reserpine into the living animal, found marked increases in synthesis and release of prolactin (MacLeod, Fontham and Lehmeyer, 1970). The net effect of reserpine on prolactin, in these animal studies in which the hormone was measured directly, was stimulation of secretion by the anterior pituitary.

Sulman (1970) reviewed the pertinent endocrine effects of reserpine and its derivatives, and noted that these drugs interfere with oestrus cycles in mice, inhibit ovulation and menstruation in monkeys, and stimulate mammary development and lactation in rats and rabbits.

Endocrinological effects in man have also been reported (McCann et al., 1972). Reserpine has mammotrophic and lactogenic effects in women, inhibits the ovarian cycle and menstruation, and has occasionally been associated with development of gynaecomastia in man (Sulman, 1970; Jarvik, 1970). Markedly increased serum prolactin levels in hypertensive patients taking reserpine for two to six weeks have been reported; untreated patients had normal levels (Turkington, 1972e).

### Alpha-methyldopa

For over a decade alpha-methyldopa (L-dopa-methyl-3,4-dihydroxy-phenylalanine) has served as a useful drug in treating essential hypertension. An effective inhibitor of dopa decarboxylase, it partially blocks synthesis of dopamine and norepinephrine and decreases the concentrations of these catecholamines in the CNS and peripheral tissues. Prolonged depression of norepinephrine in the CNS may reflect displacement by alpha-methylnorepinephrine, a metabolic product of alpha-methyldopa. This metabolite can be released at synapses by neural stimulation, and then act as a false neuro-transmitter.

Rare cases of galactorrhoea induced in women by alpha-methyldopa have been reported. In one patient both galactorrhoea and extra-pyramidal signs appeared during use of the drug (Vaidya et al., 1970), indicating that relative catecholamine deficiencies in both the hypothalamus and corpus striatum were produced by the drug. Galactorrhoea, cogwheel rigidity and tremor regressed and disappeared after cessation of alpha-methyldopa treatment. In Turkington's study (1972e) of hypertensive patients, all those placed on alpha-methyldopa for two to six weeks had markedly increased serum prolactin levels, while untreated patients had normal levels. Thus, alpha-methyldopa joins other central anti-adrenergic agents on the list of drugs demonstrated in humans to produce hyperprolactinaemia and, in some cases, galactorrhoea.

## Haloperidol

The mammotrophic effects of haloperidol and other butyrophenones have been reviewed in detail elsehwere (Mishkinsky et al., 1969; Sulman, 1970). It is believed that the drug stimulates prolactin secretion by blocking brain catecholamine stimulation of PIF release in the hypothalamus. Although hyperprolactinaemia and galactorrhoea are possible side-effects of haloperidol at high dosage levels, measurement of serum prolactin in patients on long-term therapy has not yet been reported. Experiments with parenteral administration of haloperidol to demonstrate possible acute changes in serum prolactin, akin to those performed with chlorpromazine (Kleinberg, Noel and Frantz, 1971; Turkington, 1972c), are also yet to be done.

## Tricyclic anti-depressants

Although they are phenothiazine analogues, imipramine, desipramine, amitryptyline, and nortryptyline (called tricyclic because of their triple ring structure) have no effect on agitated psychotic patients. Instead, they have clinical use as anti-depressants. Like the phenothiazines, however, they cause galactorrhoea in some patients, and produce hyperprolactinaemia even in asymptomatic subjects.

The mechanism of action of these drugs in depression is unknown, but may be related to their potentiation of CNS noradrenergic transmission or their anti-cholinergic action. Neither activity would explain the ability of the tricyclic anti-depressants to increase serum prolactin concentration. This ability may result from their potent inhibition of CNS dopamine synthesis. Experiments in which the rate of conversion of $^3$H-tyrosine to $^3$H-dopa have been estimated demonstrate that this inhibition occurs at this first step in catecholamine synthesis (Glowinski, 1970). Since dopamine may play a role as a neuro-transmitter inducing PIF secretion, potent inhibitors of dopamine synthesis, such as the tricyclic anti-depressants, might be expected to provoke prolactin release—providing they affect dopaminergic transmission in the hypothalamus.

Turkington (1972e) measured serum prolactin concentration in ten patients given imipramine hydrochloride (50 mg every eight hours) and ten given amitryptyline hydrochloride (25 mg every eight hours) for two to four weeks. Every patient developed hyperprolactinaemia. Hyperprolactinaemia was also found in a patient who developed galactorrhoea while on chronic treatment with nortryptyline hydrochloride, 25 mg three times a day. Serum prolactin levels returned to normal two weeks after the drug was stopped. Interestingly, five patients receiving lithium carbonate for manic disorders had normal serum prolactin levels: lithium has no effect on the CNS content of dopamine. The results of these experiments demonstrate that drugs capable of inhibiting CNS dopamine synthesis, release or action, are capable of producing hyperprolactinaemia.

## L-Dopa

Acute elevation of brain dopamine depresses serum prolactin in rats (Kamberi, Mical and Porter, 1971). DL-alpha-methyltyrosine, which blocks catecholamine synthesis at the rate-limiting steps of tyrosine conversion to dopa, produces a dramatic increase in plasma prolactin with 30 minutes after being injected intraperitoneally into castrated rats. It also produces continued high plasma levels of the hormone when injected regularly for several days. L-dopa administration bypasses this block in catecholamine synthesis, and marked reduction of plasma prolactin results (Donoso et al., 1971). The ability of L-dopa to decrease plasma prolactin levels is still present when conversion of dopamine to norepinephrine is selectively blocked by prior administration of diethyldithiocarbamate (Donoso et al., 1971), providing further support for the notion that dopamine plays an important role as a transmitter causing suppression of prolactin secretion—possibly by facilitating release of PIF, or by direct action on the anterior pituitary, or both (Birge et al., 1970; McCann et al., 1972).

These data from rat experiments show that prolactin secretion is inhibited by the increase in brain dopamine produced by L-dopa administration. This is the basis for testing the effects of L-dopa on human prolactin.

A single oral dose of 500 mg of L-dopa in women with galactorrhoea and elevated serum concentrations of prolactin has resulted in satisfactory lowering of the serum levels within 90 to 240 minutes. In normal women with measurable serum prolactin, serum prolactin levels have also been lowered (Malarkey, Jacobs and Daughaday, 1971; Turkington, 1972d; Friesen et al.,

1972a). In addition, chronic L-dopa administration has resulted in suppression of hyperprolactinaemia *(Figure 18.6)*, alleviation of non-puerperal galactorrhoea, increase in measurable urinary gonadotrophins, and return of cyclic menstruation in women (Turkington, 1972d). Amenorrhoea and

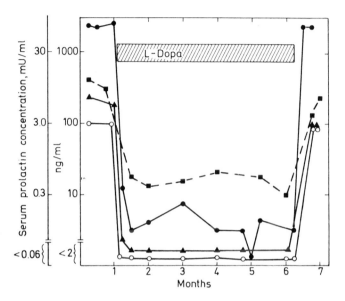

Figure 18.6. *Effect of continuous L-Dopa therapy (500 mg orally every six hours) on serum prolactin levels in four patients with idiopathic galactorrhoea. The drug was given over a five-month period* [Reproduced from Turkington (1972d) by courtesy of the Editor of *Journal of Clinical Endocrinology*]

galactorrhoea recur when the drug is stopped after as much as six months of continuous therapy.

Using L-dopa, Malarkey, Jacobs and Daughaday (1971) succeeded in lowering serum prolactin in three women with galactorrhoea associated with prolactin-secreting pituitary tumours (Forbes–Albright syndrome). A marked decrease in serum prolactin occurred 120 to 240 minutes after oral administration of 500 mg of the drug. If L-dopa, after conversion to dopamine, exerted its prolactin-suppressive effect in these patients by promoting secretion of PIF, the results suggest that at least some prolactin-secreting pituitary tumours retain their ability to respond to certain physiological stimuli—that is, some of these tumours are not autonomous. Then, as the authors suggest, 'the possibility exists that prolactin-secreting tumours result from prolonged prolactin hypersecretion secondary to disordered hypothalamic regulation.' The same range of testing techniques that revealed unsuspected non-autonomy in acromegaly can now be used in the Forbes–Albright syndrome. These include stressful stimuli and hypoglycaemia (Noel et al., 1972; Friesen et al., 1972b), central anti-adrenergic agents (Kleinberg, Noel and Frantz, 1971; Turkington, 1972c), and perhaps oral glucose loading.

## Ergot alkaloids

The ergot alkaloids are best known clinically as cranial vasoconstrictors and stimulators of uterine motility. Studies in rats showing that ergot compounds inhibit nidation and lactation—and that prolactin administration reverses these effects—have suggested that these alkaloids inhibit prolactin secretion (Shaar and Clemens, 1972). By use of a radioimmunoassay method specific for rat prolactin, several investigators have shown that various ergot alkaloids—ergocornine, ergonovine, ergotamine, and ergocryptine—are potent inhibitors of prolactin secretion (Wuttke, Cassell and Meites, 1971; Nasr and Pearson, 1971; Shaar and Clemens, 1972). A single subcutaneous injection of 0·25 to 1 mg of alkaloid resulted in complete suppression of serum prolactin levels in the rat, beginning at one hour and lasting 24 hours (Nasr and Pearson, 1971).

In one experiment, pituitary halves incubated *in vitro* with hypothalamic extract from ergocornine-treated rats released less prolactin than corresponding pituitary halves incubated with hypothalamic extract from untreated rats (Wuttke, Cassell and Meites, 1971), suggesting that hypothalamic PIF was increased by prior ergot treatment. In another experiment, hypophysectomized, pituitary-grafted rats pre-treated with ergonovine had lower serum prolactin levels than similarly treated rats without ergonovine pre-treatment (Shaar and Clemens, 1972). This indicated that ergot alkaloids acted directed on the anterior pituitary to prevent prolactin secretion. In a study of similarly prepared rats and rat anterior pituitary *in vitro,* Lu, Koch and Meites (1971) also found that ergonovine inhibited prolactin release by direct action on the pituitary. (These authors noted, in addition, that the drug counteracted the stimulatory action of oestrogen on prolactin secretion.) Thus, there is evidence that ergot compounds depress prolactin release and lower serum prolactin both by stimulating secretion of hypothalamic PIF and by direct inhibition of the pituitary.

After finding that there was a reduction in the number and granulation of acidophils in the anterior pituitaries of rats treated with ergonovine, Quadri, Lu and Meites (1972) demonstrated that both this ergot drug and ergocornine inhibited the growth of a rat pituitary tumour (MtW 15) known to secrete large quantities of prolactin and growth hormone. Prolactin secretion by the tumour was also inhibited. Since the rats were carrying the tumour as transplants unconnected to the hypothalamus, inhibition of tumour growth was independent of any action on the hypothalamus. Lehmeyer and MacLeod

(1972) also found that ergot alkaloids suppressed growth of prolactin-secreting tumours and decreased serum prolactin in rats, and reported similar results with another plant alkaloid, vincristine.

Although the effect of ergot alkaloids on human prolactin-secreting tumours has not (at this moment) been determined, two groups have used these drugs on patients with non-puerperal galactorrhoea. Lutterbeck et al. (1971) treated three women with 2-bromo-alpha-ergocryptine, using up to 9 mg daily in three divided doses. Galactorrhoea and mammary discomfort disappeared or improved considerably in the patients; dizziness, nausea and vomiting (mild acute ergotism?) appeared with higher doses. Serum prolactin levels were not measured. Lawrence and Hagen (1972) used ergonovine maleate, 0·2 mg three times a day to treat four women with non-puerperal galactorrhoea. They chose this ergot drug because it is negligibly vasoactive and unlikely to cause symptoms of peripheral vascular ischaemia due to intense vasoconstriction of blood vessels (chronic ergotism). Although serum prolactin concentrations were not measured, galactorrhoea disappeared in all patients within three months. Three of the previously amenorrhoeic women became pregnant, one after 19 years of amenorrhoea associated with galactorrhoea. Two successfully nursed and weaned their babies without recurrence of galactorrhoea. Nor did galactorrhoea return with discontinuation of ergonovine therapy. This contrasts favourably with the prompt recurrence of abnormal lactation and amenorrhoea after cessation of chronic L-dopa treatment for non-puerperal galactorrhoea (Turkington, 1972d).

Ergocornine and ergocryptine are potent anti-adrenergic drugs, but have other central and peripheral actions (Wuttke, Cassell and Meites, 1971). Indeed, their prolactin-lowering effect cannot logically be explained by any central anti-adrenergic action, since drugs with this action have been shown to stimulate prolactin release and raise serum prolactin.

## EFFECTS ON GONADOTROPHINS

Coppola (1971) has written that 'control of the involuntary act of mammalian gonadotropin secretion can be considered as one of the most important responsibilities of the autonomic nervous system', since continuity of the species depends on this secretion. Carrying the brunt of this responsibility for the autonomic nervous system are the central adrenergic fibres of its sympathetic division. It now appears that secretion of follicle-stimulating hormone (FSH) and luteinizing hormone (LH) is stimulated by a hypothalamic tonus which simultaneously restrains prolactin release (see Chapters 1 and 2).

The effect of altered brain catecholamine function on gonadotrophins has been extensively studied in the laboratory (Meyerson and Sawyer, 1968; Schneider and McCann, 1969; Kordon and Glowinski, 1969). Administration of potent central anti-adrenergic agents, including chlorpromazine, reserpine, alpha-methyldopa and tetrabenazine, results in suppression of LH release in the rat. Interestingly, in one experiment, when alpha-methyldopa was injected into the medio-basal part of the infundibulum of the rat, LH release was suppressed by a dose $2 \cdot 5 \times 10^{-5}$ of that required to achieve suppression by peripheral injection (Kordon, 1971). No effect on ovulation was noted with injections of alpha-methyldopa into other areas of the hypothalamus, nor into the pituitary. Pre-treatment, or simultaneous treatment, with monoamine oxidase inhibitors—which maintain or elevate brain catecholamine levels—prevented the drugs from suppressing LH secretion by the anterior pituitary.

Evidence of antagonism between gonadotrophin and prolactin secretion is not lacking. Amenomori, Chen and Meites (1970) observed a decline in pituitary and plasma prolactin levels after ovariectomy in rats; Ben-David, Dannon and Sulman (1971), noting the uninhibited secretion of FSH and LH that occurs in animals after ovariectomy, used a non-steroidal gonadotrophin-suppressor, methallibure, to test whether suppression of gonadotrophins by the drugs resulted in a reciprocal increase in serum prolactin in ovariectomized rats. They found that sufficient doses (20 mg/kg or more) of methallibure definitely increased serum prolactin levels. Their results further suggested that the greater the gonadotrophin suppression, the more potent the prolactin stimulation. Ben-David, Dannon and Sulman (1971) also showed that suppression of gonadotrophin hypersecretion permitted the pituitary to secrete large amounts of prolactin when the rats were challenged with injections of perphenazine.

Antagonism between gonadotrophin and prolactin secretion also exists in man. Most patients with galactorrhoea associated with hyperprolactinaemia have amenorrhoea. Serum gonadotrophin levels, normally increased by clomiphene administration, may remain unchanged in these patients. Besser et al. (unpublished observations quoted in Forsyth and Edwards, 1972) successfully exploited this gondotrophin–prolactin relationship. They used an ergot derivative, 2-bromo-alpha-ergocryptine, to suppress serum prolactin and restore the normal LH response to clomiphene.

There is little direct information on the effect of central anti-adrenergic or adrenergic drugs on gonadotrophins in humans. Amenorrhoea sometimes accompanies galactorrhoea in women treated with drugs that interfere with availability of brain catecholamines. This occurrence of amenorrhoea suggests a role for anti-adrenergic drugs in reducing gonadotrophin release. The observation that L-dopa administration results in an increase in measurable urinary gonadotrophins and a return of cyclic menstruation in some patients with non-puerperal galactorrhoea (Turkington, 1972d) supports this view. However, in one experiment in which serum FSH and LH were measured by radioimmunoassay, acute oral doses of L-dopa ranging from 250 mg to 1 g had no effect on serum gonadotrophin levels of normal men (Eddy et al., 1971). Other experiments in normal human subjects have also failed to show an effect of L-dopa on serum gonadotrophins (Mims, Stein and Bethune, 1972; Sinhamahapatra and Kirschner, 1972). These conflicting findings may be explained in two ways: (1) a difference in sensitivity to L-dopa in normal subjects and patients with amenorrhoea induced by anti-adrenergic drugs; or (2) a sex difference in response to L-dopa, since the normal subjects were men while the patients were women.

## ROLE IN THE THERAPY OF BREAST CARCINOMA

Detailed discussions of the possible role of anterior pituitary hormones, particularly prolactin, in development and growth of breast carcinoma are found in other chapters.

Until recently, little attention was given by the practising physician to the mass of experimental data indicating that commonly prescribed drugs have profound effects on the hypophysiotrophic functions of the hypothalamus. However, the present state of knowledge of hypothalamic pharmacology requires us to consider possible therapeutic indications and contra-indications of such drugs in certain human diseases, including breast carcinoma.

Now that growth hormone and prolactin have been established as discrete hormones, their mammotrophic effects have been disentangled. Laboratory and clinical observations attribute to growth hormone only a small influence on breast development and lactogenic activity (Ito, Furth and Moy, 1972; Benjamin, Casper and Kolodny 1969; Frantz and Kleinberg, 1970; Sherwood, 1971). In normal human post-partum lactation, and in various states of inappropriate lactation, serum HGH concentrations have been normal and serum prolactin elevated (Sherwood, 1971). In one instance, Forsyth et al. (1971) studied a woman with mammary hyperplasia, minimal galactorrhoea, and recurrent painful breast nodules that showed plasma cell infiltration on histological examination. The patient had high plasma prolactin activity (500 ng/ml), the level in control subjects being undetectable without evidence of other endocrine abnormalities. The authors cautiously concluded that the role of prolactin in development of breast tumours required further study. Such study is under way.

Results of animal experiments suggest that prolactin plays an important role in mammary tumorigenesis (Furth, 1968; Welsch, Clemens and Meites, 1969; Welsch, Jenkins and Meites, 1970), and that control of prolactin secretion may be necessary for successful endocrine treatment of human breast carcinoma (Stoll, 1969, 1972).

It has been shown repeatedly that elevated serum prolactin results in accelerated growth of mammary tumours induced in rats by 7,12-dimethyl-benz(a)-anthracene (DMBA). The methods of producing hyperprolactinaemia in rats have included grafting pituitary glands, grafting mammotrophic pituitary tumours, promoting prolactin secretion by hypothalamic oestrogen implantation, and producing median eminence lesions (Nagasawa and Yanai, 1970). Every method has had the same result: accelerated growth of these chemically-induced mammary carcinomas.

Prolactin alone is not sufficient to maintain the growth of mammary tumours induced in rats by DMBA; oestrogens are needed to maintain sensitivity of the tumour to prolactin effects (Sinha, Cooper and Dao, 1972). Yet ergot alkaloids, which depress serum prolactin without inhibiting ovarian oestrogens, have been successfully used to inhibit mammary tumour growth in laboratory animals.

In one study, the development and growth of chemically-induced mammary carcinomas in rats were inhibited by administration of ergocornine, which also significantly lowered serum and pituitary prolactin (Nagasawa and Meites, 1970). In another, ergocornine significantly suppressed both growth of transplanted D2 mammary tumours and pituitary prolactin levels in BALB/c agent-free mice (Singh et al., 1972). Marked increases in tumour diameter occurred when treatment was stopped. In the first study a monoamine oxidase inhibitor, iproniazid, also proved effective in inhibiting tumour growth without significantly affecting serum or pituitary prolactin. The authors suggested that ergocornine inhibited mammary tumour growth in rats by depressing secretion of pituitary prolactin, and that the mechanisms by which iproniazid acted remained unknown. The role of oestrogens in these experiments was not ascertained, and similar experiments were not done on hypophysectomized animals nor on isolated tumours to eliminate direct anti-tumour activity by ergocornine. In further experiments Yanai and Nagasawa (1972) showed that: (1) ergocornine and 2-bromo-alpha-ergocryptine inhibited tumour formation in intact C3H/He mice having a high incidence of spontaneous mammary carcinoma; and (2) prolactin secreted by pituitary isografts in adreno-ovariectomized mice promoted development of mammary carcinoma in the apparent absence of adrenal and ovarian hormones. It was concluded that prolactin is a primary hormonal factor in spontaneous mammary tumorigenesis in mice.

The prolactin-inhibiting properties of the ergot alkaloids therefore make them leading candidates for experimental treatment of human breast carcinoma. The sustained disappearance of inappropriate lactation, even after discontinuance of ergonovine maleate treatment of patients with idiopathic galactorrhoea (Lawrence and Hagen, 1972), is noteworthy. It portends early evaluation of this drug in patients with breast carcinoma.

Possible benefit of L-dopa in cases of advanced human breast carcinoma has been reported. Stoll (1972) found that L-dopa combined with oestrogen caused significant tumour regression in three of seven post-menopausal patients with soft tissue manifestations of breast carcinoma. These patients had not responded to oestrogen or L-dopa alone. Stoll suggested that L-dopa required adequate levels of exogenous or endogenous oestrogen to stimulate hypothalamic function and reduce prolactin secretion, although serum prolactin levels were not reported in his study. Dickey and Minton (1972) administered L-dopa in doses of 250–500 mg every four hours to two women with painful bone metastases, and reported relief of pain. Symptoms recurred when therapy was halted in one patient. Pain relief was again obtained by re-institution of the drug. These authors also postulated that L-dopa acted through suppression of prolactin. Although serum prolactin levels were not reported in their first communication, the same authors (Minton and Dickey, 1972) later reported decreases in serum prolactin of approximately 50 per cent, with unchanged serum FSH and LH, in both patients. A third patient had no change in prolactin levels and no clinical response. This latter report is the first to document concomitance of suppressed serum prolactin and remission of symptoms in metastatic breast carcinoma. To date, the authors have noted remission of pain in 8 of 40 patients with metastatic breast cancer treated with L-dopa (personal communication).

Serum levels of prolactin have not been determined in large series of women with breast carcinoma. In a recent symposium (Wolstenholme and Knight, 1972) Forsyth stated that she had found hyperprolactinaemia in one of six patients with advanced breast carcinoma, while Friesen reported normal serum prolactin levels in a dozen such patients. Turkington, Underwood and Van Wyk (1971) found that serum prolactin, measured by bioassay, was undetectable before pituitary-stalk section in four patients with metastatic breast cancer. Prolactin was subsequently present in high concentrations in the sera of these and other patients who experienced objective remission after operation. The authors suggested that prolactin did not stimulate growth of the carcinoma during the pre-operative or remission periods. They also suggested that hyperprolactinaemia might contribute to reactivation of the disease after the initial remission. A possible role for HGH suppression in these remissions must still be considered.

Although elevation of serum prolactin concentration has not been demonstrated in human breast carcinoma (except in a single patient), further study is essential to determine whether there may be: (1) significant differences in serum prolactin concentration in large groups of patients with this cancer compared with control groups, and (2) differences in serum prolactin dynamics—as measured by acute responses to exercise, hypoglycaemia, and pharmacological agents—between these two populations. It is possible that even 'normal' serum levels might be capable of supporting or stimulating the growth of breast carcinoma. Animal studies, and the preliminary observations of Stoll (1972), Dickey and Minton (1972) and Minton and Dickey (1972) inform us that it is necessary to determine finally whether prolactin plays a role in human breast carcinoma and whether agents capable of suppressing prolactin secretion are of therapeutic value.

There are many drugs with primarily psychotrophic effects (phenothiazines, tricyclic anti-depressants, and butyrophenones), or anti-hypertensive effects (alpha-methyldopa), or a combination of both effects (reserpine), that are capable of elevating serum prolactin in man. We need not emphasize their widespread availability and use. If prolactin plays any role in development, maintenance or spread of breast carcinoma, is non-physiological elevation of this hormone in human blood dangerous? How does the incidence of breast carcinoma in women treated chronically with these drugs for psychiatric illnesses or hypertension compare with the incidence in the general female population? Are drugs capable of elevating serum prolactin contra-indicated in patients with breast carcinoma? Are they contra-indicated in normal women with a family history of this disease?

These questions need answers.

## ACKNOWLEDGMENT

We are grateful to Joy Wendling for unstinting secretarial assistance, and to Joel Herring and Floyd Jackson for help in preparing the illustrations.

## REFERENCES

Abuzzahab, F. S. (1971). 'Effects of haloperidol and amantadine on rat brain catecholamines and behavior.' *Fedn Proc.* **30**, 381 (abst).

Amenomori, Y., Chen, C-L. and Meites, J. (1970). 'Serum prolactin levels in rats during different reproductive states.' *Endocrinology* **86**, 506.

Andén, N. E., Carlsson, A. and Häggendal, J. (1969). 'Adrenergic mechanisms.' *Ann. Rev. Pharmac.* **9**, 119.

Anton-Tay, F. and Wurtman, R. J. (1971). 'Brain monoamines and endocrine function.' In *Frontiers in Neuroendocrinology*, pp. 45–66, Ed. by L. Martini and W. F. Ganong. New York; Oxford University Press.

Apostolakis, M., Kapetanakis, S., Lazos, G. and Madena-Pyrgaki, A. (1972). 'Plasma prolactin activity in patients with galactorrhoea after treatment with psychotropic drugs.' In *Lactogenic Hormones*, pp. 349–354, Ed. by G. E. W. Wolstenholme and J. Knight. Edinburgh; Churchill Livingstone.

Ben-David, M., Dannon, A. and Sulman, F. G. (1971). 'Evidence of antagonism between prolactin and gonadotropin secretion: effect of methallibure on perphenazine-induced prolactin secretion in ovariectomized rats.' *J. Endocr.* **51**, 719.

Benjamin, F., Casper, D. J. and Kolodny, H. D. (1969). 'Immunoreactive human growth hormone in conditions associated with galactorrhea.' *Obstet. Gynec.* **34**, 34.

Birge, C. A., Jacobs, L. S., Hammer, C. T. and Daughaday, W. H. (1970). 'Catecholamine inhibition of prolactin secretion by isolated rat adenohypophyses.' *Endocrinology* **86**, 120.

Blackard, W. G. and Heidingsfelder, S. A. (1968). 'Adrenergic receptor control mechanism for growth hormone secretion.' *J. clin. Invest.* **47**, 1407.

Bloom, F. E. and Giarmin, N. J. (1968). 'Physiologic and pharmacologic considerations of biogenic amines in the nervous system.' *Ann. Rev. Pharmac.* **8**, 229.

Boris, A., Milmore, J. and Trimal, T. (1970). 'Some effects of haloperidol on reproductive organs in the female rat.' *Endocrinology* **86**, 429.

Boyd, A. E., Lebovitz, H. E. and Pfeiffer, J. B. (1970). 'Stimulation of human growth hormone secretion by L-dopa.' *New Engl. J. Med.* **283**, 1425.

Bradley, P. B., Wolstencroft, J. H., Hösli, L. and Avanzino, G. L. (1966). 'Neuronal basis for the central action of chlorpromazine.' *Nature, Lond.* **212**, 1425.

Brown, P. S. (1971). 'Pituitary follicle-stimulating hormone in immature female rats treated with drugs that inhibit the synthesis or antagonize the actions of catecholamines and 5-hydroxy-tryptamine.' *Neuroendocrinology* **7**, 183.

Cavagnini, F. and Peracchi, M. (1971). 'Effect of reserpine on growth hormone response to insulin hypoglycaemia and to arginine infusion in normal subjects and hyperthyroid patients.' *J. Endocr.* **51**, 651.

Coppola, J. A. (1971). 'Brain catecholamines and gonadotrophin secretion.' In *Frontiers in Neuroendocrinology*, pp. 129–143, Ed. by L. Martini and W. F. Ganong. New York; Oxford University Press.

Cranston, E. M. (1958). 'Effect of tranquilizers and other agents on sexual cycle of mice.' *Proc. Soc. expl Biol. Med.* **98**, 320.

Cryer, P. E., Coran, A. G., Keenan, B. S. and Sode, J. (1971). 'Cessation of growth hormone secretion associated with acute elevation of the serum free fatty acid concentration.' *Clin. Res.* **19**, 650 (abst).

Dahlström, A. and Fuxe, K. (1966). 'Monoamines and the pituitary gland.' *Acta endocr.* **51**, 301.

de Wied, D. (1967). 'Chlorpromazine and endocrine function.' *Pharmac. Rev.* **19**, 251.

Dickey, R. P. and Minton, J. P. (1972). 'Levodopa relief of bone pain from breast cancer.' *New Engl. J. Med.* **286**, 843 (letter).

Dimond, R. C., Brammer, S., Howard, W. J., Atkinson, R. L. and Earll, J. M. (1972). 'Chlorpromazine treatment of acromegaly.' *Clin. Res.* **20**, 424 (abst).

Donoso, A. O., Bishop, W., Fawcett, C. P., Krulich, L. and McCann, S. M. (1971). 'Effect of drugs that modify brain monoamine concentrations on plasma gonadotropin and prolactin levels in the rat.' *Endocrinology* **89**, 774.

Eddy, R. L., Jones, A. L., Chakmakjan, Z. H. and Silverthorne, M. C. (1971). 'Effect of levodopa (L-Dopa) on human hypophyseal trophic hormone release.' *J. clin. Endocr.* **33**, 709.

Fefferman, R. A., Costin, G. and Kogut, M. D. (1972). 'Hypothalamic gigantism.' *Clin. Res.* **20**, 253 (abst).

Forsyth, I. A. and Edwards, C. R. W. (1972). 'Human prolactin, its isolation, assay and clinical applications.' *Clin. Endocr.* **1**, 293.

— and Myres, R. P. (1971). 'Human prolactin. Evidence obtained by the bioassay of human plasma.' *J. Endocr.* **51**, 157.

— Besser, G. M., Edwards, C. R. W., Francis, L. and Myres, R. P. (1971). 'Plasma prolactin activity in inappropriate lacation.' *Br. med. J.* **3**, 225.

Frantz, A. G. and Kleinberg, D. L. (1970). 'Prolactin: evidence that it is separate from growth hormone in human blood.' *Science* **170**, 745.

Friesen, H. G. (1972). 'Prolactin: its physiologic role and therapeutic potential.' *Hosp. Pract.* **7**, 123.

— Guyda, H., Hwang, P., Tyson, J. E. and Barbeau, A. (1972a). 'Functional evaluation of prolactin secretion: a guide to therapy.' *J. clin. Invest.* **51**, 706.

— Webster, B. R., Hwang, P., Guyda, H., Munro, R. E. and Read, L. (1972b). 'Prolactin synthesis and secretion in a patient with the Forbes Albright syndrome.' *J. clin. Endocr.* **34**, 192.

Furth, J. (1968). 'Hormones and neoplasia.' In *Thule International Symposia— Cancer and Aging,* pp. 1–208. Stockholm: Nordiska Bokhandelns Forlag.

Glowinski, J. (1970). 'Release of monoamines in the central nervous system.' In *New Aspects of Storage and Release Mechanisms of Catecholamines,* pp. 237–248, Ed. by H. J. Schülmann and G. Kroneberg. New York; Springer.

Havard, C. W. H., Saldanha, V. F., Bird, R. and Gardner, R. (1972). 'The effect of diazepam on pituitary function in man.' *J. Endocr.* **52**, 79.

Himwich, W. A., Davis, J. M., Leiner, K. Y. and Stout, M. (1970). 'Biochemical effects of haloperidol in different species.' *Biol. Psychiat.* **2**, 315.

Horn, A. S. and Snyder, S. H. (1971). 'Chlorpromazine and dopamine: conformational similarities that correlate with the anti-schizophrenic activity of phenothiazine drugs.' *Proc. natn Acad. Sci. USA,* **68**, 2325.

Hornykiewicz, O. D. (1970). 'Physiologic, biochemical, and pathological backgrounds of levodopa and possibilities for the future.' *Neutrology* **20**, 1.

Hwang, P., Friesen, H., Hardy, J. and Wilansky, D. (1971). 'Biosynthesis of human growth hormone and prolactin by normal pituitary glands and pituitary adenomas.' *J. clin. Endocr.* **33**, 1.

Imura, H., Kato, Y., Ikeda, M., Morimoto, M. and Yawata, M. (1971). 'Effect of adrenergic-blocking or stimulating agents on plasma growth hormone, immunoreactive insulin, and blood free fatty acid levels in man.' *J. clin. Invest.* **50**, 1069.

Irie, M., Sakuma, M., Tsushima, T., Shizume, K. and Nakao, K. (1967). 'Effect of nicotine acid administration on plasma growth hormone concentration.' *Proc. Soc. expl Biol. Med.* **126**, 708.

Ito, A., Furth, J. and Moy, P. (1972). 'Growth hormone-secreting variants of a mammotropic tumor.' *Cancer Res.* **32**, 48.

Jarvik, M. E. (1970). 'Drugs used in the treatment of psychiatric disorders.' In *The Pharmacological Bases of Therapeutics,* 4th ed, pp. 151–203, Ed. by L. S. Goodman and A. Gilman. New York; Macmillan.

Kansal, P. C., Talbert, O. R. and Buse, M. G. (1971). 'Effect of L-dopa on serum thyroxine and growth hormone.' Endocrine Society, programme of the 53rd meeting, p. A-211 (abst).

Kim, S., Sherman, L., Kolodny, H. D., Benjamin, F. and Singh, A. (1971). 'Attenuation by haloperidol of human serum growth hormone (HGH) response to insulin.' *Clin. Res.* **19**, 718 (abst).

Kamberi, I. A., Mical, R. S. and Porter, J. C. (1971). 'Effect of anterior pituitary perfusion and intraventricular injection of catecholamines on prolactin release.' *Endocrinology* **88**, 1012.

Kleinberg, D. L. and Frantz, A. G. (1971). 'Human prolactin: measurement in plasma by in vitro bioassay.' *J. clin. Invest.* **50**, 1557.

Kleinberg, D. L., Noel, G. L. and Frantz, A. G. (1971). 'Chlorpromazine stimulation and L-Dopa suppression of plasma prolactin in man.' *J. clin. Endocr.* **33**, 873.

Kolodny, H. D., Sherman, L., Singh, A., Kim, S. and Benjamin, F. (1971a). 'Acromegaly treated with chlorpromazine. A case study.' *New Engl. J. Med.* **284**, 819.

— — — Benjamin, F. and Kim, S. (1971b). 'Chlorpromazine treatment of human acromegaly.' Endocrine Society, programme of the 53rd meeting, p. A-213 (abst).

Kordon, C. (1971). 'Blockade of ovulation in the immature rat by local micro-injection of alpha-methyl-dopa into the arcuate region of the hypothalamus.' *Neuroendocrinology* **7**, 202.

— and Glowinski, J. (1969). 'Selective inhibition of super-ovulation by blockade of dopamine synthesis during the "critical period" in the immature rat.' *Endocrinology* **85**, 924.

Lawrence, A.M. and Hagen, T. C. (1972). 'Ergonovine therapy of nonpuerperal galactorrhea.' *New Engl. J. Med.* **287**, 150 (letter).

Leymeyer, J. E. and MacLeod, R. M. (1972) 'Suppression of pituitary tumor function by alkaloids.' *Proc. Am. Ass. Cancer Res.,* 63rd annual meeting **13**, 90 (abst).

Lu, K-H. and Meites, J. (1971). 'Inhibition by L-dopa and monoamine oxidase inhibitors of pituitary prolactin release; stimulation by methyl-dopa and d-amphetamine.' *Proc. Soc. expl Biol. Med.* **137**, 480.

— Koch, Y. and Meites, J. (1971). 'Direct inhibition by ergocornine of pituitary prolactin release.' *Endocrinology* **89**, 229.

— Amenomori, Y., Chen, C-L. and Meites, J. (1970). 'Effects of central acting drugs on serum and pituitary prolactin levels in rats.' *Endocrinology* **87**, 667.

Lutterbeck, P. M., Pryor, J. S., Varga, L. and Werner, R. (1971). 'Treatment of non-puerperal galactorrhea with an ergot alkaloid.' *Br. med. J.* **3**, 228.

McCann, S. M., Kabra, P. S., Donoso, A. O., Bishop, W., Schneider, H. P. G., Fawcett, C. P. and Krulich, L. (1971). 'The role of monoamines in the control of gonadotrophin and prolactin secretion.' In *Brain–Endocrine Interaction*, pp. 224–244, Ed. by K. M. Knigge, D. E. Scott and A. Weindl. Basel: Karger.

MacLeod, R. M., Fontham, E. H. and Lehmeyer, J. E. (1970). 'Prolactin and growth hormone production as influenced by catecholamines and agents that affect brain catecholamines.' *Neuroendocrinology* **6**, 283.

Malarkey, W. M.: Jacobs, L. S. and Daughaday, W. H. (1971). 'Levodopa suppression of prolactin in nonpuerperal galactorrhea.' *New Engl. J. Med.* **285**, 1160.

Meites, J. and Nicoll, C. S. (1966). 'Adenohypophysis: prolactin.' *Ann. Rev. Physiol.* **28**, 57.

Meyerson, B. J. and Sawyer, C. H. (1968). 'Monoamines and ovulation in the rat.' *Endocrinology* **83**, 170.

Mims, R. B. and Bethune, J. E. (1972). 'Nocturnal growth hormone secretion in acromegaly.' *Clin. Res.* **20**, 219 (abst).

— Stein, R. B. and Bethune, J. E. (1972). 'The effects of a single dose of L-Dopa on plasma hormones in acromegalic, obese and normal subjects.' *Clin. Res.* **20**, 179 (abst).

Minton, J. P. and Dickey, R. P. (1972). 'Prolactin, FSH, and LH in breast cancer: effect of levodopa and oophorectomy.' *Lancet,* **1**, 1069 (letter).

Mishkinsky, J., Khazen, K., Givant, Y., Dikstein, S. and Sulman, F. G. (1969). 'Mammotropic and neuroleptic effects of butyrophenones in rat.' *Archs int. Pharmacodyn* **179**, 94.

Mühlbock, O. and Boot, L. M. (1959). 'Induction of cancer in mice without the mammary tumor agent by isografts of hypophyses.' *Cancer Res.* **19**, 402.

Müller, E. E. and Pecile, A. (Eds.) (1968). 'Studies on the neural control of growth hormone secretion.' In *Growth Hormone.* Proceedings of the First International Symposium (International Congress Series No. 158), pp. 253–266. Amsterdam: Excerpta Medica.

— Saito, T., Arimura, A. and Schally, A. V. (1967a). 'Hypoglycemia, stress and growth hormone release: blockade of growth hormone release by drugs acting on the central nervous system.' *Endocrinology* **80**, 109.

— Sawano, S., Arimura, A. and Schally, A. V. (1967b). 'Blockade of release of growth hormone by brain norepinephrine depletors.' *Endocrinology* **80**, 471.

— Pecile, A., Felici, M. and Cocchi, D. (1970). 'Norepinephrine and dopamine injection into lateral brain ventricle of the rat and growth hormone-releasing activity in the hypothalamus and plasma.' *Endocrinology* **86**, 1376.

Nagasawa, H. and Meites, J. (1970). 'Suppression by ergocornine and iproniazid of carcinogen-induced mammary tumors in rats; effects on serum and pituitary prolactin levels.' *Proc. Soc. expl Biol. Med.* **135**, 469.

— and Yanai, R. (1970). 'Effects of prolactin or growth hormone on growth of carcinogen-induced mammary tumors of adreno-ovariectomized rats.' *Int. J. Cancer* **6**, 488.

Nasr, H. and Pearson, O. H. (1971). 'Inhibition of prolactin secretion by ergot alkaloids.' Endocrine Society, program of the 53rd meeting, p. a-126 (abst).

Nickerson, M. (1970). 'Drugs inhibiting adrenergic nerves and structures innervated by them.' In *The Pharmacological Basis of Therapeutics*, 4th ed., pp. 549–584. Ed. by L. S. Goodman and A. Gilman. New York; Macmillan.

Noel, G. L., Suh, H. K., Stone, G. and Frantz, H. G. (1972). 'Prolactin response to surgery and other forms of stress in men and women.' *Clin. Res.* **20**, 435 (abst).

O'Keefe, R., Sharman, D. F. and Vogt, M. (1970). 'Effect of drugs used in psychoses on cerebral dopamine metabolism.' *Br. J. Pharmac.* **38**, 287.

Pasteels, J. L. (1970). 'Control of prolactin secretion.' In *The Hypothalamus*, pp. 385–399, Ed. by L. Martini, M. Motta and F. Fraschini. New York; Academic Press.

Quadri, S. K., Lu, K. H. and Meites, J. (1972). 'Ergot-induced inhibition of pituitary tumor growth in rats.' *Science* **176**, 417.

Roth, J., Glick, S. M., Yalow, R. S. and Berson, S. A. (1963). 'Hypoglycemia: a potent stimulus to secretion of growth hormone.' *Science* **140**, 987.

Schalch, D. S. and Reichlin, S. (1968). 'Stress and growth hormone release.' In *Growth Hormone,* Proceedings of the First International Symposium, pp. 211–225. Amsterdam; Excerpta Medica.

Schneider, H. P. and McCann, S. M. (1969). 'Possible role of dopamine as transmitter to promote discharge of LH releasing factor.' *Endocrinology* **85**, 121.

Shaar, C. J. and Clemens, J. A. (1972). 'Inhibition of lactation and prolactin secretion in rats by ergot alkaloids.' *Endocrinology* **90**, 285.

Sherman, L., Kim, S., Benjamin, F. and Kolodny, H. D. (1971). 'Effect of chlorpromazine on serum growth hormone concentration in man.' *New Engl. J. Med.* **284**, 72.

Sherman, L. and Kolodny, H. D. (1971). 'The hypothalamus, brain catecholamines, and drug therapy for gigantism and acromegaly.' *Lancet* **1**, 682.

—— Singh, A., Deutsch, S. and Benjamin, F. (1972). 'Suppressive effect of a single dose of L-dopa on serum growth hormone in acromegaly.' *Clin. Res.* **20**, 86 (abst).

Sherwood, L. M. (1971). 'Human prolactin.' *New Engl. J. Med.* **284**, 774.

Singh, D. V., Meites, J., Halmi, L., Kortright, K. H. and Brennan, M. J. (1972). 'Suppression of pituitary prolactin level and transplanted mammary tumor growth in mice by ergocornine.' *Proc. Am. Ass. Cancer Res.* 63rd annual meeting, **13**, 8 (abst).

Sinha, D., Cooper, D. and Dao, T. L. (1972). 'The relationship of estrogen and prolactin in mammary tumorigenesis in rats.' *Proc. Am. Ass. Cancer Res.,* 63rd annual meeting **13**, 10 (abst).

Sinhamahapatra, S. B. and Kirschner, M. A. (1972). 'Effect of L-Dopa on testosterone and luteinizing hormone production.' *J. clin. Endocr.* **34**, 756.

Stoll, B. A. (1969). *Hormonal Management of Breast Cancer,* pp. 6–12, 15–16. Philadelphia; Lippincott.

— (1972). 'Brain catecholamines and breast cancer: a hypothesis.' *Lancet* **1**, 431 (letter).

Strauch, G., Modigliani, E. and Bricaire, H. (1969). 'Growth hormone response to arginine in normal and hyperthyroid females under propranolol.' *J. clin. Endocr.* **29**, 606.

Sulman, F. G. (1959) 'The mechanism of the "push and pull" principle. II. Endocrine effects of hypothalamus depressants of the phenothiazine group.' *Archs Int. Pharmacodyn.* **118**, 298.

— (1970). 'Pharmacological regulation of lactation.' In *Hypothalamic Control of Lactation,* pp. 59–161. New York; Springer.

Thomas, L. (1971). 'Notes of a biology-watcher: On societies as organisms.' *New Engl. J. Med.* **285**, 101.

Turkington, R. W. (1971a). 'Measurement of prolactin activity in human serum by the induction of specific milk proteins in mammary gland *in vitro*.' *J. clin. Endocr.* **33**, 210.

— (1971b). 'Ectopic production of prolactin.' *New Engl. J. Med.* **285**, 1455.

— (1972a). 'Serum prolactin levels in patients with gynecomastia.' *J. clin. Endocr.* **34**, 62.

— (1972b). 'Secretion of prolactin in patients with pituitary and hypothalamic tumors.' *J. clin. Endocr.* **34**, 159.

— (1972c). 'Phenothiazine stimulation test for prolactin reserve: the syndrome of isolated prolactin deficiency.' *J. clin. Endocr.* **34**, 247.

— (1972d). 'Inhibition of prolactin secretion and successful therapy of the Forbes-Albright syndrome with L-dopa.' *J. clin. Endocr.* **34**, 306.

— (1972e). 'Prolactin secretion in patients treated with various drugs.' *Archs intern. Med.* **130**, 349.

— (1972f). 'Human prolactin: an ancient molecule provides new insights for clinical medicine.' *Am. J. Med.* **53**, 389.

Turkington, R. W. and MacIndoe, J. H. (1972). 'Hyperprolactinemia in sarcoidosis.' *Ann. intern. Med.* **76**, 545.

— Underwood, L. E. and van Wyk, J. J. (1971). 'Elevated serum prolactin levels after pituitary-stalk section in man.' *New Engl. J. Med.* **285**, 707.

Vaidya, R. A., Vaidya, A. B., Van Woert, M. H. and Kase, N. G. (1970). 'Galactorrhoea and Parkinson-like syndrome: an adverse effect of alpha-methyl-dopa.' *Metabolism* **19**, 1068.

Van Loon, G. R. (1971). 'Growth-hormone secretion.' *New Engl. J. Med.* **284**, 616 (letter).

Welsch, C. W., Clemens, J. A. and Meites, J. (1969). 'Effects of hypothalamic and amygdaloid lesions on development and growth of carcinogen-induced mammary tumors in the female rat.' *Cancer Res.* **29**, 1541.

— Jenkins, T. W. and Meites, J. (1970). Increased incidence of mammary tumors in the female rat grafted with multiple pituitaries.' *Cancer Res.* **30**, 1024.

Werrbach, J. H., Gale, C. C., Goodner, C. J. and Conway, M. J. (1970). 'Effects of autonomic blocking agents on growth hormone, insulin, free fatty acids and glucose in baboons.' *Endocrinology* **86**, 77.

Wolstenholme, G. E. W. and Knight, J. (Eds.) (1972). *Lactogenic Hormones*, p. 195. Edinburgh; Churchill Livingstone.

Wuttke, W., Cassell, E. and Meites, J. (1971). 'Effects of ergocornine on serum prolactin and LH, and on hypothalamic control of PIF and LRF.' *Endocrinology* **88**, 737.

Yanai, R. and Nagasawa, H. (1972). 'Inhibition of mammary tumorigenesis by ergot alkaloids and promotion of mammary tumorigenesis by pituitary isografts in adreno-ovariectomized mice.' *J. natn Cancer Inst.* **48**, 715.

York, D. H. (1972). 'Dopamine receptor blockade—a central action of chlorprom-azine on striatal neurones.' *Brain Res.* **37**, 91.

# 19

# Psychoendrocrine Factors and Breast Cancer Growth

## Basil A. Stoll

For many years it has been suggested that there may be a relationship between the growth and spread of cancer on the one hand, and personality, emotional stress or affective disorders in the patient on the other. Although personal impressions and anecdotal evidence on this topic are abundant, so far no scientific evidence has been provided to prove such a connection. However, recent research suggests that a mechanism exists for such a relationship in the case of breast cancer.

It has been established that, although the activity of the anterior pituitary gland may be modified by direct stimuli, it is mainly regulated by the brain through the agency of the hypothalamus (see Chapters 7 and 8). The hypothalamus in turn has widespread connections with the limbic system, globus pallidus and forebrain, so that stimuli originating in those regions can modify the release of pituitary secretion. Immediate responsibility for the release of pituitary trophic hormones lies in centres in the median eminence of the hypothalamus, and activity of these centres is thought to involve the synthesis and release of catecholamines such as dopamine. The catecholamines act as neuro-transmitters to release specific releasing factors for each individual trophic hormone, and the releasing factors then pass through the portal plexus to the anterior pituitary secretory tissue.

In addition to controlling the release of pituitary trophic hormones, the hypothalamus is thought to exert control over the response both to acute and chronic stress, by the stimulation of catecholamine or ACTH secretion. Hypothalamic function may also influence the immune response mechanism which determines the rate and extent of local and metastatic spread of cancer in the body. It appears, therefore, that dysfunction of the hypothalamus may, in several ways, play an essential part in deciding the prognosis of human mammary cancer.

## HYPOTHALAMIC DYSFUNCTION AND BREAST CANCER

For most of the pituitary trophic hormones the hypothalamus produces releasing factors, but in the case of prolactin an inhibiting factor is produced. As a result, either interference with the transmission of the factors to the pituitary gland, or their decreased production by the hypothalamus may lead to over-release of prolactin and under-release of gonadotrophin, corticotrophin, thyrotrophin and growth hormone. This type of hypothalamic dysfunction can result from the presence of a pituitary tumour or from some form of hypopituitarism as discussed below, and the hormonal changes resulting may well affect the activity of an existing hormone-sensitive mammary cancer.

Another way in which hypothalamic dysfunction may manifest is by a rise in the hypothalamic threshold to stimulation by specific hormones. This may occur either as a result of advancing age (see Chapter 10), or due to the presence of long continued stress (see Chapter 5). If the raised hypothalamic threshold to feedback leads to high circulating levels of steroids such as oestrogens and corticosteroids, as has been suggested, this also could influence the growth of existing hormone-sensitive mammary cancer.

Another possible cause of hypothalamic dysfunction is suggested here. There may be a common aetiology both for hypothalamic dysfunction and for affective disorders, particularly peri-menopausal endogenous depression. A rising hypothalamic threshold to feedback may result from decreased dopamine transmission at central adrenergic receptor sites (see Chapter 16), while there is evidence that endogenous depression is associated with high levels of monoamine oxidase in the brain, and this also can lead to decreased dopamine transmission. There are indeed recent observations that endogenous depression may be associated with a raised hypothalamic threshold to feedback (Kastin et al., 1972; Prange et al., 1972). Increased levels of corticosteroids in the plasma are common in endogenous depression (Beumont, 1972), and this may be one manifestation of the hypothalamic dysfunction. It thus seems likely that the not uncommon presence of endogenous depression in women around the time of the menopause may be associated with hypothalamic dysfunction, and this could affect the prognosis of existing hormone-sensitive mammary cancer.

The evidence that monoamine oxidase is a major regulator of brain levels of catecholamines is mainly indirect (Kopin, 1964; Sandler and Youdin, 1972), and derived from observations of the pharmacological effects of agents such as reserpine, amphetamines, tricyclic anti-depressants, and monoamine oxidase inhibitors (Schildkraut, 1965). Plasma monoamine oxidase levels are significantly higher than normal in pre-menopausal women with endogenous depression (Klaiber et al., 1972), and peripheral MAO levels are thought to reflect central MAO levels. The latter authors also noted that the serum level of monoamine oxidase in these patients could be restored to normal by administration of oestrogen in the form of Premarin 5 mg daily, and that the oestrogen administration also relieved the symptoms of depression in almost all cases. The effect of oestrogen administration upon the rate of catecholamine turnover in the brain is uncertain (see Chapter 7) but it may be relevant to the mechanism of oestrogen responsiveness by breast cancer.

It has also been noted that monoamine oxidase levels are markedly increased in women both after oophorectomy and after the natural menopause (Kobayashi, Kobayashi and Kato, 1964; Tryding, Tufvesson and Nilsson, 1972). A rise in the monoamine oxidase level in both brain tissue and plasma is seen also with advancing age (Robinson et al., 1972), and this could lead to decreased dopamine transmission in the brain. This may be the cause of the observation mentioned above that the hypothalamic threshold to feedback tends to rise with advancing age (see Chapter 10).

## OVER-RELEASE OF PROLACTIN

It is a generalization that changes in the blood level of prolactin are inversely related to those of pituitary gonadotrophin. Such a relationship has been shown in the rat (see Chapter 16) and amenorrhoea is frequently found to be associated with galactorrhoea in hypothalamo-hypophyseal dysfunction in the human. It is also found that suppression of prolactin over-release in such cases is usually followed by a return to normal gonadotrophin levels in the blood. Three syndromes of non-puerperal galactorrhoea have been described in the literature. The Argonz–del Castillo syndrome occurs in nulliparous women while the Chiari–Frömmel syndrome occurs after normal pregnancy and lactation. Both are associated with high serum prolactin levels, low gonadotrophin levels and a normal-sized sella turcica. The Forbes–Albright syndrome into which the other two syndromes may progress is, on the other hand, associated with an enlarged sella turcica, and usually also evidence of a pituitary tumour.

In the cases where no pituitary tumour is found, it is assumed that either hypopituitarism or a disturbance of hypothalamic neuro-transmission causes increase in prolactin release with galactorrhoea, and decrease in gonadotrophin release with amenorrhoea (see Chapter 9). Such a disturbance may result either from a lesion in the hypothalamus itself, or one affecting the portal system surrounding the pituitary stalk, so that the hypothalamo-hypophysiotropic factors fail to reach the pituitary tissue. Whatever the cause, the hormonal change described might well influence the growth of existing hormone-sensitive mammary cancer.

403

It is of considerable interest that over-release of prolactin associated with galactorrhoea and amenorrhoea has been occasionally reported following the cessation of long continued usage of oral contraceptives (Shearman, 1971). The cause of such functional disturbance is uncertain, but a clue may be provided by the observation that the incidence of depression is five times as high as normal in women taking oral contraceptives and, moreover, is more likely the greater the progestogenic component (Annotation, 1970). If endogenous depression is evidence of increase in monoamine oxidase levels in the brain, it could be associated with decreased dopamine transmission in the hypothalamus. This would reduce the production of prolactin-inhibiting factor and result in prolactin over-release, while reducing the gonadotrophin releasing factor and causing amenorrhoea.

Evidence of prolactin over-release may be seen also in conjunction with other hormonal abnormalities (see Chapter 9). Thus galactorrhoea may follow evidence of primary hypothyroidism. Such an association may be explained by the over-production of thyrotrophin releasing hormone which is able to increase the release of both prolactin and TSH. The prolactin level in the blood may also be found to rise parallel with the growth hormone level, in response to insulin-induced hypoglycaemia, but the hypothalamic mechanism involved here is unknown.

## PSYCHOTROPIC AGENTS AND HYPOTHALAMIC FUNCTION

Considerable anxiety has been expressed in the past over the administration of oestrogenic agents to peri-menopausal or post-menopausal women, because of the possible danger of causing breast pathology or of increasing the predisposition to mammary cancer. (Most authorities are still agreed on the inadvisability of administering oestrogen to women with a history of breast cancer.) Similar anxiety is now being expressed over the administration of other agents which are able to increase serum prolactin levels (see Chapter 18). There are many psychotropic drugs in common use which depress dopamine transmission in the brain and thus lead to elevated serum prolactin levels which are usually associated with decreased gonadotrophin levels. Drugs of this type include neuroleptic agents such as reserpine, phenothiazines such as chlorpromazine, antihistamines such as meclizine and perphenazine, and anti-hypertensive agents such as α-methyl-dopa and phentolamine. There is no need to emphasize the rapid increase in the use of such agents recently both in psychiatry and general medicine. Their possible effects on the development or aggravation of human mammary cancer must be considered.

It is commonly assumed that an increase in prolactin level must inevitably favour the growth of mammary cancer in the human. This concept derives from the stimulating effect exerted by prolactin on the growth of spontaneous or carcinogen-induced hormone-sensitive mammary carcinoma in rodents. However, it should be noted that tumour stimulation occurs only when prolactin levels are elevated *after* the appearance of such tumours. If prolactin levels are elevated *before* or concurrently with the administration of a carcinogen such as dimethylbenzathracene, this will cause the mammary gland to be protected from the action of the carcinogen (see Chapter 2). Such an effect has been demonstrated after elevation of serum prolactin levels either by injection of reserpine or by placement of a median eminence lesion. A protective effect has also been shown from the early administration of oestrogen or progesterone, or of oestrogen–progesterone combinations as in oral contraceptives (Meites, 1972).

All of these methods undoubtedly act, at least in part, by stimulating prolactin secretion and release. If used after the DMBA-induced tumour is established, they promote its growth, yet used before administration of the carcinogen, they protect the mammary tissue. The different effect suggests that stimulation of functional activity in mammary tissue by prolactin can interfere with the action of a carcinogen. If these observations in rats can be extrapolated to the human being, it is possible that the administration of agents capable of causing increase in blood prolactin levels (and this includes oral contraceptives), may protect the breast against malignancy rather than predispose to malignant change. Until this is proven, however, caution in the use of such agents is still advisable in the presence of a history of breast cancer, in spite of the tumour regression reported in some pre-menopausal patients from treatment with oral contraceptive combinations (see Chapter 13).

## CEREBRAL INFLUENCES ON BREAST CANCER GROWTH

The suckling stimulus has been shown capable of inducing proliferation of lobulo-alveolar tissue in the breast, and even of causing milk secretion in non-pregnant, non-parturient women (see Chapter 1). This response is mediated by a neuroendocrine reflex passing through the hypothalamus and enhancing prolactin release from the anterior pituitary gland. The prolactin release pathway which is activated by suckling has been traced in the rabbit to the lateral preoptic area, just in front of the lateral hypothalamus (Tindal and Knaggs, 1972). The same group have reported that stimulation of a specific area in the orbito-frontal area of the cerebral cortex can cause marked release of prolactin, probably mediated by the centre in the lateral preoptic area.

Since the orbitofrontal area in the human receives a considerable sensory input, it is possible that the mental state of the patient may play a part in the regulation of prolactin secretion. By this means, it can influence not only normal mammary growth and lactation, but may also play a part in the development of breast pathology associated with abnormal prolactin activity.

For very many years, the belief has been expressed that the personality of a patient is a factor in the development of cancer. Even Galen suggested that the melancholy type of woman suffered from cancer more frequently than the sanguine type! It has also frequently been suggested that psychological or emotional experiences of the patient may affect the growth of established breast cancer, but such reports have been mainly anecdotal. Thus, it has often been observed that recurrence of breast cancer after a long free interval may follow closely upon an emotional upheaval, such as the death of a very close relative. It would now seem that such an effect is possible through endocrinological or immunological channels.

It is well known that the pituitary–adrenal axis is very sensitive to stressful stimuli—both acute and chronic. Urinary excretion of catecholamines is very considerably raised by emotional arousal. Significant changes in glucocorticoid levels also are associated with emotional disturbances, and increased adrenocortical activity has been noted, particularly in patients with endogenous depression and anxiety states (see review by Beumont, 1972). There are also variations in the release of both growth hormone and prolactin in response to psychologically stressful situations (see Chapter 18), and gonadotrophin release also may be interfered with by psychologically traumatic situations and by anxiety.

For such reasons, investigation has been suggested of the relationship between personality patterns, stress reactions and psychoneurotic disorders on the one hand, and the incidence and growth of breast cancer on the other. The likelihood of breast cancer developing is probably decided 10–30 years previously, and possibly even at the time of the first pregnancy according to Cole and MacMahon (1969). However, it is possible also that a modifying factor may affect its onset in later years. This has been suggested to explain the protective effect of castration, and might apply also to other factors capable of causing severe endocrinological upset. A recent survey carried out by Snell and Graham (1971) investigated the effect of psychological factors, but showed that there was no evidence of an increased incidence of psychological trauma in the five years prior to the *diagnosis* of breast cancer in a group of patients compared to the normal population. More extensive surveys are necessary to investigate a possible link between psychological factors and cancer *recurrence*, particularly the role of severe emotional upset in precipitating recurrence of breast cancer after a long free interval.

## THE IMMUNE PROCESS AND BREAST CANCER GROWTH

It has recently become clear that the survival and growth of tumours in the body is a matter of balance between the immune process and the growth potential of the particular tumour. It has been suggested also that endocrinological and immunological mechanisms may overlap in the control of breast cancer growth. It is suggested by Stein, Schiavi and Luparello (1969) that hypothalamic changes may modify the immune response to cancer by three possible mechanisms. The first is by a change in neuroendocrine activity. Thus, stimulation by ACTH of corticosteroid and androgen secretion, and stimulation by TSH of thyroxine secretion, are both said to be necessary for maintaining antibody formation. Other possible mechanisms by which the hypothalamus can influence the immune response to cancer are by an effect on the activity of the autonomic nervous system and by an effect on the anaphylactic response.

It is noted in Chapter 5 that there is in patients with breast cancer a correlation between poor prognosis and a high 17-OHCS level in the plasma. The latter is associated with evidence of an abnormally high hypothalamic threshold to adrenal steroid feedback. It is suggested that this can lead to excessive stimulation by ACTH of adrenal oestrogen secretion, which may in turn have a deleterious effect upon the growth of established breast cancer. It has also been shown by Mackay et al. (1971) that in breast cancer patients, a rise in the 17-OHCS level in the blood is associated with evidence of depression of the immune mechanism, and both changes are generally found among the more advanced tumours.

It is therefore especially interesting that Katz et al. (1969) have noted that high levels of hydrocortisone production are associated not only with a poor defence against breast cancer, but also with a poor psychological attitude to the disease. Thus, patients with symptoms of apprehension, worry or depression have a higher hydrocortisone production than those who are more fatalistic or stoic. It has also been noted that in ovariectomized women, the oestrogenic index of the vaginal smear can be increased as a result of psychological stress causing stimulation of ACTH secretion (see Chapter 5). It seems highly likely, therefore, that personality factors may be able to influence the prognosis in breast cancer.

The presence of a raised hypothalamic threshold to adrenal and ovarian steroids in breast cancer patients is suggested also in Chapter 10. However, it is there suggested that the abnormality is part of a generalized failure of the homeostatic mechanism caused by ageing, and that the process may encourage the development in women of cancer either in the breast or in the uterus.

Steroid excretion in breast cancer patients was first used to distinguish those more likely to respond to endocrine ablation therapy and was later found to reflect the prognosis of the tumour (Bulbrook, Hayward and Thomas, 1964). Patients with a low aetiocholanolone excretion relative to 17–OHCS were shown to have a worse prognosis. A similar discriminant based upon ACTH-stimulated levels of 17-oxosteroids and 17-OHCS has been found of value in predicting response to adrenalectomy (Wilson and Moore, 1968). In the case of lung cancer patients also, it has been noted that the mean ratio of androsterone to 17-OHCS levels is significantly lower than normal especially in those with a poor prognosis (Rao and Hewit, 1970). The androgenic abnormality in either tumour is not a result of the tumour's presence, because it does not improve after resection of the tumour in the latter case, or after endocrine ablation has caused tumour regression in the former case.

It appears that both in the case of breast cancer and lung cancer, survival is worse in patients with a low androgen level. It is therefore suggested that like corticosteroid levels, androgen levels may relate to the patients' resistance to the growth and spread of the tumour (Rao and Hewit, 1970; Mackay et al., 1971). It is suggested that at least some of the androgen abnormality in these cases may stem from a pre-clinical genetically determined abnormality.

One way in which the immune response may affect established cancer may also be concerned with the control of cell differentiation. If the cancer process can be regarded as a defect of growth and differentiation, the multipotential cell can become more differentiated by the loss of specific genetic information. It is suggested by Bennette (1967) that the cell may not be genetically committed to its neoplastic condition, but is subject to influences which can modify the effect of genetic information. Such an influence may be the immune response of the patient. This may be the mechanism responsible for the increasing functional differentiation which has been observed in mammary cancer, leading to the carcinostatic effect described in Chapter 3. The carcinostatic effect is seen following the administration of high dosage of oestrogen and as is shown below, oestrogen therapy may provide an example of overlap between endocrine therapy and immunotherapy in the control of tumour growth.

Several reports suggest that the immunological competence of the lymphoid system is markedly stimulated by the administration of natural or synthetic oestrogens of high potency (Nicol et al., 1964; Magarey and Baum, 1971). This is said not to apply to the administration of progestin or androgen (Nicol and Bilbey, 1957). If oestrogen can stimulate the immune response it has been suggested that the concomitant administration of oestrogen may help to counteract the immunosuppressive effect of cytotoxic agents—an effect which could promote the acceleration or dissemination of tumour growth (Magarey and Baum, 1971).

It has been observed that the administration of cyclophosphamide concurrently with oestrogen leads to less complete regression of human mammary cancer than is seen from oestrogen therapy alone (Firat and Olshin, 1968), presumably as a result of cyclophosphamide diminishing the immunological competence of the host. The role of *local* immunological mechanisms in the control of breast cancer is also currently the focus of considerable interest, but at this time, it is not possible to evaluate its significance in relation to the control of tumour growth. Its relationship to therapy by ovarian steroids is discussed in Chapter 3.

# CONCLUSIONS

Although not proven, a relationship is possible between the growth and spread of breast cancer, and personality, emotional stress and affective disorders in the patient. The hypothalamus, which has widespread connections with the limbic system and forebrain, controls not only the release of pituitary trophic hormones, but also the response of the organism to acute and chronic stress. Moreover, it is able to influence the immune response mechanism controlling the rate and extent of spread of cancer in the body. In these several ways, hypothalamic dysfunction may determine the prognosis of breast cancer.

There are specific syndromes of hypothalamo-hypophyseal dysfunction, associated with prolactin over-release and low circulating gonadotrophin levels, which could influence the mitotic activity of hormone-sensitive breast cancer. More commonly seen is evidence of a rising hypothalamic threshold to feedback. When seen in patients with endogenous depression, it may be ascribed to increased monoamine oxidase levels in the brain, and it is possible that a similar change is responsible for the increased hypothalamic threshold found to be associated with advancing age or with long-continued stress, either physical or mental. Whatever the cause, a resulting rise in the circulating corticosteroid and oestrogen levels may affect the progress of hormone-sensitive breast cancer.

Endocrinological and immunological mechanisms may overlap in the control of breast cancer. Hypothalamic dysfunction may modify the immune response to cancer by different channels—by an effect on corticosteroid, thyroxine and androgen secretion, by an effect on the activity of the autonomic nervous system and by an effect on the anaphylactic response. It is difficult to evaluate the significance of the low androgen level found to be associated with a poor prognosis in patients with breast cancer. It may relate to the patient's resistance to the spread of the tumour and probably antedates the clinical appearance of the tumour. On the other hand, a raised corticosteroid level can be the result of a raised hypothalamic threshold, due either to the presence of long-standing and widespread disease or to long-continued anxiety or depression. Anxiety and stress can also cause temporary fluctuations in the release of ACTH, prolactin, growth hormone and gonadotrophin from the anterior pituitary gland, and these also may affect the growth of existing hormone-sensitive breast cancer.

## REFERENCES

Annotation (1970). 'Depression and oral contraceptives.' *Br. med. J.* **4**, 127.
Bennette, G. (1967). 'Second Conference on Psychophysiological Aspects of Cancer.' *Ann. N.Y. Acad. Sci.* **164**, 454, 595.

Beumont, P. J. V. (1972). 'Endocrines and psychiatry.' *Br. J. hosp. Med.* **8**, 458.

Bulbrook, R. D., Hayward, J. L. and Thomas, B. S. (1964). 'The relation between the urinary 17 hydroxycorticosteroids and 11 deoxy 17 oxosteroids and the fate of patients after mastectomy.' *Lancet* **1**, 945.

Cole, P. and MacMahon, B. (1969). 'Oestrogen fractions during early reproductive life in the aetiology of breast cancer.' *Lancet* **1**, 604.

Firat, D. and Olshin, S. (1968). 'Treatment of metastatic carcinoma of the female breast with combinations of hormones and other chemotherapy.' *Cancer Chemother. Rep.* **52**, 743.

Kastin, A. J., Ehrensing, R. H., Schalch, D. S. and Anderson, M. S. (1972). 'Improvement in mental depression with decreased thyrotrophin response after administration of TRH.' *Lancet* **2**, 740.

Katz, J., Gallagher, T., Hellman, L., Sachar, E., and Weiner, H. (1969). 'Psychoendocrine considerations in cancer of the breast.' *Ann. N. Y. Acad. Sci.* **164**, 509.

Klaiber, E. L., Kobayashi, Y., Broverman, D. M., Vogel, W. and Moriarty, D. (1972). 'Effects of oestrogen therapy on plasma monoamine oxidase activity and E.E.G. driving responses of depressed women.' *Am. J. Psychiat.* **128**, 1492.

Kobayashi, T., Kobayashi, Y. and Kato, R. (1964). 'Effects of sex steroids on the choline acetylase activity in the hypothalamus of female rats.' *Endoc. Jap.* **11**, 9.

Kopin, I. J. (1964). 'Storage and metabolism of catecholamines—the role of monoamine oxidase.' *Pharmac. Rev.* **16**, 179.

Mackay, W. D., Edwards, M. H., Bulbrook, R. D. and Wang, D. Y. (1971). 'Relation between plasma androgen sulphates and immune response in women with breast cancer.' *Lancet* **2**, 1001.

Magarey, C. J. and Baum, M. (1971). 'Oestrogen as reticuloendothelial stimulant in patients with cancer.' *Br. med. J.* **2**, 367.

Meites, J. (1972). In *Prolactin and Carcinogenesis* (4th Tenovus Workshop), p. 54, Ed. by A. R. Boyns and K. Griffiths. Cardiff; Alpha Omega Alpha.

Nicol, T. and Bilbey, D. L. J. (1957). 'Reversal by diethylstilboestrol of the depressant effects of cortisone on the phagocytic activity of the R.E. system.' *Nature, Lond.* **179**, 1137.

—— Charles, L. M., Cordingley, J. L. and Vernon Roberts, B. (1964). 'Oestrogen, the natural stimulant of the body defences.' *J. Endocr.* **30**, 277.

Prange, A. J., Wilson, J. C., Lara, P. P., Alltop, L. B. and Breese, G. R. (1972). 'Effects of TRH in depression.' *Lancet* **2**, 999.

Rao, L. G. S. and Hewit, M. L. (1970). 'Prognostic significance of a steroid discriminant function in patients with inoperable lung cancer.' *Lancet* **2**, 1063.

Robinson, D. S., Davis, J. M., Nies, A., Colburn, R. W., Davis, J. N., Bourne, H. R., Bunney, W. E., Shaw, D. M. and Coppen, A. J. (1972). 'Ageing, monoamines and monoamine oxidase levels.' *Lancet* **1**, 290.

Sandler, M. and Youdin, M. B. H. (1972). 'Multiple forms of monoamine oxidase.' *Pharmac. Rev.* **24**, 331.

Schildkraut, J. J. (1965). 'Catecholamine hypothesis of affective disorders—review of supporting evidence.' *Am. J. Psychiat.* **122**, 509.

Shearman, R. P. (1971). 'Prolonged secondary amenorrhoea after oral contraceptive therapy.' *Lancet* **2**, 64.

Snell, L. and Graham, S. (1971). 'Social trauma as related to cancer of the breast.' *Br. J. Cancer* **25**, 721.

Stein, M., Schiavi, R. C. and Luparello, T. J. (1969). 'The hypothalamus and the immune process.' *Ann. N. Y. Acad. Sci.* **164**, 464.

Tindal, J. S. and Knaggs, G. S. (1972). 'Pathways in the forebrain of the rabbit concerned with the release of prolactin.' *J. Endocr.* **52**, 253.

Tryding, N., Tufvesson, G. and Nilsson, S. (1972). 'Ageing, monoamines and monoamine oxidase levels.' *Lancet* **1**, 489.

Wilson, R. E. and Moore, F. D (1968). 'Biochemical and clinical factors in the selection of patients for endocrine surgery.' In *Prognostic Factors in Breast Cancer*, p. 339, Ed. by A. P. M. Forrest and P. B. Kunkler. Edinburgh; Livingstone.

# Index

ACTH (*see* Corticotrophin)
Adrenal metastasis in breast cancer, 107
Adrenalectomy,
    comparison with hypophysectomy
        in breast cancer, 328
    effect on gonadotrophin excretion
        in breast cancer, 127
Adrenergic blocking agents, 374
Adrenocorticotrophic hormone (*see*
    Corticotrophin)
Ageing,
    effects on mammary parenchyma, 8
    hypothalamic sensitivity changes in,
        197–228
Alpha-methyldopa, effects on prolactin
    secretion, 384
Amines, biogenic, role in prolactin
    secretion, 166
Amphibians, prolactin functions in, 230
Anahormones to reduce secretion of
    protein hormones, 221
Androgens,
    effect on gonadotrophin
        production, 127
    urinary, hypophyseolysis and, 299
Anti-depressants, tricyclic, effects on
    prolactin secretion, 385
Anti-oestrogens,
    clinical trials in breast cancer, 91
    definition and scope, 84
    initiation of mammary cancer, and, 86
    treatment of experimental mammary
        cancer, in, 88
    treatment of mammary cancer, in,
        82–100

Birds, prolactin functions in, 231
Bone metastases in breast cancer,
    effect of pituitary ablation therapy,
        295

Brain lesions, effect on mammary
    tumorigenesis in mice and rats, 33
Breast cancer (*see* Mammary cancer)

Carcinoma, mammary (*see* Mammary
    cancer)
Carcinostatic mechanism in oestrogen
    therapy, 64
Catecholamines,
    effect on prolactin secretion, 41
    involvement in prolactin secretion,
        139, 166
    pituitary regulation by, 139–159
    role in treatment of mammary
        cancer, 326–348
Cell division in mammary gland, 9
Cerebral control of prolactin secretion,
    405
Chlormadinone, clinical trial in
    breast cancer, 268
Chlorpromazine,
    effect on growth hormone secretion,
        371
    effect on prolactin levels, 167, 168,
        382
Clomiphene in treatment of experimental
    mammary cancer, 89, 93
Corticosteroid–progestin–oestrogen
    combinations in treatment of
    mammary cancer, 265–282
Corticotrophin,
    action on breast cancer, 101
    estimation, 314
        in relation to glycogenic steroids,
            101
        in relation to oestrogens, 102
        radioimmunoassay, 314
    releasing factor, 31
    role in maintenance of mammary
        cancer, 328

413